NUTRITION and HEART DISEASE

Edited by

Herbert K. Naito, Ph.D.
The Cleveland Clinic Foundation
and
Department of Chemistry
Cleveland State University
Cleveland, Ohio

MTP PRESS LIMITED
International Medical Publishers

Proceedings of the 19th Annual Meeting of the American College of Nutrition (Monographs of the American College of Nutrition, Vol. 5)

Published in the UK and Europe by
MTP Press Limited
Falcon House
Lancaster, England

Published in the US by
SPECTRUM PUBLICATIONS, INC.
175-20 Wexford Terrace
Jamaica, N.Y. 11432

Softcover reprint of the hardcover 1st edition 1982

ISBN-13: 978-94-011-6694-2 e-ISBN-13: 978-94-011-6692-8
DOI: 10.1007/978-94-011-6692-8

Contributors

Gerald S. Berenson, M.D.
Section of Cardiology
Louisiana State University Medical Center
New Orleans, Louisiana

Nicholas J. Birch, Ph.D., A.F.A.C.N.
Department of Biological Sciences
The Polytechnic
Wolverhampton, England

Henry Blackburn, M.D.
Laboratory of Physiological Hygiene
School of Public Health
and
School of Medicine
University of Minnesota
Minneapolis, Minnesota

Henry Buchwald, M.D., Ph.D.
Department of Surgery and Biomedical Engineering
University of Minnesota Hospitals
Minneapolis, Minnesota

D.L. Clough, M.D.
Department of Physiology
Uniformed Services University
Bethesda, Maryland

Philippe Collery, M.D., F.A.C.N.
Faculté de Médecine de Reims
and
Hôpital de la Maison Blanche
Reims, France

Pierre Coudoux, M.D.
Faculté de Médecine de Reims
and
Hôpital de la Maison Blanche
Reims, France

Jean Davignon, M.D., M.Sc., F.R.C.P. (C.), F.A.C.P., F.A.C.N.
Department of Lipid Metabolism and Atherosclerosis Research
Clinical Research Institute of Montreal
and
Section of Vascular Medicine
Hôtel-Dieu Hospital
and
Faculty of Medicine
University of Montreal
Montreal, Canada

Francis L. Earl, D.V.M.
Division of Toxicology, Bureau of Foods
Food and Drug Administration
Laurel, Maryland

M. Ernst, M.D.
Med.-Univ.-Poliklinik
Münster, West Germany

Eric J. Essman, Ph.D.
Department of Biochemistry
Queens College
City University of New York
Flushing, New York

Walter B. Essman, M.D., Ph.D., F.A.C.N.
Department of Biochemistry
Queens College
City University of New York
Flushing, New York

Gail C. Frank, R.D., M.P.H.
Department of Medicine
Specialized Center of Research–Arteriosclerosis
Louisiana State University Medical Center
New Orleans, Louisiana

Henri Geoffroy, M.D.
Faculté de Médecine de Reims
and
Hôpital de la Maison Blanche
Reims, France

David M. Grischkan, M.D.
Huron Road Hospital
University Heights, Ohio

Francis J. Haddy, M.D., Ph.D.
Department of Physiology
Uniformed Services University
Bethesda, Maryland

Felix P. Heald, M.D.
Department of Pediatrics
University of Maryland School of Medicine
Baltimore, Maryland

Fran Hoerrmann, R.D.
Department of Nutritional Services
The Cleveland Clinic Foundation
Cleveland, Ohio

Michael P. Holden, B.M., B.Ch.
Northern Regional Health Authority
and
The University of Newcastle-upon-Tyne
Department of Cardiothoracic Surgery
Freeman Hospital
Newcastle-upon-Tyne, England

Jeng M. Hsu, D.V.M., Ph.D.
Veterans Administration Medical Center
Bay Pines, Florida

H.L. Johansen, M.D.
B. of Epidemiology
National Health and Welfare
Ottawa, Canada

Mushtaq A. Khan, Ph.D.
Metabolism Branch, Division of Toxicology
Bureau of Foods, Food and Drug Administration
Beltsville Research Facility
Laurel, Maryland

Leslie M. Klevay, M.D., S.D. in Hyg.
Grand Forks Human Nutrition Center
P.O. Box 7166, University Station
Grand Forks, North Dakota

O. Knoll, M.D.
Med.-Univ.-Poliklinik
Münster, West Germany

David Kritchevsky, Ph.D.
The Wistar Institute
Philadelphia, Pennsylvania

A. Lison, M.D.
Med.-Univ.-Poliklinik
Münster, West Germany

Suzanne Lussier-Cacan, M.Sc., Ph.D.
Department of Lipid Metabolism and
Atherosclerosis Research
Faculty of Medicine
University of Montreal
Montreal, Canada

R. Martin, M.D.
Med.-Univ.-Poliklinik
Münster, West Germany

Herbert K. Naito, Ph.D.
Lipid-Lipoprotein Laboratories
Division of Laboratory Medicine
and
Division of Research
The Cleveland Clinic Foundation
and
Department of Chemistry
Cleveland State University
Cleveland, Ohio

Luciano C. Neri, M.D.
Department of Epidemiology and
Community Medicine
Ottawa, Canada

M.B. Pamnani, M.D.
Department of Physiology
Uniformed Services University
Bethesda, Maryland

Donna B. Rosenstock, R.D.
Department of Nutritional Services
The Cleveland Clinic Foundation
Cleveland, Ohio

Richard D. Rucker, M.D.
University of Minnesota Hospitals
Minneapolis, Minnesota

Thomas J. Schaffner, M.D.
Pathologisches Institute
Bern, Switzerland

Colin J. Schwartz, M.D.
Department of Pathology
University of Texas
San Antonio, Texas

Mildred S. Seelig, M.D., M.P.H.,
F.A.C.N.
Goldwater Memorial Hospital
New York University Medical Center
New York, N.Y.

Raymond J. Shamberger, Ph.D.
Enzyme Laboratory
Division of Laboratory Medicine
The Cleveland Clinic Foundation
Cleveland, Ohio

Ezra Steiger, M.D., F.A.C.S.
Department of General Surgery
The Cleveland Clinic Foundation
Cleveland, Ohio

Alexander J. Steiner, M.D., F.A.C.N.,
A.C.C.P.
Department of Internal Medicine
Missouri Baptist Hospital
St. Louis, Missouri

Richard L. Varco, M.D., Ph.D.
University of Minnesota Hospitals
Minneapolis, Minnesota

Dragoslava Vesselinovitch, D.V.M., M.S.C.
Department of Pathology
and
The Specialized Center of Research in Atherosclerosis
University of Chicago
Chicago, Illinois

Larry S. Webber, Ph.D.
Planning and Analysis Section
Specialized Center of Research–Arteriosclerosis
Department of Medicine
Louisiana State University Medical Center
New Orleans, Louisiana

Robert W. Wissler, Ph.D., M.D.
The Specialized Center of Research in Atherosclerosis
University of Chicago
Chicago, Illinois

H. Zumkley, M.D.
Med.-Univ.-Poliklinik
Münster, West Germany

Contents

Preface

Entering the 1980's, coronary heart disease (CHD) still remains the major cause of death in the United States and ranks second in the world in terms of CHD mortality rates. However, CHD mortality and morbidity rates in the United States have declined significantly since the 1950's. There are many reasons for this positive and encouraging change, one of which is the increasing awareness of the importance of the role of nutrition in health and disease. Diet has been identified as an important factor contributing to hyperlipidemia in individuals and populations. Dietary modification has become a routine means of treating patients with lipid disorders. The relationship between diet and chronic disease is, however, far from simple and at the present time, needs further intensive research.

Many significant advances have recently taken place in our understanding of the effect of different nutritional components on blood lipids and lipoproteins and on the initiation progression and regression of atherosclerotic processes. This symposium (The 19th annual meeting of the American College of Nutrition: Cardiovascular Disease and Nutrition held at Bloomington, Minn. on June 1-2, 1978) addressed many of the important questions concerning the association of diet and CHD. We have not restricted the topic to hyperlipidemia and CHD, *per se* but have considered cardiovascular disease in general. This monograph should be of interest to the dietitian, nutritionist, pediatric clinician, cardiologist, physicians in general, and researchers in the field of cardiovascular disease.

Herbert K. Naito, Ph.D.
1982

1

A Review of Atheroma

HERBERT K. NAITO
COLIN J. SCHWARTZ

INTRODUCTION

Atheroma is a disease of tremendous importance in contemporary society, not only because of its associated mortality, but also because of its considerable morbidity. Although intensive research efforts have begun to elucidate various facets of its etiology and pathogenesis, in order to provide improved diagnostic procedures and more useful approaches to intervention, long-term objectives must logically continue to be those of disease prevention, based upon a thorough understanding of the origin and development of the atheromatous process.

Intermediate objectives could realistically relate to at least two important areas; first, initiation and evaluation of intensive attempts to induce significant lesion regression in patients with severe diffuse disease; and second, further therapeutic attempts to minimize intravascular thrombosis, a process responsible in many patients for the rapid conversion of latent atheroma to events of overt clinical significance, such as cerebral or myocardial infarction.

This chapter highlights selected aspects of the pathology and clinicopathologic implications of atheroma, and presents, in an overview format, the present status of our understanding of etiologic and pathogenic mechanisms. It is clearly neither possible nor desirable to examine the minutiae of atherogenesis in this review.

PATHOLOGY OF HUMAN ATHEROMA

Lesions are most prevalent in large- and medium-sized arteries, and may extend into arteries of smaller caliber, particularly in hypertensive diabetics.

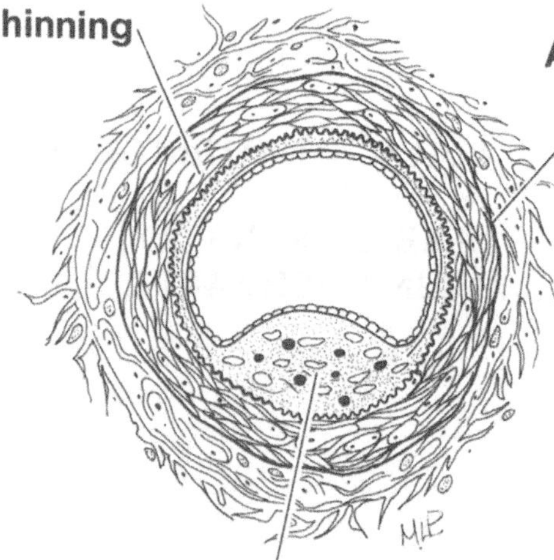

Fig. 1. Summary of the events that occur during the development of the atheromatous plaque.

Histologic Features of the Atheromatous Plaque

The histologic features of human atheroma are summarized in Fig. 1. Intimal changes, traditionally regarded as characteristic of the raised or fibrous plaque, include a dense collagenous cap which is covered by endothelium on the luminal surface and which overlies and partially encases a necrotic, pultaceous, lipid-rich core. The cellularity of the intimal plaque may vary considerably. Cells that have some of the morphological criteria of smooth muscle cells are copious. Other cells can be identified as macrophages, lymphocytes, and polymorphonuclear leucocytes.

As might be expected, the identity or origin of some cells remains uncertain, even at the ultrastructural level. Lipid-rich macrophages or foam cells occur most consistently around the periphery of the central lipid core but may also be observed toward and on the surface of the collagenous cap, particularly toward the edges of a lesion. These cells appear to be derived from smooth muscle cells, macrophages, and possibly blood-borne mononuclear cells.

Fibrous proteins, a category which includes collagen, elastin, and fibrin, are important constituents of the plaque. Collagen, predominantly of Types I and III, is the major component of the fibrous cap. Fibrin can be observed both superficially and in the depths of plaques, and may be derived from circulating fibrin or fibrinogen directly, or from the organization and incorporation of mural thrombi. In this context, it is important to recognize the laminated, almost sedimentary structure of many plaques, a structure which in all likelihood results from the successive organization and incorporation of episodically occurring mural thrombi. There is little doubt that mural thrombosis contributes significantly to plaque growth. Inasmuch as thrombosis and atherosclerosis are so closely associated, risk factors for clinical arterial disease usually do not differentiate between atherogenesis and thrombogenesis. Coronary heart disease (CHD) risk factors may enhance the risk for CHD through thrombogenic mechanism(s) (Schwartz et al., 1978).

Most atheromatous plaques contain Schiff-positive material and exhibit varying degrees of metachromasia. These staining reactions reflect the glycosaminoglycan content of lesions and in particular the complex sulfated polysaccharides such as chondroitin sulfate A and C, dermatan sulfate, hyaluronic acid, and heparitin sulfate.

Medial thinning, characteristic of the advanced raised or fibrous plaque, is largely the result of atrophic loss of smooth muscle cells. Adventitial changes associated with fibrous plaque but not with fatty streaks, include fibrosis, an increased vascularity, and in the majority of patients, a mononuclear infiltrate which is predominantly lymphocytic.

This triad of histologically identifiable changes in the arterial adventitia is consistent with a chronic inflammatory reaction which, because of the considerable lymphocytosis, may have an immune or autoimmune basis. These changes are readily apparent to the vascular surgeon and make adventitial dissection of severely diseased arteries relatively difficult because of thickening and adhesions. The ultimate significance of this adventitial lymphocytosis remains uncertain; studies on the possible role of immune mechanisms in both atherogenesis and thrombogenesis are long overdue.

Definitions of Atherosclerotic Lesions

The term *raised atherosclerotic lesion* is sometimes used to indicate the sum of fibrous plaques, complicated lesions, and calcified lesions. Raised lesions are contrasted with fatty streaks which typically show little or no elevation above the surrounding intimal surface.

It should be emphasized that the use of the word *atheroma* is not consistent among investigators. Some use it for the lesion described as a plaque with a pool of degenerated or necrotic lipid-rich debris. Others use *atheroma* to refer to the process of atherosclerosis or arteriosclerosis. Still others have used the term to refer to various lesions–from a fatty streak to a complicated lesion. To avoid ambiguity when one uses the term, it should be qualified or modified so that its meaning is perfectly clear.

Strong et al. (1978) described working definitions for different types of atherosclerotic lesions detectable (grossly); although this classification implies a pathogenetic sequence, it can be used as a descriptive classification regardless of the ideas of pathogenetic interrelationships among the lesions.

This classification of lesions based on gross examination does not permit distinction between those plaques with and without a core of degenerated or necrotic lipid-rich debris. Those plaques with necrotic lesions and ulceration of the surface would of course be classified as complicated lesions. The plaques with necrotic centers and intact intimal surfaces (atheroma according to some classifications) would be classified as fibrous plaques. Microscopic examination is usually necessary to distinguish various subtypes of fibrous plaques:

1. Fatty streak: A fatty intimal lesion that is stained distinctly by Sudan IV and shows no other underlying change. Fatty streaks are flat, or only slightly elevated, and do not significantly narrow the lumina of blood vessels.
2. Fibrous plaque: A firm elevated intimal lesion which in the fresh state is gray white, glistening, and translucent. The surface of the lesion may be sudanophilic, but usually is not.

Human fibrous plaques characteristically contain fat. Often a thick fibrous connective tissue cap containing varying amounts of lipid covers a more concentrated core of lipid. If a lesion also contains hemorrhage, thrombosis, ulceration, or calcification, that lesion is classified according to one of the next two categories.

3. Complicated lesion: An intimal plaque in which there is hemorrhage, ulceration, or thrombosis with or without calcium.
4. Calcified lesion: An intimal plaque in which insoluble mineral salts of calcium are visible or palpable without overlying hemorrhage, ulceration, or thrombosis.

Topographic Distribution

The topographic distribution of atherosclerotic lesions has been described qualitatively (Duff et al., 1951; Schwartz and Mitchell, 1962; Glagov and Ozoa, 1968), and it appears that lesions occur earliest and most extensively in the aorta. Lesions develop later and less extensively in the coronary and cerebral arteries, and the renal, mesenteric, and pulmonary arteries are the least susceptible to atherosclerotic lesions.

The arteries are involved by atherosclerosis in a definite sequence. The aorta is first involved beginning in infancy with fatty streaks which increase rapidly during puberty. Fatty streaks begin in the coronary arteries during puberty, but begin to increase significantly and become converted into fibrous plaques in the third decade of life in high-risk populations. The carotid arteries begin to be involved with fatty streaks at approximately the same age as the aorta, and the other cerebral arteries begin at approximately the same age as the coronary arteries. Raised lesions develop in the carotid arteries at roughly the same age as in the aorta, but do not develop in the vertebral and intracranial arteries until much later. Detailed quantitative or morphometric description on the distribution of lesions within the aorta, coronary arteries and arteries in the brain can be obtained elsewhere (Schwartz et al., 1978).

Sequence of Events

Atherosclerosis develops and progresses through stages involving a certain sequence of events (Strong et al., 1974; Haust, 1978). The lesions may begin in infancy as one of the three earliest forms, that is, the fatty dot and streak, microthrombus, or gelatinous elevation. In the first two decades of life only the early lesions are encountered. The second stage of the lesions, that is, the fibrous atherosclerotic plaque, may develop at the end of the second but is usually established at the beginning of the third decade of life. The so-called complicated third-stage lesions (Morgan, 1956; Haust and More, 1972) develop in the fourth and subsequent decades. Since the clinical manifestations of the disease are preceded by stages in the evolution of the lesion over at least two to three decades, it is understandable that attention has been directed recently toward early life in the hope of retarding the conversion of the earliest lesions to the advanced, instrumental in this conversion thus becomes important in the study of atheroma, particularly in view of the fact that at present we are not capable of preventing the inception of the early lesion, or of treating the advanced lesions and their sequelae.

In humans, the difficulty in unraveling the above problems is compounded by many factors, which may be minimized or eliminated in experimental animals. One cannot study serially the evolution of the emerging, complex human lesion at various time intervals. A given population, no matter how similar the constituent subjects, can never be as homogeneous in a biological sense as inbred animals of the same litter. The reactions of the highly individualistic *Homo sapiens* to his or her environment and to the factors considered to be important in atherosclerosis; for example, food, occupation, stress, genetic predisposition to CHD, cultural background, physical activities, other habits, and geography, are expected to vary from one person to another, as do the lesions, even of the same type. It is, therefore, doubtful whether it will ever be possible to provide answers to questions and problems raised in the introduction, at least with respect to the human lesion. Notwithstanding these limitations, and on the basis of our knowledge of general tissue reactions, it is reasonable to postulate the following course of events in the natural history of the atherosclerotic lesion.

Various factors relating to the makeup of the arterial wall, the prevailing hemodynamic conditions, and the status of the circulating blood may be injurious either to the endothelium or to the elements in the underlying intima (Haust, 1970; Haust and More, 1972). Injury to the endothelium may be followed by an influx (insudation) of plasma constituents into the intima to form a gelatinous elevation, or by deposition of a microthrombus, or both (Haust and More, 1970). Both processes may induce fatty metamorphosis of the smooth muscle in the underlying intima, and in addition the insudation may cause mechanical damage to the intimal connective tissues. The failure to remove or organize the insudate and/or the thrombus may furnish substances that induce further lipid accumulation and provide stimuli for smooth muscle cells (SMCs) to proliferate in the area. The latter phenomenon may be enhanced in part by platelet factors (Rutherford and Ross, 1976) and by the nature of the lipoproteins in the insudate (Fischer-Dzoga et al., 1974).

The native SMCs accumulating lipid droplets may continue on that course beyond their ability to survive. Necrosis follows and the intracellular lipids, released into the extracellular space, contribute to the lipid component of the lesion. Once established, lesions of any one of the three basic types appear to promote the development of some or all features of the two other forms. The tendency to repeated episodes of mural thrombosis and insudation, and the simultaneously ongoing proliferative and reparative phenomena in the area contribute further to the complexity of the process.

Present knowledge of the morphogenesis of the lesions, while not sufficiently advanced to permit the prevention of their inception, may be considered to be at a stage that provides some basis for rational intervention of their growth, or retardation of their progression to fibrous atherosclerotic plaques and their complicated forms, according to Wissler (1978). There are three stages in the reversal of the atherosclerotic process: (1) *regression* (decreased lipid content, cells, collagen, elastin, and calcium); (2) *remodeling* (condensation and reorientation of collagen and elastin); and (3) *healing* (decreased evidence of endothelial cell damage, increased cell proliferation, etc.).

RISK FACTORS AND ATHEROSCLEROSIS

Epidemiologic investigation of living populations has disclosed characteristics of persons which are associated with increased risk of developing clinically manifest disease due to atherosclerosis–myocardial infarction, sudden death, angina pectoris, stroke, or peripheral vascular disease. These characteristics are known as *risk factors*, a descriptive but noncommittal term which avoids the question of whether these characteristics are causative agents, intervening variables, early manifestations of disease, or secondary indicators of an underlying disturbance.

The primary risk factors also are associated with more severe and more extensive atherosclerotic lesions as well as with more frequent clinical disease. We have various degrees of knowledge about the mechanisms of their effects on atherogenesis, but relatively little knowledge about whether they affect thrombosis as a terminal occlusive episode, and if so, how.

Age

Of all risk factors, age has the strongest and most consistent association with lesions. As with so many chronic diseases, the incidence rates of all atherosclerotic diseases increase with age. The simplest explanation of this association is an accumulation of responses to injury as exposure to injury increases. This explanation may be true in middle-aged and older persons, but the early stages of atherogenesis during adolescence show more specific age-dependent changes. Aortic fatty streaks increase rapidly in extent between 8 and 18 years and fibrous plaques begin to form from fatty streaks in the coronary arteries at about 20 years (McGill, 1968). These age trends suggest that the artery wall undergoes a systematic change with maturation, that the artery wall is exposed to distinctive atherogenic agents at those ages.

The concept of aging as a degenerative change after attaining adult growth is not yet sufficiently refined to explain progression of the advanced lesions of atherosclerosis in biochemical and physiologic terms (Bierman and Ross, 1977). The cumulative effect of repeated injuries and the associated scarring seem to account for most of the age effects on lesions in adulthood, but a more precise definition of aging of smooth muscle cells may change this view.

Male Sex

Except for age, male sex is one of the best documented and strongest risk factors for *coronary* heart disease, but not for the other forms of atherosclerotic disease. Furthermore, the sex differential in coronary heart disease is most marked in whites and is greatly attenuated or absent in nonwhites. The sex differential also is much attenuated in populations with low overall incidence rates of atherosclerotic disease, and is reduced or eliminated among diabetics. Despite the attractiveness of the hypothesis that the estrogenic hormones of the female are responsible for her protection from coronary artherosclerosis, it has become clear that exogenous estrogen administration does not protect the male and may even be atherogenic or thrombogenic. Neither does it appear that exogenous estrogens, as in oral contraceptives, add to the natural protection of the female. Females have slightly lower levels of three major risk factors (serum cholesterol, blood pressure, and cigarette smoking) between the menarche and the menopause, but the lower levels of risk factors do not seem sufficient to account for the differences in coronary heart disease. Male sex in whites remains the most puzzling of all of the risk factors, and the one for which we have the least coherent hypothesis regarding mechanism.

Hypercholesterolemia

Until recently total serum cholesterol concentration was recognized as the strongest and most consistent risk factor for atherosclerotic disease other than age and sex, and reduction in serum cholesterol has received much attention as a means of preventing disease. Serum cholesterol concentration can be elevated in many animal species by feeding a humanlike high-fat, high-cholesterol diet, and these animals develop intimal lipid deposits resembling human fatty streaks. Cholesterolemia maintained in the range of 200 to 400 mg/dl for several years leads to experimental lesions that are reasonable facsimiles of human fibrous plaques. However, in both humans and animals, there remains a high degree of individual variation in cholesterolemic response to an atherogenic diet; and at any level of serum cholesterol, there is wide variation in the response of the arterial wall in forming atherosclerotic lesions.

Knowledge about the cellular metabolism of low-density lipoprotein (LDL), which carries most of the plasma cholesterol, provides an attractive hypothesis for the mechanism by which hypercholesterolemia initiates intimal lipid deposits and causes some of them to progress to fibrous plaques (Goldstein and Brown, 1975). Cells (including fibroblasts and smooth muscle cells) possess specific receptors which bind LDL and promote internalization. The uptake of LDL suppresses synthesis of cholesterol in the cell. Internalized LDL is degraded, and the cholesterol is hydrolyzed and reesterified as cholesteryl oleate. The cell thus obtains cholesterol for membrane structures at lower energy cost than by synthesis. In the presence of excess LDL, lipoprotein is internalized by a nonspecific process which does not suppress cholesterol synthesis, and cholesteryl ester accumulates within the cell in excess (Fig. 2). Prolonged accumulation leads to cell death, extravasation of cholesterol esters and other debris, and a consequent chronic inflammatory and reparative reaction which results in the fibrous plaque.

Since elevated serum cholesterol levels can be lowered by diet modification, exercise, weight reduction or drugs, a major question now is whether

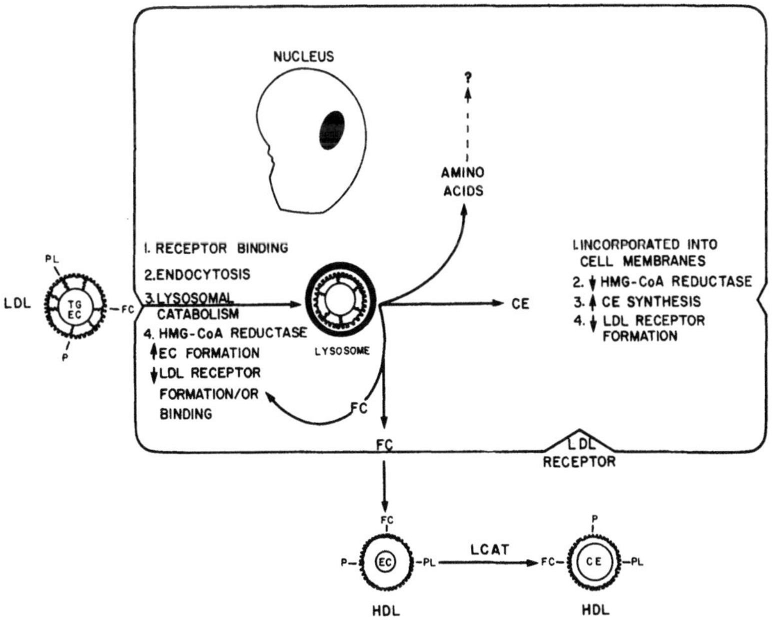

Fig. 2. Schematic diagram representing the cellular metabolism of lipoproteins.

reduction in serum cholesterol slows progression or permits regression of advanced atheroslerosis. Clinical trials of lipid-lowering agents in postmyocardial infarction patients (secondary prevention) have shown no benefit, and early trials of lipid-lowering regimens in relatively small numbers of apparently healthy middle-aged or elderly persons (primary prevention) have yielded suggestive but not conclusive results. Currently, large-scale trials are underway (Rifkind, 1977). It may never be possible to conduct a controlled trial of maintaining low serum cholesterol levels from childhood, but much circumstantial evidence suggests that control in childhood is likely to be more effective than in adults.

The relationship of serum cholesterol concentration to atherosclerotic disease has been strengthened by the recent demonstration of an inverse association with high-density lipoprotein (HDL) cholesterol (Gordon et al., 1977). This epidemiologic observation is consistent with current hypotheses that the metabolic function of HDL is to transport cholesterol from peripheral tissues to the liver for eventual degradation and excretion. However, it now appears that serum total cholesterol levels do not correlate as well as HDL-cholesterol and LDL-cholesterol when studying CHD prevalence in population studies. The data suggests that the virtue of partitioning total cholesterol into the various lipoprotein fractions assessing CHD risk appears to be a more reasonable approach for biochemical profiling. If one fraction (HDL-cholesterol) has a negative association with the risk for CHD while the other two (VLDL- [very-low-density] and LDL-cholesterol) have positive associations with CHD risk, then the arithmetic sum (i.e., total cholesterol) must be a less sensitive indicator of risk than an appropriately weighted algebraic sum.

Thus, knowledge of lipoprotein metabolism supports the link between serum cholesterol concentration and atherogenesis by suggesting biochemical mechanisms for the relationship. Whether elevation of serum cholesterol or a specific lipoprotein concentration contributes to the risk of coronary heart disease by other mechanisms, such as, for example, by predisposing to thrombosis, remains a possibility that may provide additional information.

Hypertension

Like serum cholesterol concentration, increase in blood pressure in all ranges is associated with increased risk of atherosclerotic disease (Lewis and Naito, 1978), and particularly of cerebrovascular disease (Stemmerman et al., 1980). The risk increases progressively with higher levels of blood pressure and is demonstrable in both systolic and diastolic pressure (Freis, 1973). When diastolic pressures are in the range 85 to 94 mm Hg, the incidence of events is significantly increased above that of men whose diastolic pressure falls below 85 mm Hg. There is doubling of incidence if diastolic pressures are in the range 95 to 104 mm Hg, and a quadrupling of this rate with still higher diastolic pressure. Comparable risks attach to these groupings of diastolic pressure when assessed by death rates for CHD. When hypertension coexists along with hypercholesterolemia or cigarette smoking, there is additional risk for the first major coronary events. For all levels of diastolic blood pressure, the risk is increased by a factor of 2 when the persons are also cigarette smokers. In addition to its contribution of risk for CHD, hypertension is an important determinant of the occurrence of other life-threatening illnesses, that is, renal failure, stroke, and congestive heart failure. Elevation of blood pressure is one of the most commonly occurring physical abnormalities in adults, and very probably in adolescents (Londe and Golding, 1976). Hypertension selectively augments cerebral atherosclerosis (Solberg and McGarry, 1972). The most obvious mechanisms of action of hypertension on atherogenesis are by increasing filtration of lipoprotein-rich plasma through the intima, or by increasing the work load of SMCs of the artery wall. Less obvious is the potential effect of humoral mediators of blood pressure on the artery wall, as, for example, angiotension II, norepinephrine, serotonin, and bradykinin (Hollander, 1976; Lewis and Naito, 1978). Since some antihypertensive drugs lead to increased levels of these mediators, such drug regimens may augment rather than ameliorate the atherogenic effect of hypertension. The beneficial effects of antihypertensive drug therapy on stroke and congestive heart failure are not in question, but whether such therapy reduces coronary heart disease incidence is still doubtful. Not to be neglected is the fact that hypertension also may affect thrombosis as well as atherogenesis.

Cigarette Smoking

As the association between cigarette smoking and atherosclerotic disease was developed in epidemiologic studies, there was initial uncertainty as to whether cigarette smoking accelerated atherogenesis or whether it only predisposed to the terminal episode by precipitating thrombosis or arrhythmia. It now appears certain that cigarette smoking augments atherogenesis in the coronary arteries and the abdominal aorta (Strong and Richards, 1976), and it probably has a similar effect on the peripheral arteries. In essence, the greater the daily usage, the larger the risk. Similarly, the person who characteristically smokes most of each cigarette, and discards but little, increases the hazard of the habit. The age at which cigarette smoking is adopted as a habit is also of importance; the younger the age, the greater the eventual risk of experiencing the clinical manifestations of the disease. The length of the period of habitual smoking in years and the total number of cigarettes smoked are potent determining factors as well. All of these factors seem to pertain only to the use of tobacco in the form of cigarettes. The same risks do not apply to the smoking of a pipe or cigars. Since inhaling of cigarette smoke is a common practice, whereas inhaling of tobacco smoke from cigars or pipes is not, it has been suspected that the process of inhaling is an important determinant (Doll and Hill, 1974).

A number of reports have brought evidence that once the habit of cigarette smoking is discarded, the relative risk of developing manifestations of CHD is reduced. Following an interval of ten or more years of abstinence, the ex-smoker enters a risk category comparable to that of the person who has never smoked (Report of Intersociety Commission for Heart Disease Resources, 1970; Rode et al., 1972; Stamler, 1973; Rosenman et al., 1975; Telecom Health Research Group, 1977). The experience of those who stop smoking suggests that it also affects the terminal occlusive episode since the risk of ex-smokers begins to drop more rapidly after cessation than we would expect from regression of advanced atherosclerosis alone (Kannel et al., 1980).

We do not know what component of cigarette smoke is responsible for the acceleration of atherosclerosis nor the hypothesized effect on thrombosis. Carbon monoxide is widely suspected, but its role is not proven. Cigarette smoke contains about 3000 identified chemicals and probably more unidentified ones, and therefore many possibilities remain.

Of all the risk factors, cigarette smoking seems the most likely to be thrombogenic as well as atherogenic. Scattered reports indicate that it affects several coagulation tests. A promising new lead is that a tobacco glycoprotein activates Factor XII (Becker and Dubin, 1977).

Family History

Familial aggregation of atherosclerotic disease has long been recognized, but only a small beginning has been made in isolating the strictly genetic basis for this aggregation, in contrast to the common environment shared by family members. The only specific progress has been in identifying genetic hyperlipidemias. Genetic bases for hypertension and diabetes are suspected. Undoubtedly, a portion of the residual variability in atherosclerosis not explained by the known risk factors lies in unidentified genetic traits, perhaps programmed characteristics of the artery wall. Genetically determined variations in susceptibility to atherosclerosis have been demonstrated in animals (Wagner et al., 1973; Malinow et al., 1976) and undoubtedly exist in humans as well.

In view of the numerous genetic defects in the coagulation system and the presumed important role of thrombosis in atherosclerotic disease, it is remarkable that no genetic coagulation abnormality has been found associated with atherosclerotic disease.

Obesity

The precise role of obesity in atherosclerotic disease remains uncertain, despite nearly universal recommendations that obesity should be avoided in order to reduce risk of atherosclerotic disease. Obesity appears well established as a risk factor for hypertension, hyperlipidemia, and diabetes, and undoubtedly influences atherosclerosis indirectly through these mechanisms; but, in their absence, no clear association of obesity with either atherogenesis or with atherosclerotic disease has been demonstrated.

The Framingham, Massachusetts data demonstrate a definite and independent risk for sudden death and the development of angina pectoris in men and a smaller, more indefinite risk in women (Kannel et al., 1967). In this evaluation, obesity was assessed by assigning a relative weight for each individual, derived by comparison of the weight on initial observation with the median weight in the Framingham sample of persons of the same sex and height. Obese persons were defined as having a relative weight of 120% or above. The rate of occurrence of angina pectoris was compared in obese and nonobese men who either did or did not have elevation in systolic blood pressure (i.e., 160 mm Hg or above) or serum cholesterol (i.e., 250 mg/dl or greater). The risk of angina was similarly enhanced (by a factor of about 2.7) in obese men, whether or not there was coexisting hypertension or hypercholesterolemia. However, the existence of one or both of the complicating major risk factors increased the risk for both the nonobese and obese. The morbidity ratio in nonobese men was increased from 0.7, when neither blood pressure or cholesterol was elevated, to 1.15, when either or both were increased. Comparable ratios in obese men were 1.9 without, and 3.29 with these associated major risk factors. The same measures in women show little difference between obese and nonobese individuals when neither blood pressure nor cholesterol was elevated; but, with increase in either, the morbidity ratio was increased from 1.13 in nonobese to 1.76 in obese women. Another assessment of the possible effect of obesity was provided by relating gain in body weight after the age of 25 years to the rate of development of angina pectoris. The observed increase in risk was proportional to the weight gained. Other evidence indicates that the extent of obesity is an important consideration in assessing risk (Kagan et al., 1975) but that moderate obesity without coexistent hypercholesterolemia, hypertension, or cigarette smoking produces only a modest increase of coronary disease (Truett et al., 1967; Report of Intersociety Commission for Heart Disease Resources; 1970).

Physical Activity

Many benefits are derived from regular physical activity, and it has been widely recommended for preventing atherosclerotic disease (Paffenbarger and

Hale, 1975; Naito, 1976). There is some evidence that extreme physical activity is associated with less risk of coronary heart disease (Wagner et al., 1973), but the level of activity required is difficult to attain in our present society. While exercise directly increases cardiovascular fitness, increased physical activity is known to lower total serum cholesterol (Naito, 1976; Wood et al., 1976) and LDL-cholesterol, yet raise HDL-cholesterol (Wood et al., 1976).

Part of the anticoronary effect of exercise might be through relationships between physical activity and other risk factors. Certainly, relative inactivity and characteristic sedentary modes of living contribute importantly to the occurrence of obesity. Although, as noted above, obesity is not in itself a major risk factor, loss of weight is often accompanied by lessening of other risks, that is, reduction in serum cholesterol and blood pressure and improvement in glucose tolerance. An important part of effective programs of weight reduction for obese persons is planned and ongoing exercise to achieve increased and moderate energy expenditure. Animal experiments have found that exercise may suppress rather than increase appetite (Oscai and Holloszy, 1969; Naito, 1976). Moreover, the physical training brings physiologic and metabolic adaptations that may improve cardiovascular and other organ system function.

Fasting plasma lipids (especially elevated triglycerides) are responsive to physical activity. They are lower in physically trained men as contrasted to others who are sedentary, and these levels are reduced by programs of planned exercise (Bjorntoys et al., 1972; Scheuer and Tipton, 1977). A bout of vigorous activity will reduce elevated levels of triglycerides in plasma. In contrast, the total cholesterol content of plasma is not as responsive to increased physical activity, especially if the concentration is already normal or low-normal or the exercise program is of not sufficient intensity, duration, and frequency. It is likely that reports of reduced cholesterol levels with exercise have been influenced by modification of diet and loss of body weight. A fact of potential significance, however, is the recent demonstration that the cholesterol content of plasma lipoproteins is quite different in very active men when compared to a randomly selected control group of comparable age (Wood et al., 1976). Specifically, HDL-cholesterol concentration was greater and LDL-cholesterol concentration less in the active group, a situation previously reported as favorable for reduced risk of CHD.

Renal Failure Patients on Chronic Hemodialysis

It is well known that patients with renal failure on chronic hemodialysis die of premature CHD. According to Lindner et al. (1974) more than 60 percent of hemodialysis patients died of arteriosclerotic cardiovascular complications. The mechanism by which this occurs has not been resolved. There is sufficient documentation that hyperlipidemia and dyslipoproteinemia occurs in this group of subjects (Wada et al., 1975; Handa, 1978; Miamisono et al., 1978). More specifically, 58 percent of the hemodialysis patients have elevated levels of intermediate-density lipoprotein (IDL), which suggests a defect in VLDL catabolism due to a decreased postheparin lipoprotein activity (Miamisono et al., 1978).

Diabetes Mellitus

Cardiovascular disease, particularly atherosclerotic disease, remains the major health hazard for the diabetic. According to the study done by Palumbo et al. (1976), 39 percent of the diabetic patients died because of CHD, a rate 1.7 times that expected. Forty percent of the patients were obese and with relative weight of 125 percent or more. The rates of occurrence of other CHD risk factors, such as hypercholesterolemia, hypertriglyceridemia, hypertension, and cigarette smoking were not given. A comparable mortality experience was reported for a group of 21,447 diabetic patients cared for at the Joslin Clinic in Boston during the period from 1930 to 1960, in which the overall mortality was higher than in the population at large by a factor of 1.93 and the standardized mortality ratio for coronary artery disease was 1.84 (Kessler, 1971).

The University Group Diabetes Study (UGDS) was undertaken to determine if the use of hypoglycemic agents and the control of blood sugar influenced the rate of occurrence of vascular complications in patients with adult-onset diabetes (University Group Diabetes Program, 1977). Among the findings of this investigation was the fact that all efforts to control hyperglycemia, as measured by fasting blood sugar levels, failed to reduce mortality or morbidity from cardiovascular causes. Moreover, the number and proportion of deaths due to myocardial infarction and other cardiovascular diseases was significantly greater in patients provided treatment with the hypoglycemic agents.

The atherogenic effect of diabetes has not been linked to the capillary basement membrane thickening characteristic of diabetes. Both vascular lesions may have as a common basis a fundamental defect affecting connective tissue, but such a link is speculative. Diabetics have higher serum lipid levels, especially of triglycerides, than do nondiabetics, but the differences do not account for the increased risk of atherosclerotic disease. Diabetes reduces greatly the sex differential in mortality from coronary heart disease, but does not change the sex differential in angina pectoris (Gordon and Shurtleff, 1973). A diabetic effect on the terminal episode would be consistent with this observation. Neither insulin nor oral hypoglycemic agents protect diabetics from the increased risk of atherosclerotic disease, and the findings of the UGDS indicate that oral hypoglycemic drugs increase the probability of cardiovascular death for the diabetic (University Group Diabetes Program, 1977). As with other complex metabolic diseases, it seems likely that diabetes also may influence thrombosis.

Hypothyroidism

It has long been known both from clinical observations and animal experiments that the metabolism of lipids is influenced by hormones, particularly thyroxine. Among the lipids, serum cholesterol levels show the greatest regularity in response to the circulating level of thyroid hormone, but other lipid components may be affected (see review by Naito and Kumar, 1980). Our results (Naito and Kumar, 1980), indicated that the serum total cholesterol concentration of the hypothyroid patients is higher than the euthyroid group. On the other hand, the hyperthyroid patients have slightly lower levels of total cholesterol. The serum triglyceride and phospholipid levels of the hypothyroid group are slightly higher than the eu- or hyperthyroid groups, which is in agreement with past reports.

The serum lipoprotein electrophoresis study indicates that there is a higher percentage of β-lipoprotein in the hypothyroid group when compared to the euthyroid patients. This agrees with the elevated serum total cholesterol content seen in the hypothyroid individuals. While there is a reduction in the total cholesterol in the hyperthyroid group, there was no reduction in the distribution of lipoproteins in the β-lipoprotein class. There is, however, less cholesterol (45 ± 3 mg/dl) in the HDL of the hyperthyroid group when compared to the hypothyroid group (53 ± 4 mg/dl). HDL cholesterol concentration for the euthyroid group was 50 ± 4 mg/dl. It is interesting that the slight elevation of serum triglycerides seen in the hypothyroid group did not result in a concomitant rise in the pre-β-lipoprotein area. Whether the increased proportion of β-lipoprotein in the hypothyroid group resulted in more cholesterol and triglycerides carried in that moiety is not clear. Only when serum triglycerides were markedly elevated (>200 mg/dl) did we see a concomitant rise in the pre-β-lipoprotein fraction.

Gout

A common metabolic disorder associated with gout is hyperlipidemia. The high incidence of atherosclerosis as a complication of gout has been recognized for about 100 years. However, the precise relationships of gout or hyperuricemia to coronary artery disease have not been clear. The relationship of primary gout to dysmetabolism of lipids and lipoproteins is also not clear.

A review (Naito et al., 1980) indicated that, although there is much discrepancy in published data on the relationship between increased serum uric acid and blood lipid concentrations, there appears to be a high correlation between the two variables, particularly between hypertriglyceridemia and hyperuricemia. However, the relationship between serum uric acid and triglyceride concentrations is not always predictable (Feldman and Wallace, 1964). However, according to Naito and Mackenzie (1979), about 73 percent of the asymptomatic gout patients had hypertriglyceridemia in their studies, 1.6-fold the frequency found in the control group. Types IV and IIb lipoprotein electrophoretic patterns were most prevalent in the gout group. Neither alcohol intake nor hyperuricemia per se seems to be the cause of the lipid and lipoprotein disorder, which cannot be related to liver or kidney dysfunctions. Obesity was the major underlying factor associated with lipidemia. The study suggested that diet and, possibly, defective clearance of triglycerides may be etiologic factors associated with the abnormal serum triglyceride and lipoprotein concentrations in these individuals.

Oral Contraceptive Agents

The introduction and wide use of oral contraceptive agents has brought significant health and social advantages for women. However, it has become increasingly apparent that there are health hazards involved in their use. Most important among these are morbidity and mortality from cardiovascular diseases. The physiologic and metabolic effects of these agents are dependent on the type and quantity of steroid contained, whether synthetic estrogens or derivatives of nortestosterone and progesterone. These effects cannot be examined in detail here, but a comprehensive review of the subject is available (Beck, 1973).

Metabolic side effects of the contraceptive steroids include changes in plasma cholesterol and triglyceride concentrations, which are related to the specific steroids used, dosage, and duration of treatment (Ferrari and Naito, 1978). In general, the effects are small, and nortestosterone derivatives counteract the triglyceride-increasing effect of synthetic estrogens. The effects on triglycerides are greater than those on cholesterol, and persist through the middle fifties. These hormones generally modify the age-related changes in plasma cholesterol and triglyceride levels. There appears to be a small increase in hypercholesterolemia among hormone users up to age 49, after which there was decreased risk among users (Wallace et al., 1977). Similar analysis of the triglyceride data demonstrated a five-fold increase in hypertriglyceridemia in the youngest women, aged 15 to 19, who used contraceptive steroids, with persistently higher rates up through the 45- to 49-year-old group, when the risk of developing the hyperlipidemia was twice that of nonusers. The significance of the elevation in plasma triglyceride levels is uncertain, since the relation of this hyperlipidemia and VLDL with CHD is inconclusive. Other reports have demonstrated that in postmenopausal women synthetic estrogens increase HDL-cholesterol content and decrease the LDL-cholesterol content (Furmon et al., 1967; Gustafson and Svanborg, 1972), effects which should reduce risk.

Oral contraceptives have been reported to produce elevation of blood pressure in hypertensive women (Yang and Van Stallie, 1976). In other instances, hypertensive blood pressures have been observed to fall when women discontinued using the hormones (Crane et al., 1971). The frequency and extent of blood pressure elevation has been studied in 13,358 women who were currently using, had discontinued use, or had never used oral contraceptives (Fisch and Frank, 1977). Mean systolic and diastolic blood pressures were given by age in these three groups of women. In all age groups, mean values for both systolic and diastolic pressures were greatest in women who were current users. The overall contribution of the oral contraceptive was to increase systolic pressure by 5 to 6 mm Hg and diastolic pressure by 1 to 2 mm Hg. There was an increased proportion of women users with elevated blood pressure, with this risk greatest for women older than 35 years but independent of relative weight.

An increased risk of fatal myocardial infarction in older women using oral contraceptives has been reported (Mann and Inman, 1976). The use of oral contraceptives has been shown to increase the risk of stroke, independent of the effects of smoking and hypertension (Collaborative group for study of stroke in young women, 1975). This may result from the thrombogenic activity of the contraceptive steroids. The search for the responsible mechanism has been undertaken, and a decrease in plasma of activated Factor X inhibitory activity has been reported by Wessler and associates (1976).

Stress

The term *stress* means many different things to different individuals. Thus, there is no common denominator that equivocally links stress to CHD.

There is a large body of literature that has sought to examine and describe the various psychologic, social, cultural, and behavioral characteristics of individuals and their relationship with the incidence of CHD. A review of this area has recently been published (Jenkins, 1976). The interest in the area derives from the fact that only a portion of the total risk for CHD can be ascribed to the major risk factors. In addition, there is a widely held notion that certain individuals are coronary prone because of behavioral and psychologic factors. Such characteristics are also seen to be important determinants of whether an individual smokes cigarettes, selects foods appropriate to health, or responds to external stimulus in a way in which blood pressure is increased. Accordingly, psychosocial factors may be of such potency as to determine whether major risk factors exist in the individual and whether they can be dealt with effectively in programs of risk-factor reduction.

Much attention has been given to the claim that persons are at higher risk if they have Type A coronary-prone behavior patterns (Friedman and Rosenman, 1971). This is described as a style of behavior that includes some of the following characteristics: intense striving for achievement, competitiveness, easily provoked impatience, time urgency, abruptness of gesture and speech, overcommitment to vocation and profession, and excess of hostility and drive. In contrast, Type B behavior is relaxed, calm, and unhurried. Most investigations utilizing this characterization of behavior have found higher CHD morbidity and mortality associated with Type A persons. The significance of this finding and its relationship to other risk variables needs further elaboration.

ETIOLOGY AND PATHOGENESIS

In reviewing the complex subject of the etiology and pathogenesis of atheroma we shall endeavor to adopt a synthetic or holistic approach, rather than subscribe preferentially to one or more of the mutually exclusive hypotheses. Hopefully it will become apparent that the etiology of atheroma is not the sole domain of the platelet, lipoproteins, high blood pressure, lysosome, or smooth cell, but rather that each of these factors is an essential piece for the sequential assembly of an exceedingly complex mosaic to which we ascribe the term *atherogenesis.*

Initiating Factors

It is not unreasonable to make the basic and probably correct assumption that the essential event or sine qua non of atherogenesis is enhanced transendothelial transport of macromolecules, resulting either from frank endothelial injury or, alternatively, from more subtle modifications in endothelial structure and function. The factors that enhance this transendothelial permeability to macromolecules, including low-density lipoprotein, which results in a net influx or retention within the subendothelium and media, may be conveniently considered as initiating factors. Retention may result not only from an enhanced influx but also from a decreased efflux. Decreased efflux may reflect binding of the macromolecules to components of the arterial wall or, alternatively, molecular modifications that occur within the arterial wall and render the molecules less able to tranverse the endothelium to the lumen.

Focal hemodynamically induced endothelial injury with enhanced permeability is the probable determinant of the consistent and discrete localization of the atheromatous process. Hemodynamic effects may be mediated by shear, stretch, vibration, or pressure. Additional initiating factors, other than those associated with focal hemodynamics, include the release of platelet constituents, hypertension, carbon monoxide, antigen-antibody complexes, and hyperlipidemia. Cigarette smoking may prove to be an important initiating factor which exerts its effects either directly through an immune mechanism or indirectly through released platelet constituents or carbon monoxide.

Accelerating Factors

Factors that influence the nature or rate of lesion development at all subsequent stages are conveniently classified under the generic term *accelerating factors*. Accelerating factors of note include hypercholesterolemia with an associated excess of low-density lipoprotein and disturbances in platelet function, hemostasis, and thrombosis. These accelerating factors, namely, LDL and platelet factors, may influence the nature and rate of plaque development by stimulating the proliferation of smooth muscle cells and by stimulating to varying degrees the synthesis by smooth muscle cells (SMC) of collagen, elastin, and the glycosaminoglycans. In addition, lipoproteins may significantly influence SMC lipid metabolism, including cholesterol synthesis, and the uptake and accumulation of lipids within smooth muscle cells.

Interaction between initiating and accelerating factors: As might be anticipated, there may be several levels of complex interaction, not only among differing accelerating factors, but also between accelerating and initiating factors. For example, platelets, through the release of their constituents, including 5-hydroxytryptamine, histamine, thromboxane A_2, and lysosomal enzymes, may directly cause endothelial injury or modify endothelial permeability. This modification of endothelial permeability will serve to enhance the entry of accelerating factors, such as LDL, and certain platelet proteins, which subsequently stimulate SMC proliferation.

In addition, platelets may directly contribute to plaque growth by serving as components of mural thrombi. LDL may directly induce a spectrum of changes consistent with endothelial injury. In Type II hyperlipoproteinemia, LDL has been shown as well to be associated with modified platelet function which might influence the risk of thrombus formation.

Other Pathogenic Processes

Other processes not yet discussed which are of importance in pathogenesis include the concept of a monoclonal origin of the cells in atheroma, and also the concept that atheroma is a lysosomal storage disease, with the marked accumulation of cholesterol esters resulting from an overload of the lysosomal enzyme systems. Both the monoclonal explanation for the cellular monotypism, which in essence implies that atheromatous lesions are benign smooth muscle cell tumors, and the possible role of a lysosomal enzyme deficit in the accumulation of arterial lipids are compatible with the overview presented. Just how important each of these mechanisms is in the pathogenesis of atheroma has yet to be established.

There remain many unanswered questions and unresolved issues. For example, the precise relationship between fatty streaks and fibrous plaques in the evolution of atheroma has still to be clarified. Furthermore, how does the fibrous atherosclerotic plaque begin and progress, are the earliest lesions as characteristic of the disease as is the atherosclerotic plaque, and what extramural factors directly or indirectly influence the composition of the precursor lesions and the rate of their progression to the plaque? Other important questions relate to the time scale for the development or regression of clinically significant disease, the reasons for the striking sex-associated differences in disease prevalence and severity, and the mechanisms underlying the consistently greater frequency of clinical disease in patients with diabetes mellitus.

Finally, there may exist risk factors that so far have not been recognized and therefore are not measured. Identification of measurable characteristics associated with the probability of atheroma would make possible testing their relationship to coronary heart disease.

REFERENCES

Beck, P. Progress in endocrinology and metabolism–Contraceptive steroids: Modifications of carbohydrate and lipid metabolism. *Metabolism* 22, 841–855 (1973).

Becker, C.G., and Dubin, T. Activation of factor XII by tobacco glycoprotein. *J. Exp. Med.* 146(2), 457–467 (1977).

Bierman, E.L., and Ross, R. *Atherosclerosis Reviews,* Vol. 2. A.M. Gotto, and R. Paoletti, eds. Raven Press, New York (1977), pp. 79–111.

Bjorntoys, P., Fahlen, M., Grimby, G., Gustafson, A., Holm, J., Renstrom, P., and Schersten, T. Carbohydrate and lipid metabolism in middle-aged physically well-trained men. *Metabolism* 21, 1037–1044 (1972).

Collaborative group for the study of stroke in young women, Oral contraceptives and stroke in young women–Associated risk factors. *J. Am. Med. Assoc.* 231, 718–722 (1975).

Crane, M.G., Harris, J.J., and Winsor, W. III. Hypertension, oral contraceptive agents, and conjugated estrogens. *Ann. Intern. Med.* 74, 13–21 (1971).

Doll, R., and Hill, A.B. Mortality in relation to smoking: Ten years' observations of British doctors. *Br. Med. J.* 1, 1399–1410 (1964).

Duff, G.L., and McMillan, G.C. Pathology of atherosclerosis. *Am. J. Med.* 11, 92–108 (1951).

Feldman, E.B., and Wallace, S.L. Hypertriglyceridemia in gout. *Circulation* 29, 508–513 (1964).

Ferrari, L., and Naito, H.K. Effect of estrogens on rat serum cholesterol concentrations; consideration of dose, type of estrogen, and treatment duration. *Endocrinology* 102(5), 1621-1627 (1978).

Fisch, I.R., and Frank, J. Oral contraceptives and blood pressure. *JAMA* 237, 2499-2503 (1977).

Fischer-Dzoga, K., Jones, R.M., Vesselinovich, D., and Wissler, R.W. Increased mitotic activity in primary cultures of aortic medial smooth muscle cells after exposure to hyperlipemic serum, in *Atherosclerosis III*. G. Schettler, and A. Weizel, eds. Springer-Verlag, Berlin (1974), pp. 193-195.

Freis, E.D. Age, race, sex, and other indices of risk in hypertension. *Am. J. Med.* 55, 275-280 (1973).

Friedman, M., and Rosenman, R.H. Type A behavior pattern–its association with coronary heart disease. *Ann. Clin. Res.* 3, 300-312 (1971).

Furman, R.H., Alaupovic, P., and Howard, R.P. Effects of androgens and estrogens in serum lipids and the composition and concentration of serum lipoproteins in normolipemic and hyperlipemic states. *Prog. Biochem. Pharmacol.* 2, 215-249 (1967).

Glagov, S., and Ozoa, A.K. Significance of the relatively low incidence of atherosclerosis in the pulmonary, renal, and mesenteric arteries. *Ann. N.Y. Acad. Sci.* 149(2), 940-955 (1968).

Goldstein, J.L., and Brown, M.S. Lipoprotein receptors, cholesterol metabolism, and atherosclerosis. *Arch. Path.* 99(4), 181-184 (1975).

Gordon, T., and Shurtleff, D. *An Epidemiological Investigation of Cardiovascular Disease,* Section 29. Department of Health, Education, and Welfare Pub. No. 74-478. National Institutes of Health, Washington, D.C. (1973).

Gordon, T., Castelli, W.P., Hjortland, M.C., Kannel, W.B., and Dawber, T.B. High density lipoproteins as a protective factor against coronary heart disease. The Framington Study. *Am. J. Med.* 62(5), 707-714 (1977).

Gustafson, A., and Svanborg, A. Gonadal steroid effects on plasma lipoproteins and individual phospholipids. *J. Clin. Endocrin. Metab.* 35, 203-207 (1972).

Handa, Y. Studies on a dyslipoproteinemia in hemodialysis patients. *Jap. Heart J.* 19, 236-251 (1978).

Haust, M.D. Injury and repair in the pathogenesis of atherosclerotic lesions, in *Atherosclerosis.* R.J. Jones, ed. Springer-Verlag, New York (1970), pp. 12-20.

Haust, M.D. Light and electron microscopy of human atherosclerotic lesions, in *The Thrombic Process in Atherogenesis.* A.B. Chandler, K. Eurenivs, G.C. McMillan, C.B. Nelson, C.J. Schwartz, and S. Wissler, eds. Plenum Press, New York (1978), pp. 33-60.

Haust, M.D., and More, R.H. Significance of the smooth muscle cell in atherogenesis, in *The Pathogenesis of Atherosclerosis.* R.W. Wissler, and J.C. Geer, eds. Williams and Wilkins Co. (1972), Baltimore, pp. 1-19.

Hollander, W. Role of hypertension in atherosclerosis and cardiovascular disease. *Am. J. Cardiol.* 38, 786-800 (1976).

Jenkins, C.D. Recent evidence supporting psychologic and social risk factors for coronary disease. *N. Eng. J. Med.* 294, 987-994, 1033-1038 (1976).

Kagan, A., Gordon, T., Rhoads, G.G., and Schiffman, J.C. Some factors related to coronary heart disease incidence in Honolulu Japanese men: The Honolulu Heart Study. *Int. J. Epidem.* 4, 271-279 (1975).

Kannel, W.B., LeBauer, E.J., Dawber, T.R., and McNamara, P.M. Relation of body weight to development of coronary heart disease. *Circulation* 35, 734-744 (1967).

Kannel, W.B., Sorlie, P., Brand, F., Castelli, W.P., McNamara, P.M., and Gheradi, G.J. Epidemiology of coronary atherosclerosis: Postmortem vs. clinical risk factor correlations. The Framingham Study, in *Atherosclerosis V.* A.M. Gotto, Jr., L.C. Smith, and B. Allen, eds. Springer-Verlag, New York (1980), pp. 54–56.

Kessler, I.I. Mortality experience of diabetic patients. A twenty-six year follow-up study. *Am. J. Med.* 51, 715–724 (1971).

Lewis, L.A., and Naito, H.K. Relation of hypertension, lipids, and lipoproteins to atherosclerosis. *Clin. Chem.* 24, 2081–2098 (1978).

Lindner, A., Charra, B., Sherrard, D.J., and Scribner, B.H. Accelerated atherosclerosis in prolonged maintenance hemodialysis. *N. Eng. J. Med.* 290, 697–701 (1974).

Londe, S., and Golding, D. High blood pressure in children: Problems and guidelines for evaluation and treatment. *Am. J. Card.* 37, 650–657 (1976).

McGill, H.C., Jr. (ed.) *The Geographic Pathology of Atherosclerosis.* Williams and Wilkins, Baltimore (1968).

Malinow, M.R., McLaughlin, P., Papworth, L., Naito, H.K., Lewis, L., and McNulty, W.P. A Model for therapeutic interventions on established coronary atherosclerosis in a nonhuman primate, in *Atherosclerosis Drug Discovery.* C.E. Day, ed. Plenum Press, New York (1976), pp. 3–31.

Mann, J.I., and Inman, W.H.W. Oral contraceptives and death from myocardial infarction. *Br. Med. J.* 2, 245–248 (1976).

Miamisono, T., Wada, M., Akamatsu, A., Okabe, M., Handa, Y., Morita, T., Asagami, C., Naito, H.K., Nakamoto, S., Lewis, L.A., and Mise, J. Dyslipoproteinemia (a remnant lipoprotein disease) in uremic patients on hemodialysis. *Clin. Chem. Acta* 84, 163–172 (1978).

Morgan, A.D. *The Pathogenesis of Coronary Occlusion.* Blackwell Scientific Publications, Oxford (1956).

Naito, H.K. Effects of physical activity on serum cholesterol metabolism: A review. *Cleveland Clin. Q.* 43, 21–49 (1976).

Naito, H.K., and Kumar, M.S. Serum lipids and lipoproteins and their relationship with thyroid function, in *CRC Handbook of Electrophoresis, Volume II: Lipoproteins in Disease.* L.A. Lewis, and J.J. Oppit, eds. Chemical Rubber Co. Press, Boca Raton, Florida (1980), pp. 197–215.

Naito, H.K., and Mackenzie, A.H. Secondary hypertriglyceridemia and hyperlipoproteinemia in patients with primary asymptomatic gout. *Clin. Chem.* 25, 371–375 (1979).

Naito, H.K., Mackenzie, A., Willis, C.E., and Olnyk, M. Effect of gout on serum lipids and lipoproteins, in *CRC Handbook of Electrophoresis, vol. II: Lipoprotein in Disease.* L.A. Lewis, and J.J. Opplt, eds. Chemical Rubber Co. Press, Boca Raton, Florida (1980), pp. 185–196.

Oscai, L.B., and Holloszy, J.O. Effects of weight changes produced by exercise, food restriction, or overeating on body composition. *J. Clin. Invest.* 48, 2124–2128 (1969).

Paffenbarger, R.S., Jr., and Hale, W.E. Work activity and coronary heart mortality. *N. Eng. J. Med.* 292(11), 545–550 (1975).

Palumbo, P.J., Elveback, L.R., Chu, C.P., Connolly, D.C., and Kurland, L.T. Diabetes mellitus: Incidence, prevalance, survivorship, and causes of death in Rochester, Minnesota, 1945–1970. *Diabetes* 25, 566–573 (1976).

Report of the Intersociety Commission for Heart Disease Resources. Primary Prevention of the Atherosclerotic Diseases. *Circulation* 62, A-55–A-95 (1970).

Rifkind, B.M., in *Atherosclerosis Reviews,* vol. 2. A.M. Gotto and R. Paoletti eds. Raven Press, New York (1977), pp. 67–78.

Rode, A., Ross, R., and Shepard, R.J. Smoking withdrawal programme: Personality and cardiorespiratory fitness. *Arch. Env. Health* 24, 27–36 (1972).

Rosenman, R.H., Brand, R.J., Jenkins, C.D., Friedman, M., Strauss, R., and Wurm, M. Coronary heart disease in the Western collaborative group study. *JAMA* 233, 872–877 (1975).

Rutherford, R.B., and Ross, R. Platelet factors stimulate fibroblasts and smooth muscle cells quiescent in plasma serum to proliferate. *J. Cell Biol.* 69(1), 196–203 (1976).

Scheuer, J., and Tipton, C.M. Cardiovascular adaptations to physical training. *Ann. Rev. Physiol.* 39, 221–251 (1977).

Schwartz, C.J., and Mitchell, J.R.A. Observations on the localization of arterial plaques. *Circ. Res.* 11, 63–73 (1962).

Schwartz, C., Chandler, A.B., Gerrity, R.G., and Naito, H.K. Clinical and pathological aspects of arterial thrombosis and thromboembolism, in *The Thrombic Process in Atherogenesis,* A.B. Chandler, K. Eurenivs, G.C. McMillan, C.B. Nelson, C.J. Schwartz, and S. Wissler, eds. Plenum Press, New York (1978), pp. 111–126.

Solberg, L.A., and McGarry, P.A. Cerebral atherosclerosis in Negroes and Caucasians. *Atherosclerosis* 16, 141–154 (1972).

Stamler, J. Epidemiology of coronary heart disease. *Med. Clin. N. Am.* 57, 5–46 (1973).

Stemmermann, G.N., Rhoads, G.G., and Hayashi, T. Atherosclerosis and its risk factors among Hawaii Japanese, in *Atherosclerosis V.* A.M. Gotto, Jr., L.C. Smith, and B. Allen, eds. Springer-Verlag, New York (1980), pp. 63–66.

Strong, J.P., and Richards, M.L. Cigarette smoking and atherosclerosis in autopsied men. *Atherosclerosis* 23(3), 451–476 (1976).

Strong, J.P., Eggen, D.A., and Oalmann, M.C. The natural history, geographic pathology, and epidemiology of atherosclerosis, in *The Pathogenesis of Atherosclerosis.* R.W. Wissler, and J.C. Geer, eds. Williams and Wilkins, Baltimore (1974), pp. 20–40.

Strong, J.P., Eggen, D.A., and Tracy, R.E. The geographic pathology and topography of atherosclerosis and risk factors for atherosclerotic lesions, in *The Thrombotic Process in Atherogenesis.* A.B. Chandler, K. Eurenivs, G.C. McMillan, C.B. Nelson, C.J. Schwartz, and S. Wissler, eds. Plenum Press, New York (1978), pp. 11–31.

Telecom Health Research Group. Cardiovascular risk factors among Japanese and American telephone executives. *Int. J. Epidem.* 6, 7–15 (1977).

Truett, J., Cornfield, J., and Kannel, W. A multivariate analysis of the risk of coronary heart disease in Framingham. *J. Chron. Dis.* 20, 511–524 (1967).

University Group Diabetes Program, A study of the effects of hypoglycemic agents on the vascular complications on patients with adult onset diabetes. *J. Am. Diab. Assoc.* 19, 747–830 (1970).

Wada, M., Minamisono, T., Fujii, H., Morita, T., Akamatsu, A., Mise, J., Nakamoto, S., and Naito, H.K. Studies on the effects of hemodialysis on plasma lipoproteins. *Trans. Am. Soc., Artif. Int. Org.* XXI, 464–71 (1975).

Wagner, W.D., Clarkson, T.B., Feldner, M.A., and Pritchard, R.W. The development of pigeon strains with selected atherosclerosis characteristics. *Exp. Mol. Path.* 19, 304–319 (1973).

Wallace, R.B., Hoover, J., Sandler, D., Rifkind, B.M., and Tyroler, H.A. Altered plasma-lipids associated with oral contraceptive or estrogen consumption. *Lancet* 2, 11–14 (1977).

Wessler, S., Gitel, S.N., Wan, L.S., and Pasternack, B.S. Estrogen-containing oral contraceptive agents, a basis for their thrombogenicity. *JAMA* 236, 2179–2182 (1976).

Wissler, R.W. Progression and regression of atherosclerotic lesions, in *The Thrombic Process in Atherogenesis.* A.B. Chandler, K. Eurenivs, G.C. McMillan, C.B. Nelson, C.J. Schwartz, and S. Wissler, eds. Plenum Press, New York (1978), pp. 77–110.

Wood, P.D., Haskell, W., Klein, H., Lewis, S., Stern, M.P., and Farquhar, J.W. The distribution of plasma lipoproteins in middle-aged male runners. *Metabolism* 25, 249–1257 (1976).

Yang, M.U., and Van Stallie, T.B. Composition of weight lost during short-term weight reduction. *J. Clin. Invest.* 58, 722–730 (1976).

2

Factors in Childhood and Adolescence Leading to Premature Atherosclerotic Vascular Disease

ALVIN L. SCHULTZ

INTRODUCTION

It is becoming apparent that by the time overt atherosclerotic vascular disease becomes manifest in adult life, damage to vital arteries (coronary, cerebral, renal, and aortic) is usually so extensive that preventive measures at that point in time have little to offer for improving prognosis. There is increasing interest and emphasis directed at identifying those persons in the population who, for a variety of reasons, are at increased risk for the premature development of atherosclerotic vascular disease at an early age, and beginning management at that time. This requires an understanding of the factors currently known to be associated with risk of premature vascular disease, screening children and young adults for the presence of these factors, and promptly instituting what remedial and preventive measures we now have available.

The following factors have been shown to be associated with an increased risk of premature vascular disease:

1. Family history of coronary artery or cerebrovascular disease before age 50 years
2. Presence of Type II (familial) hyperlipidemia
3. Presence of hypertension
4. End-stage renal disease requiring chronic hemodialysis or renal allograft transplantation
5. Primary hypothyroidism with associated hypercholesterolemia
6. Diabetes mellitus
7. Corticosteroid excess
8. Oral contraceptive pills

At the time of writing there is no way of changing one's genetic configuration and its associated risk to life. However, it is still important to identify young persons with high risk factors related to genetic makeup, so that all other risk factors can be minimized. Children with a family history of myocardial infarction in close relatives before age 50 years, with or without a history of familial hyperlipidemia, should be screened early in life and closely followed for occurrence of other risk factors (smoking, obesity, hypertension, diabetes, etc.). Dietary and other means of eliminating or minimizing these additive risk factors should be instituted as early in life as possible.

Although controversy still continues in regard to the relationship of serum lipid levels within the so-called normal range and the occurrence of atherosclerotic vascular disease, there is no question that there is greatly accelerated atherosclerosis in individuals with chronically elevated serum cholesterol levels, particularly if on a familial basis. It is this group of individuals whom we hope to identify early in life and modify their lipid levels. One of the problems in identifying this high-risk group is the establishment of an upper limit of normal for use as a reference. A fasting serum cholesterol of 240 mg percent at five years of age is considered by some to be an upper limit of normal (Freis, 1976). In a study (Morrison et al., 1977) of 6775 schoolchildren aged 6–17 years, the ninety-fifth percentiles for serum lipids were as follows:

	Ninety-fifth Percentile (mg%)			
	Males		*Females*	
Age	*White*	*Black*	*White*	*Black*
Plasma cholesterol (mg%)				
6–11 years	204	214	204	219
12–17 years	200	208	198	213
Plasma triglyceride (mg%)				
6–11 years	102	88	113	94
12–17 years	154	106	133	114

In adults between 35 and 44 years of age, a serum cholesterol level of 265 mg percent or higher appears to carry a fivefold increase in the risk of coronary artery disease compared to a level of 220 mg percent or less (Kannel et al., 1971). Once a child is identified with an increased risk due to family history of accelerated vascular disease or hyperlipidemia, he or she and his or her siblings should be carefully screened for serum lipid abnormality and closely followed thereafter. Hyperlipidemia in childhood and adolescence is usually asymptomatic and will be recognized only by lipid measurement.

Childhood and adult patients on chronic hemodialysis and those who have received a renal allograft tend to have increased levels of serum cholesterol and triglyceride and an increased mortality from coronary artery disease. In the renal transplant patients, the hyperlipidemia appears to be related to corticosteroid therapy, and the use of low-dose, alternate-day, steroid administration seems to decrease serum lipid levels (Pennisi et al., 1976).

Several hormonal disorders are associated with an increased risk of accelerated vascular disease. Sexually active teenaged girls and young women are using contraceptive pills in increasing numbers. Studies (Beral and Kay, 1977) indicate that the risk of death from myocardial infarction and hypertension in women taking oral contraceptives is almost five times the rate observed in paired women who have never taken "the pill." The mortality rate becomes almost ten times greater in women 35 to 49 years of age who have been on the pill for five years or longer. Whether the mortality occurs in a selected group of women with other underlying risk factors cannot be answered at this time. However, the present recommendation is that women with a family or personal history of cardiovascular disease, stroke, diabetes mellitus, hypertension, or lipid abnormality should not be placed on oral contraceptives. Women taking oral contraceptives should not smoke cigarettes and should restrict saturated fat intake in their diet. It is advisable that no young woman remain on oral contraceptives for longer than five years.

Screening newborns for hypothyroidism by means of serum thyroxine measurement indicates that as many as 2 percent have primary thyroid failure. The hypercholesterolemia secondary to untreated hypothyroidism is associated with premature atherosclerosis. The routine screening of newborns and children for hypothyroidism is now being widely applied with prompt treatment of the thyroid deficiency when established.

Diabetes mellitus afflicts at least 5 percent of the population and about 15 percent of all diabetes occurs in childhood and adolescence. Accelerated and premature atherosclerotic vascular disease causing myocardial infarction, diabetic retinitis, stroke, and renal failure is common in juvenile diabetes, with death from vascular complications occurring in the age range of 20 to 40 years (Crall and Roberts, 1978). Poor diabetic control and frequent bouts of ketoacidosis appear to be important factors in the occurrence of vascular lesions. The hyperlipidemia associated with diabetes mellitus is also probably an important factor. Early recognition of diabetes mellitus, control of the carbohydrate intolerance, prevention of ketoacidosis, and dietary management of the hyperlipidemia are all usually attainable and effective in extending life expectancy and diminishing crippling vascular disease in the young diabetic.

Adrenal corticosteroid excess is associated with hyperlipidemia, hypercoagulability, and accelerated atherosclerosis. Cushing's disease is usually readily recognized and controlled. However, it is frequently necessary to place children and young adults on cortisol and its analogues for long periods of time in the treatment of asthma, systemic lupus erythematosus (SLE), rheumatoid arthritis, and other serious diseases requiring steroid treatment for control. It should be recognized that a vascular risk to these patients exists, and the lowest steroid dosage should be used, as well as eliminating any other factors which may be associated with arterial damage.

REFERENCES

Beral, V., and Kay, C.R. Mortality among oral contraceptive users. *Lancet* 2, 727–731 (1977).

Crall, F.V., and Roberts, W.C. Extramural and intramural coronary arteries in juvenile diabetes mellitus. *Amer. J. Med.* 64, 221–230 (1978).

Freis, P.C. Atherosclerosis and the pediatrician. *Mil. Med.* 141, 771–776 (1976).

Kannel, W.B., Castelli, W.P., Gordon, T., and McNamara, P.M. Serum cholesterol, lipoproteins, and the risk of coronary heart disease. *Ann. Int. Med.* 74, 1–12 (1971).

Morrison, J.A., de Groot, I., Edwards, B.K., Kelly, K.A., Rauh, G.L., Mellies, M., and Glueck, C.J. Plasma cholesterol and triglyceride levels in 6775 school children, ages 6–17. *Metabolism* 26, 1199–1211 (1977).

Pennisi, A.J., Heuser, E.T., Mickey, M.R., Lyssey, A., Malekzadeh, M.H., and Fine, R.N. Hyperlipidemia in pediatric hemodialysis and renal transplant patients. *Am. J. Dis. Child.* 130, 957–961 (1976).

3

Early Nutritional Roots of Cardiovascular Disease

MILDRED S. SEELIG

INTRODUCTION

The cardiovascular diseases of infancy and childhood that are common enough to require specialty medical care and surgical correction are a development of the past 30 to 40 years, as is the epidemic of sudden death of men under 50 from ischemic heart disease (IHD). Less widely recognized is the evidence that sudden death from IHD has also occurred in infancy and childhood, with increasing frequency during the same period of time, as has generalized arteriosclerosis in very young infants, and atherosclerosis, hyperlipemia, and hypertension in older infants and children (Seelig, 1980). The initiating cardiovascular lesion can begin very early in life (in some individuals during gestation; in many during early infancy). The years during which cardiovascular diseases of all ages have increased in incidence correlate with the years during which major dietary changes were made in the industrialized countries. The amount of magnesium consumed has slowly declined; the consumption of vitamin D and phosphates (both substances that decrease magnesium retention) have risen sharply in the period from the 1920s to the present. It is thus important to note that experimental magnesium deficiency causes arterial and cardiac lesions much like those reported in thousands of infants under 2½ years of age (Seelig, 1980), and that excesses of vitamin D or phosphate, or both, intensify the abnormalities (reviews: see Seelig, 1980; and Haddy, 1980).

Table 1. Arterial Abnormalities in Infants Dead at Birth or in the First Month of Life (From Published Data, Tabulated by Seelig, 1980)

	Individual Cases (154)	*Pathology Surveys (>500)*
Arterial Pathology		
Affected Arteries:		
Coronaries (Small; Medium*	16	>170
Major)	25	
Aorta	27	?
Pulmonary	11	?
Cerebral	1	?
Visceral (Renal, Pancreatic, etc.)	12	?
Generalized	13	?
Pathologic Changes:		
Intimomedial Thickening	15	124 (18 of 54 Autopsied**)
Intimomedial, Elastica Degeneration	13	51
Intimomedial, Elastica Calcification	14	?
Lipid Infiltration	0	15
Thrombi	13	2
Atresia, Coarctation (Aorta, Pulmonary)	25	(in 140 with EFE: 36% of 1580 Autopsied)**

*Rarely examined.
**In 1 series.

Table 2. Cardiac Abnormalities Suggestive of Myocardial Hypoxia in Infants Dead at Birth or Dying Within First Month (From Published Data, Tabulated by Seelig, 1980)

	Individual Cases (154)	*Pathology Surveys (>500)*
Myocardial Damage:		
Mural	36	?
Subendocardial, Papillary Muscle	34	?
Multifocal, Disseminated	26	?
Massive Infarct	14	5
Pathologic Changes:		
Myocardial Necrosis, Cell Infiltration	41	?
Myocardial Calcification	28	?
Myocardial Fibrosis	37	?
Myocardial Lipid Infiltration	2	?
Endocardial Fibroelastosis	80	206
Conduction System Abnormality*	7	33
Outflow Obstruction:		
Supra-, Sub-, and Valvular Stenosis (Coarctation; Atresia on Artery Table)	25	>3

*Rarely examined.

Table 3. Arterial and Associated Abnormalities in Infants >1 Month to 2½ Years with Ischemic Heart Disease (Mostly Autopsy) (From Published Data, Tabulated by Seelig, 1980)

	Individual Cases (251)	*Pathology Surveys (About 2500)*
Arterial Pathology		
Arteries Affected:		
Coronaries (Small, Medium*	41	70*
Large)	69	>600
Aorta	17	>350
Pulmonary	22	
Visceral (Renal, Pancreatic, etc.)	30	
Generalized	34	>150*
Pathologic Changes:		
Intimomedial Thickening	67	>300*
Intimomedial, Elastica Degeneration	35	> 50*
Intimomedial, Elastica Calcification	45	> 50*
Lipid Infiltration, Atheroma	2	50 (Late)
Thrombi	24	
Atresia, Coarctation	20	>350

*Rarely reported.

Table 4. Cardiac Abnormalities Suggestive of Myocardial Hypoxia in Infants >1 Month to 2½ Years (Mostly Autopsy) (From Published Data, Tabulated by Seelig, 1980)

	Individual Cases (251)	*Pathology Surveys (About 2500)*
Myocardial Damage:		
Mural	35	?
Subendocardial; Papillary Muscle	48	?
Multifocal, Disseminated	39	> 50*
Massive Infarct	20	28
Pathologic Changes:		
Myocardial Necrosis; Cell Infiltration	63	?
Myocardial Calcification	26	?
Myocardial Fibrosis	40	?
Myocardial Lipid Infiltration	5	?
Myocardial Cellular (Enlargement)	2**	
(Early Change)	1**	<100**
Endocardial Fibroelastosis	111	>600
Conduction System Abnormality*	18	
Outflow Obstruction	40	About 800
Supra-, Sub-, and Valvular–Stenosis		About 250

*Rarely examined.
**UM–Ultramicroscopy or special stain.

FETAL AND INFANTILE CARDIOVASCULAR DAMAGE IN WHICH HYPOXIA OR ISCHEMIA IS IMPLICATED

Analysis of the literature (Seelig, 1980) has disclosed over 150 individually described infants and more than 500 listed in surveys of autopsied infants who had been stillborn or died in the first month of life with arterial or cardiac lesions or both–such as have been associated with hypoxia (Tables 1 and 2). The literature analysis also revealed over 250 individually reported cases and about 2500 in pathology surveys of infants dying after one month to 2½ years of age (Tables 3 and 4). Among those who were stillborn, or who died within the first few days of life, the lesions must be assumed to have occurred during gestation or perinatally. As indicated in the top portions of Tables 5 and 6, data on the condition or history of the mother have been given infrequently. When cited, the conditions were generally those that predispose to fetal malnutrition and hypoxia and resultant intrauterine growth retardation (IUGR), reflected by infants that are small for gestational age (SGA). The early necrotic changes found in arteries of myocardium of infants born with severe perinatal hypoxia (Gruenwald, 1949), and the endocardial fibroelastosis (EFE) found in infants with neonatal hemolytic disease (Hogg, 1962), suggest that placental abnormalities that interfere with fetal oxygenation earlier in gestation might play a role in some of the grosser congenital cardiac anomalies (Johnson, 1952), as well as in the arteriosclerosis found at birth and early infancy. Scrutiny of individual case reports and pathology surveys shows that, although infrequently examined, involvement of the small- and medium-sized coronary arteries was reported almost as frequently as was disease of the major coronaries. Blanc et al. (1966), whose group had observed coronary disease in only 0.6 percent of 6000 consecutive autopsies of neonates to 12-year-old children, found that when the small (e.g., terminal) branches of the coronaries were examined, the incidence of coronary disease and associated myocardial infarction (MI) rose to 12 percent of 153 consecutive autopsies. They stated that the myocardial fibrosis and calcification found in some cases suggested that the myocardial necrosis might have been prenatal. Lesions of the subendocardium and of the papillary muscles (the most frequently involved sites in early infancy), and disseminated multifocal lesions (which probably reflect disease of the small intramyocardial arteries (for a review, see Seelig and Haddy, 1980) were more frequently reported than were massive infarctions. However, that as many as 19 infants under a month of age, and that 48 more from one month to 2½ years should have died of massive MIs is startling. It should be noted that infantile MI was reported to be occurring with increasing frequency (Sabiston et al., 1960), particularly in association with anomalous origin of coronary arteries–a group excluded from the tabulation referred to here.

Table 5. Abnormalities During Gestation and Antemortem in Infants Stillborn or Dead in <1 Month with Pathologic Evidence of Ischemic Heart Disease (From Published Data, Tabulated by Seelig, 1980)

	Individual Cases (Data on ½ of 154)	*Pathology Surveys (Rarely Reported: >500)*
Pre-Eclampsia, eclampsia, diabetes mellitus Mother >38 years old	11	D.M.: 1/20–1/43* >38:1/84
Maternal immaturity; multiple; frequent births	17	9% (multiple) of 97 with cardiomegaly
Abnormal gestation; RH incompatibility	28	43 with EFE**
Fetal distress (Cardiac; ECG)	35	34
Difficult; Caesarian deliveries	10	?
Placenta praevia; abnormality	8	12
Low birth weight	10	37% of 620 LBW had cardiomegaly
Infantile cyanosis, respiratory distress	56	21 noted
Tachycardia; arrhythmia; block; other ECG abnormalities	15	10 noted
Cardiomegaly; congestive heart failure	31	?
Sudden death	10	?

*With congenital heart disease.
**EFE = Endocardial fibroelastosis.

Marked intimomedial hypertrophy, sometimes with necrosis and calcification, has been described in coronary and other arteries of very young infants. The incidence of such arterial changes cannot be ascertained from a retrospective survey of the literature, since some studies include sites of intimal proliferation and fibrosis ("cushions") as precursors of atheromata (Dock, 1946; Fangman and Hellwig, 1947), whereas others specifically exclude them as normal variants (Schornagel, 1956; Robertson, 1960; Oppenheimer and Esterly, 1967). More generalized intimal and medial proliferation and fibrosis is being increasingly considered an early manifestation of infantile arterial disease, that in a severe form has been termed "occlusive infantile arteriopathy" (Witzleben, 1970). Such infantile arterial disease might be the early form of adult atherosclerosis (Danilevicus, 1974). The most definitive pathology studies in this area are those by Neufeld and Vlodaver (1968, 1971). Their findings indirectly implicate nutritional, more than genetic, factors in the different susceptibilities to atherosclerosis of different racial groups, by analyzing the thickness of the arterial walls of infants and children of three

Table 6. Abnormalities During Gestation and Infancy in Infants >1 Month to 2½ Years with Evidence of Ischemic Heart Disease (Mostly Autopsy) (From Published Data, Tabulated by Seelig, 1980)

	Individual Cases (251)	*Pathology Surveys (About 2500)*
Pre-eclampsia, eclampsia*	9	?
Maternal immaturity; multiple; frequent births*	37	?
Fetal distress, placental abnormality*	6	?
Low birth weight*	19	?
Infantile cyanosis, respiratory distress (excluding pre-terminal)	93	?
Growth and mental retardation	35	>150**
Irritability, seizures, tremors	31	Occasional*
Apathy, atony, apnea	20	?
Syncope	16	> 70
Deafness	9	(Occasional labyrinth calcific*)
Cardioeachs	10	<700
Cardiomegaly, murmurs, failure	97	(Antemortem ?)
Tachycardia, bradycardia, block, other arrhythmia, ECG abnormality	76	>200
Hypertension	19	>750***
Hyperlipemia*	11	?
Hypercalcemia*	20	?
Sudden death (including sudden onset of short terminal illness)	87	(At Least 100)

*Rarely reported.
**In outflow obstructive disease; sometimes with ↑ Ca; vitamin D toxicity.
***All with coarctation.

Semitic groups in Isräel: Ashkenazim (Jews of European derivation), Yemenite Jews, and Bedouins. It was among the male Ashkenazim, the group with the highest incidence of early IHD, that there was the most intimomedial thickening (Fig. 1). Although it was present in the earliest months, the difference became marked in the Ashkenazi males as age progressed, as graphed for 3- to 12-month-old infants and >1- to 10-year-old boys.

Endocardial fibroelastosis is the condition reported most often in the cases tabulated: the localized or patchy forms are more frequent in the younger group (Table 2) and the diffuse thick form is more frequent in the

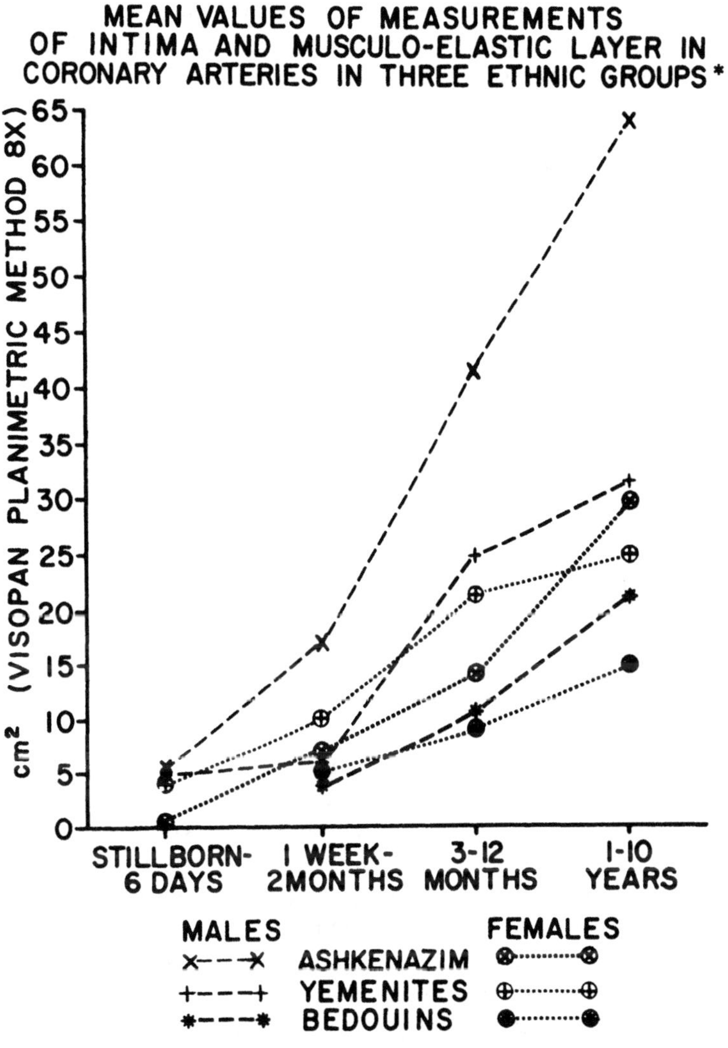

*Adapted from Neufeld and Vlodaver, 1971; from Seelig, 1980.

Fig. 1

older infants (Table 4). These lesions are included because they have been attributed to hypoxia and to ischemia (Craig, 1949; Johnson, 1952; Horley, 1955; Elliott and Elliott, 1973). Gross (1941) noted the similarity of the myocardial lesions associated with early EFE to that of adult bland MI. Elliott and Elliott (1973) remarked that endomyocardial scars of young infants are generally in areas most remote from the coronary blood supply and thus most vulnerable to hypoxia. Intimomedial thickening of the intramyocardial coronaries, that might well be responsible for inadequate blood supply to the terminal arterioles, has been reported in EFE (Craig, 1949).

It is provocative that many of the infants with luminal narrowing of the small coronaries, EFE or myocardial necrosis, whose antemortem histories had been reported, had had conduction or ECG abnormalities and not a few were reported to have died suddenly (Tables 5, 6). Tachycardia, atrial fibrillation, depressed or inverted T waves, prolonged P-R intervals, ST depression, and partial to complete heart block have all been reported, some even *in utero* (Blumberg and Lyon, 1952; Kelly and Andersen, 1956; Moller et al., 1964; Oppenheimer and Esterly, 1967). An infant born with A-V block died at two months of age with degeneration and calcification of the conducting tissue (Miller et al., 1972). Young infants with EFE were found to have involvement of the purkinjeal zone (Elliott and Elliott, 1973), a possible clue to the frequency of conduction abnormalities that have led to sudden infant death (SID) associated with EFE. Degenerative changes have also been found to be frequent in portions of the A-V node and bundle of His in infants–both in those who had died of the SID syndrome (unknown cause) and in those with identified causes of death (Anderson et al., 1970). Similar lesions were found in a baby who developed normally until a conduction defect suddenly appeared at 12½ months, leading to death a month later (Lev et al., 1967). SIDS is commonly thought to occur in infants who had been completely well; Naeye et al. (1976) have reported histories of symptoms in many resembling those listed on Tables 5 and 6. Kastor (1973) has proposed that the cause of many electrical disturbances of the heart is unknown, and that some–such as A-V block and the Wolff-Parkinson-White syndrome–might be forms of congenital heart disease. He consideres fibrosis of the peripheral bundle branches to be probably "acquired"; the foregoing data suggest that the acquisition can be very early in life.

It has been suggested that fibrosis and elastic tissue changes, seen both in coronary arteries and endocardial lesions of infants and children with EFE might be similarly caused (Esterly and Oppenheimer, 1967). Metabolic defects leading both to coronary lesions and to EFE have been considered plausible (Kelly and Andersen, 1956; Davies and Coles, 1960). Hypoxia and mechanical factors (Moller et al., 1964; Franciosi and Blanc, 1968), or predominantly outflow-obstruction (Bryan and Oppenheimer, 1969) have been implicated. Outflow-obstruction, commonly caused by great-vessel coarctation or valvular stenosis, has been considered part of the metabolic condition that increases susceptibility to hypervitaminosis D. It has been suggested that the specific malformation might depend on the magnitude, time, and extent of overdosage or degree of susceptibility (Taussig, 1965, 1966; Beuren et al., 1964, 1966), but that all of the outflow-obstructions and possibly other cardio-

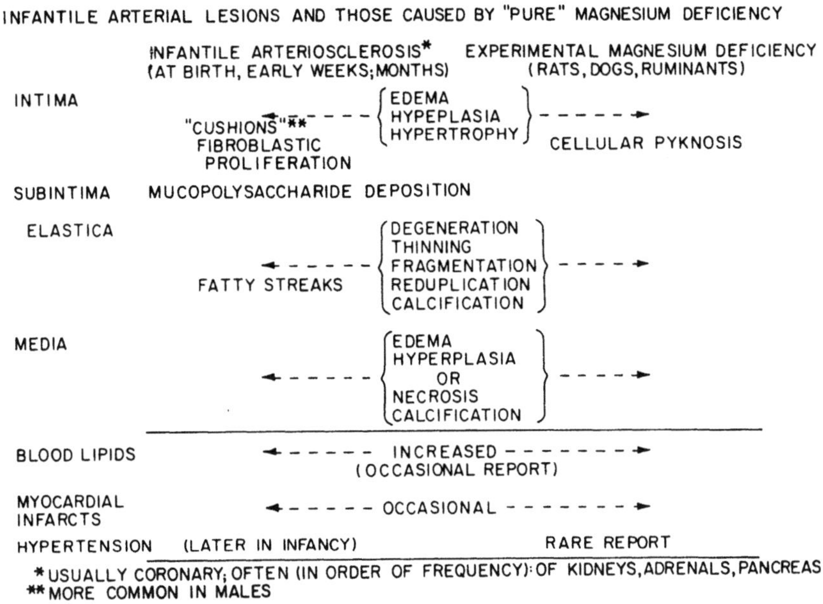

Fig. 2

vascular abnormalities might be part of the same disease process (Beuren, 1978 [personal communication]). This concept suggests that at least some of the major cardiac arterial anomalies that had been excluded from the tabulations (Seelig, 1980) from which the cited figures were derived might justifiably have been included—as possibly resulting from fetal malnutrition and hypoxia caused by maternal nutritional imbalances and placental damage.

It is important to note, in considering the damage caused by excess vitamin D to heart and arteries (Seelig, 1969b), that vitamin D excess causes magnesium loss (review: see Seelig, 1980; Seelig and Haddy, 1980), and that vitamin D excess and dietary magnesium deficiency have each been implicated in hyperlipemia and hypertension (reviews: see Linden, 1977; Seelig, 1980; Seelig and Haddy, 1980; Haddy and Seelig, 1980).

IS MAGNESIUM DEFICIENCY A FACTOR IN INFANTILE CARDIOVASCULAR DISEASE?

The coronary and cardiac lesions of stillborn and very young infants resemble those of experimental animals maintained on diets that are notable, predominantly, for magnesium deficiency (Seelig and Haddy, 1980); (Fig. 2). That this may be more than a fortuitous finding is suggested by the evidence that magnesium insufficiency is likely, both during gestation and infancy.

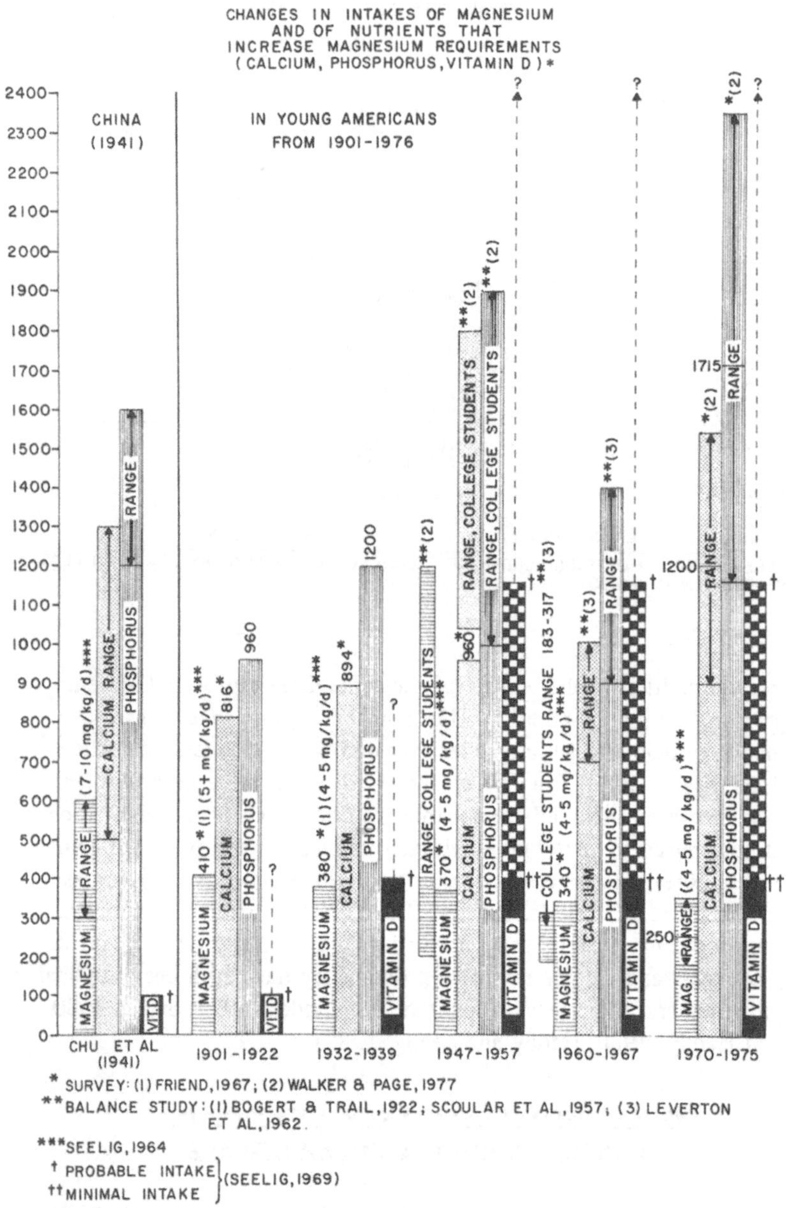

*From Seelig, 1980.

Fig. 3

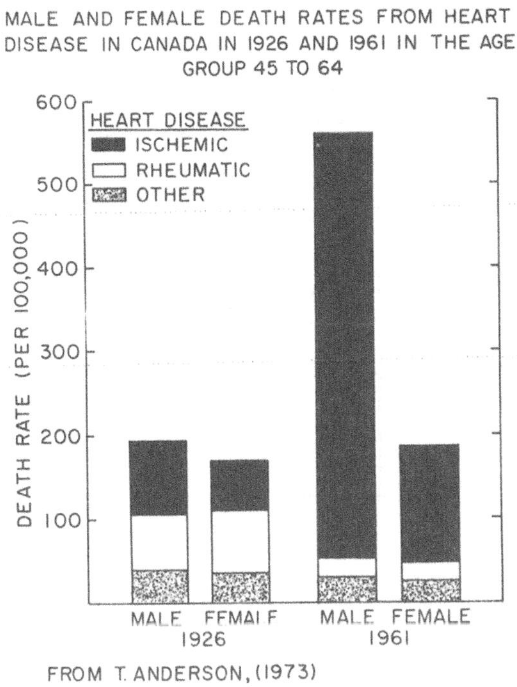

Fig. 4

Decreased Magnesium Intake and Availability

Figure 3 depicts the contrast in dietary intakes by a prerevolution middle-class population in China (Chu et al., 1941) (as representative of the Orient, where the incidence of cardiovascular disease has long been accepted as lower than it is in the Occident) and those during this century in the United States (Bogert and Trail, 1922; Leverton et al., 1962; Friend, 1967; Scoular et al., 1957; Seelig, 1969b; Walker and Page, 1977). The graph depicts the decline in magnesium intakes and the steep rises in intakes of vitamin D and phosphate, each of which increases magnesium requirements either by increasing its urinary excretion (vitamin D) or by interfering with its absorption (phosphate): the vitamin D from the mid 1920s on, and the phosphate (largely in soft drinks) from the 1940s on. It is thus important to note that both vitamin D and sodium phosphates have been used to produce or intensify experimental cardiomyopathy, and that magnesium (often with potassium and chloride) has been protective (Selye, 1958; Lehr and Krukowski, 1963; Lehr, 1965; Sos, 1965; Seelig, 1972; Seelig and Heggtveit, 1974; Seelig and Haddy, 1980).

INFLUENCE OF SEX ON MAGNESIUM BALANCE AND ON PERCENTAGE OF INTAKE EXCRETED AT DIFFERENT INTAKES OF MAGNESIUM

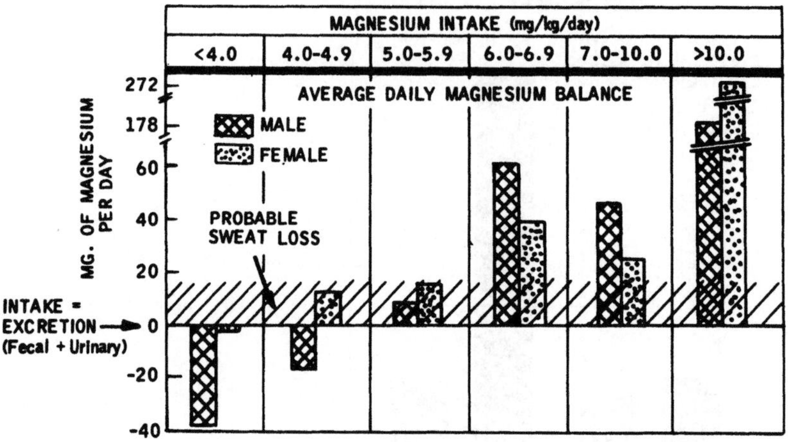

Fig. 5

SCHEMATIC REPRESENTATIONS OF ELECTROCARDIOGRAMS OF MODERATE AND SEVERE HYPOMAGNESEMIA COMPARED TO THOSE CAUSED BY HYPER- AND HYPOKALEMIA AND CALCEMIA

(FROM SEELIG, 1969)

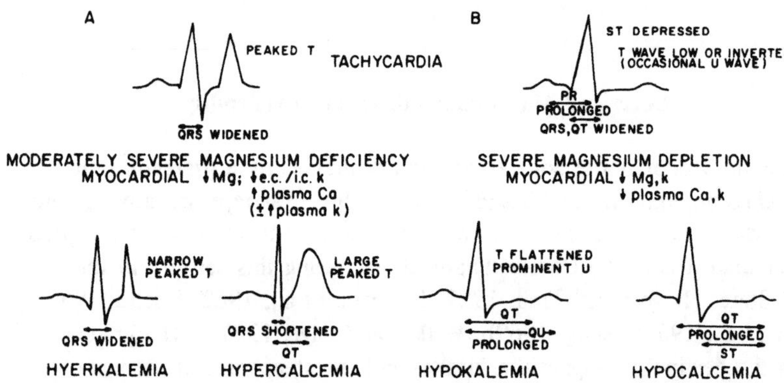

Fig. 6

Correlation of Decreased Magnesium and Increased Cardiovascular Disease

Sudden Death from IHD

It is possible that the combination of declining intakes of magnesium with sharp increases in vitamin D and phosphate intakes might have contributed to the sharp rise in incidence of IHD in men from 1926 to 1961 (Fig. 4; Anderson, 1973). The difference in retention of magnesium by young men and women on marginal intakes of magnesium (Fig. 5) first suggested to the author that a common denominator between the lower incidence of IHD in young women than young men, and in the Orient than in industrialized countries, might be the magnesium retained or ingested (Seelig, 1964). The similarity of abnormal ECGs of infants to those of magnesium deficiency (Fig. 6; Seelig, 1969a; Burch and Giles, 1977) and the similarity of arterial damage caused by magnesium deficiency to that reported in arteries supplying the conduction system of infants, many of whom died suddenly (*supra vide*), is further inferential evidence that magnesium deficiency should be considered in sudden death.

Inadequate Magnesium During Gestation

Superimposing ranges of magnesium intakes during pregnancy on a graph depicting the average calcium intake and the probable range of vitamin D intakes (Fig. 7; Seelig, 1978, 1980), shows that magnesium needs of pregnant women, and thus of their unborn babies, are unlikely to be met by the typical American diet. The Food and Nutrition Board (1980) has recommended that pregnant and lactating women ingest 450 mg of magnesium a day, an amount not even approached in the most recent surveys of the dietary intakes of midwestern American women (Ashe et al., 1979; Johnson and Philipps, 1980). Hummel et al. (1936, 1937) published long-term balance studies of two pregnant women that suggest that the optimum intake during pregnancy might be even higher than 450 mg/day. Although we cannot draw general conclusions from even long-term studies of only two subjects, it is noteworthy that the mother of three very healthy children consistently consumed a diet that provided about 600 mg of magnesium daily during her fourth pregnancy, whereas a teenaged primipara with a poor nutritional history, whose magnesium intake approached that recommended, retained only half as much magnesium as did the multipara (Table 7). The compilation of published data (Fig. 8; Coons et al., 1935) confirms the much greater retention of magnesium by pregnant women on higher than on lower intakes.

Effect of Gestational Magnesium Deficiency on Incidence of Eclampsia and on Placenta and Fetus

Two groups of investigators studied the increase in magnesium present in human fetuses as they grew and matured (Table 8; Coons et al., 1935; Widdowson and Dickerson, 1962). The amount of magnesium acquired by the fetus increases markedly towards the end of gestation. On the other hand, pregnant rats kept on a magnesium-poor diet retained their own tissue mag-

MAGNESIUM INTAKES DURING PREGNANCY AND CHANGING AVERAGE INTAKES OF MAGNESIUM, CALCIUM, VITAMIN D DURING THE 20th CENTURY
(Derived from Friend, 1967; Seelig, 1969, 1971; Johnson & Phillips, 1976; Ashe et al, 1979)

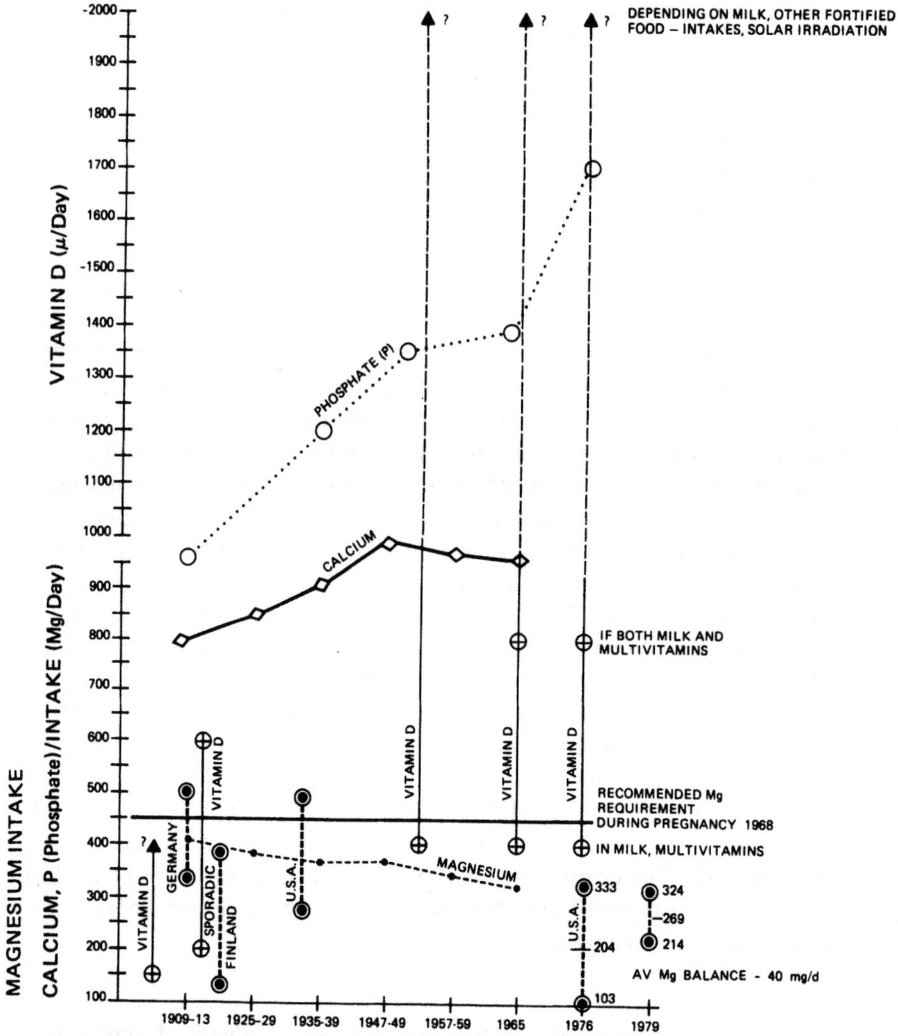

CALCULATED AVERAGE Ca INTAKE, ADULT

P INTAKE, ADULT

AVERAGE Mg INTAKE

RANGE OF VITAMIN INTAKE

Mg INTAKES, PREGNANT WOMEN

Fig. 7

Table 7. Magnesium Retentions During Last Months of Pregnancy

	Average Daily Intake and Retention			
	Healthy Quadripara (With Successful Pregnancies)*		*18 Year-Old Primipara** (Poor Nutritional History)*	
Month of Pregnancy	*Intake (mg Mg/day)*	*Retention*	*Intake (mg Mg/day)*	*Retention*
>6–7	614	+128	403	+ 58
>7–8	590	+ 85	392	+102
>8–9	615	+104	375	+ 25
>6–9 Total retention		9.6 grams		4.2 grams

*From Hummel et al., 1936.
**From Hummel et al., 1937.

COMPILATION OF PUBLISHED DATA ON THE RETENTION OF MAGNESIUM DURING HUMAN PREGNANCY SHOWING RELATION OF STORAGE TO INTAKE

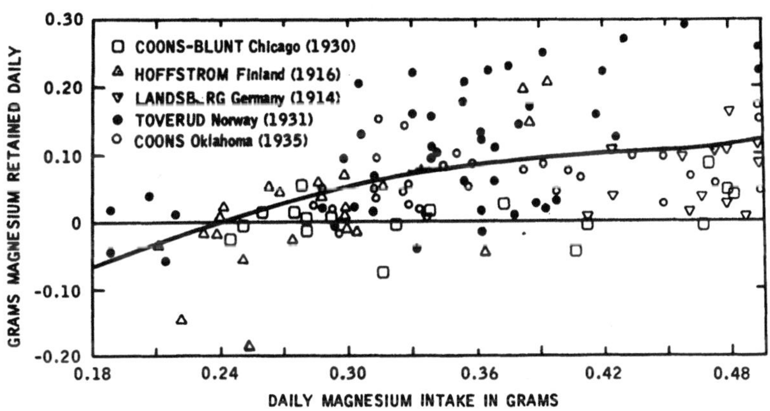

From Coons, C.M., Oklahoma Agric. & Expt'l Station Bull., 223, 1935.

Fig. 8

nesium fairly well, whereas the amount of magnesium acquired by their fetuses was less than one-fifteenth that of controls (Table 9; Dancis et al., 1971). The magnesium-deficient pregnant rats and their fetuses were comparably hypomagnesemic.

Women with toxemic pregnancies retain high percentages of therapeutic parenteral doses of magnesium (Pritchard, 1955; Kontopoulos et al., 1980) and require large amounts to maintain pharmacologic levels of plasma magnesium (Fig. 9) (Pritchard, 1955; Hall, 1957; Flowers et al., 1962; Hutchinson et al., 1963; Harbert et al., 1968). These observations, and low pretreatment serum magnesium levels, have been interpreted as possibly pointing toward

Table 8. Increase in Total Body Magnesium with Fetal Growth

*Body Weight (Grams)	mg of Mg/kg (Dry Fat-Free Fetal; Infant)	Total mg of Mg in Fetus; Baby (Dry, Fat-Free)	**Age: Fetus, Baby (Lunar Months)	(#)	Average Mg (mg) Content in Fetus, Baby	Average Mg Uptake (mg/Day)
11.1	.09	0.9				
175	.14	24	3	(7)	15	0.5
400	.15	60	4	(3)	58	1.5
737	.21	165	7	(6)	173	2.6
1500	.21	320	8	(8)	306	4.7
2500	.23	580	9	(7)	512	7.4
3500	.22	760	10	(10)	703	9.0

*From Widdowson and Spray, 1951; Coons et al., 1935.
**From Widdowson and Dickerson, 1962.

Table 9. Magnesium Levels in Maternal and Fetal Tissues (From Magnesium Deficient and Control Rats)*

	(mEq/L or kg ± SE) Magnesium Deficient	Control
Maternal plasma	0.33 ± 0.03	1.6 ± 0.04
Maternal bone	176.0 ± 12.1	213 ± 0.8
Maternal muscle	24 ± 0.5	23 ± 0.8
Fetal plasma	0.31 ± 0.02	2.4 ± 0.07
Fetus	8.9 ± 0.22	142 ± 0.39

*From Dancis et al., 1971.

magnesium deficiency as a factor in preeclampsia and eclampsia (Flowers et al., 1965; McGanity, 1965; Lim et al., 1969; Muller, 1968; Muller et al., 1974; Hurley, 1971; Seelig and Bunce, 1972; Kontopoulos et al., 1980; Seelig, 1980; Weaver, 1980). The low levels of magnesium and high levels of calcium in placentas from women who had toxemic pregnancies or borne twins (Table 10; Charbon and Hoekstra, 1962) parallels that seen in placentas of magnesium-deficient rats (Dancis et al., 1971). Is the fact that both toxemic women and magnesium deficient rats have young that are SGA another indication of IUGR in magnesium-poor mothers? Johnson and Phillips (1980) reported a direct correlation between low magnesium intakes by the pregnant Wisconsin women surveyed, and low-birth-weight infants. Abnormalities during pregnancy were not reported.

It is possible that hypervitaminosis D during gestation might be contributory to abnormal placentas, as well as to the congenital heart disease cited earlier. Scarred, small, calcified placentas were produced in rats given excess vitamin D during pregnancy (Potvliege, 1962; Ornoy et al., 1968).

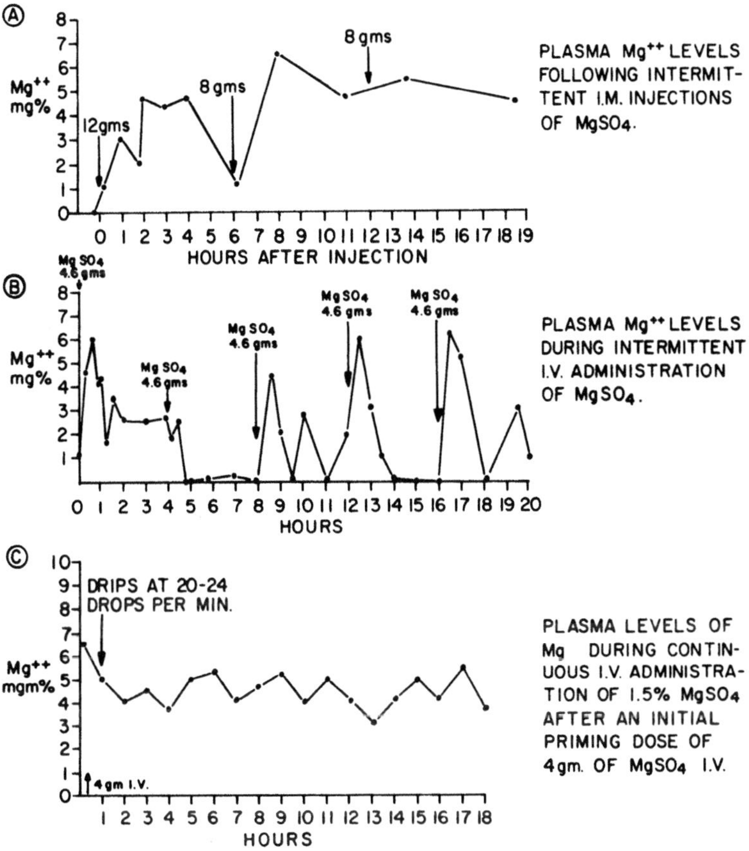

(FROM FLOWERS ET AL., 1962)

Fig. 9

Table 10. Calcium and Magnesium Content of Placentas (Tabulated by Charbon and Hoekstra, 1962)*

	Normal	*Twins*	*Pre-eclampsia*	*Eclampsia*
Magnesium (mg %)	8.87	6.94	6.49	4.30
Calcium (mg %)	86.4	124.6	942	134.6

*From Mischel, 1957.

Supravalvular aortic stenosis and EFE were produced in rabbits born to dams overdosed with vitamin D during gestation (Coleman, 1965; Friedman and Roberts, 1966). IUGR is a product of scarred placentas (Warkany et al., 1961; Scott and Usher, 1966; Wigglesworth, 1966), and there is a greater likelihood of its occurring in immature primiparas, mothers who have had previous SGA-infants or who have had six or more pregnancies. It is associated with a 16-fold increase of incidence of congenital heart disease (Scott and Usher, 1966). Required is investigation of the magnesium and vitamin D status of mothers suffering from toxemic pregnancy, who have had histories of abnormalities during pregnancy, or have had stillbirths, SGA-infants, or children with congenital heart disease.

Better insight into the magnesium status of pregnant and postpartum mothers and infants is likely to be obtained by determination of percentage-retention of a parenteral load of magnesium than by determining serum magnesium levels (Harris and Wilkinson, 1971; Caddell, 1975; Byrne and Caddell, 1975; Caddell et al., 1975a, b), assuming essentially normal renal handling of magnesium (Freeman and Pearson, 1966). It may now be difficult to ascertain whether relative or absolute vitamin D excess during human gestation affects the health of the mother, the placenta, or the infant, because vitamin D supplementation is normally unavoidable. This is particularly true in the United States and Canada, where milk, breakfast foods, and prenatal vitamins each usually provide all or some of the 400 I.U. of vitamin D recommended as both the recommended daily allowance and the maximal permitted amount (Committee on Nutrition, 1963; Seelig, 1970), an interesting situation for a substance to which there is an enormous variation in response (Fanconi, 1956; Seelig, 1969b, 1970). During the 1930s, when vitamin D-supplementation gained in popularity, and when it was starting to be given (usually with calcium salts) to pregnant women, two studies were undertaken that indicated that such supplementation might not be uniformly safe. Brehm (1937) found extensive placental calcification in two groups of 90 women each, who were given vitamin D_2 (one with and one without calcium lactate) during pregnancy. Such placental calcification was not seen in the four other groups of 90 women each, who were given (1) only calcium lactate, (2) cod liver oil, (3) both, or (4) neither. This study was undertaken when the incidence of calcified placentas, fused sutures and decreased size of fontanels, and difficult labors, was found to have increased in incidence after the practice of vitamin D supplementation had been instituted in an obstetrical clinic. Another group of investigators, also concerned about the possible effect of vitamin D supplementation during pregnancy on increased bone density, and on cranial suture closure of infants that might contribute to difficult labors, found that in several instances, in which women received vitamin D_2 and calcium phosphate, maternal and cord blood levels of calcium

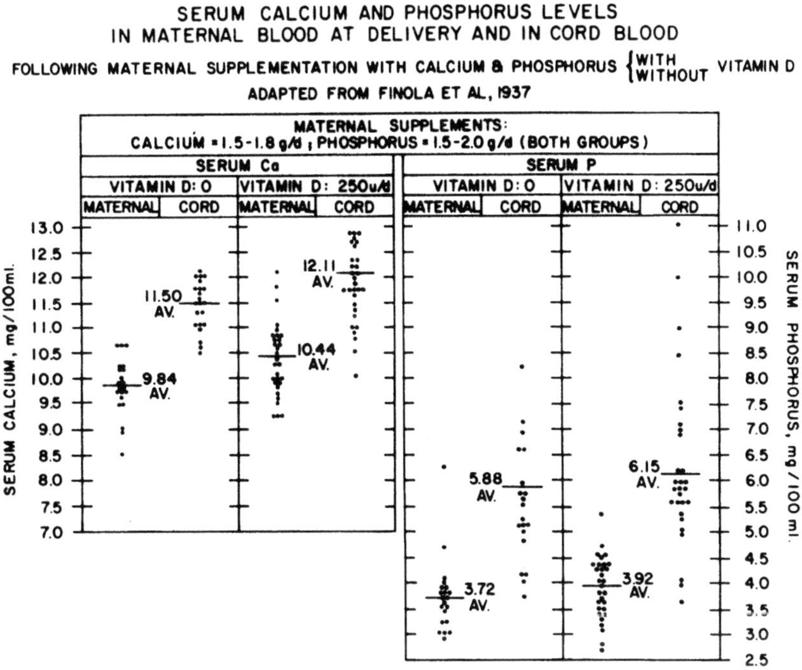

Fig. 10

were at pathologically high levels (Fig. 10; Finola et al., 1937). Although the average cord phosphorus levels were almost the same in the supplemented and nonsupplemented groups, a few infants born to supplemented mothers were hyperphosphatemic. Magnesium levels were not measured.

Vitamin D During Infancy; Human Versus Cows' Milk

Another common change during most of this century was the shift from breast- to bottle-feeding. Cows' milk has a much higher P/Mg ratio that does human milk: 7.5/1 versus 1.9/1 (Cockburn et al., 1973). Thus, it is not surprising that hyperphosphatemia is more prevalent in formula-fed than in breast-fed infants, with and without vitamin D supplements (Figs. 11, 12; Pincus et al., 1954). The same investigators also measured the serum calcium levels of the same groups of infants, and reported an unexpected finding: among the formula-fed infants, despite the higher concentrations of calcium in cows' than in human milk, the serum calcium levels of several infants were lower than in any of the breast-fed infants (Fig. 12). The lowest calcium levels were in several infants given the larger amount of vitamin D. Adapting

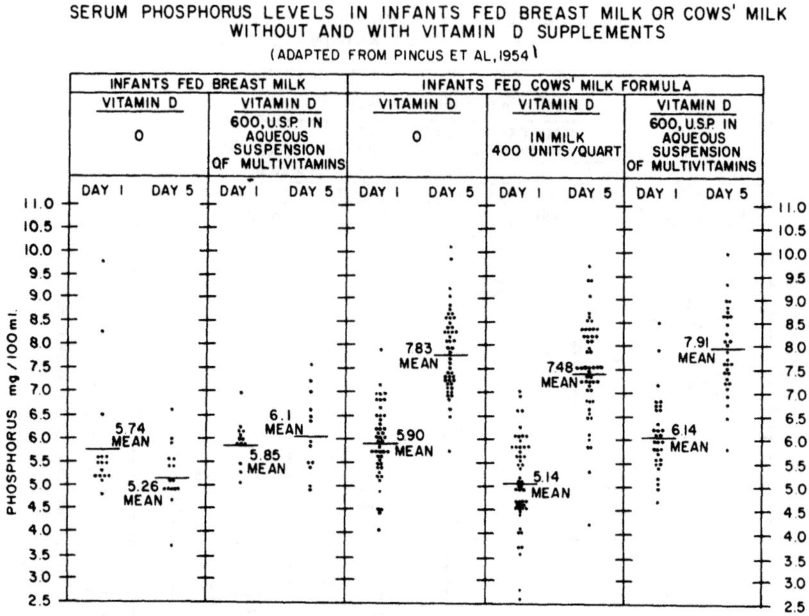
SERUM PHOSPHORUS LEVELS IN INFANTS FED BREAST MILK OR COWS' MILK WITHOUT AND WITH VITAMIN D SUPPLEMENTS
(ADAPTED FROM PINCUS ET AL, 1954)
INFANTS FED BREAST MILK
INFANTS FED COWS' MILK FORMULA
VITAMIN D 0
VITAMIN D 600, U.S.P. IN AQUEOUS SUSPENSION OF MULTIVITAMINS
VITAMIN D 0
VITAMIN D IN MILK 400 UNITS/QUART
VITAMIN D 600, U.S.P. IN AQUEOUS SUSPENSION OF MULTIVITAMINS
DAY 1
DAY 5
PHOSPHORUS mg / 100 ml
5.74 MEAN
5.26 MEAN
6.1 MEAN
5.85 MEAN
7.83 MEAN
5.90 MEAN
7.48 MEAN
5.14 MEAN
7.91 MEAN
6.14 MEAN

Fig. 11

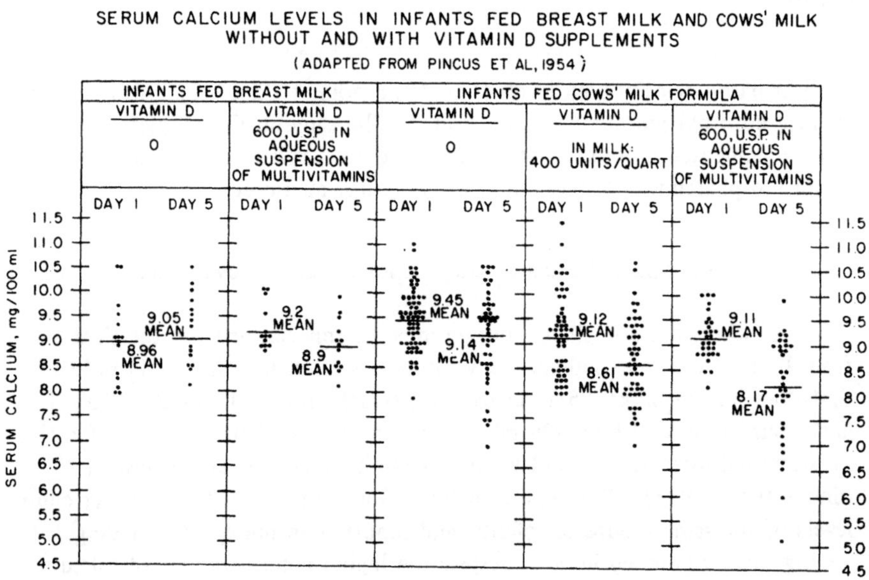
SERUM CALCIUM LEVELS IN INFANTS FED BREAST MILK AND COWS' MILK WITHOUT AND WITH VITAMIN D SUPPLEMENTS
(ADAPTED FROM PINCUS ET AL, 1954)
INFANTS FED BREAST MILK
INFANTS FED COWS' MILK FORMULA
VITAMIN D 0
VITAMIN D 600, U.S.P. IN AQUEOUS SUSPENSION OF MULTIVITAMINS
VITAMIN D 0
VITAMIN D IN MILK: 400 UNITS/QUART
VITAMIN D 600, U.S.P. IN AQUEOUS SUSPENSION OF MULTIVITAMINS
DAY 1
DAY 5
SERUM CALCIUM, mg/100 ml
9.05 MEAN
8.96 MEAN
9.2 MEAN
8.9 MEAN
9.45 MEAN
9.14 MEAN
9.12 MEAN
8.61 MEAN
9.11 MEAN
8.17 MEAN

Fig. 12

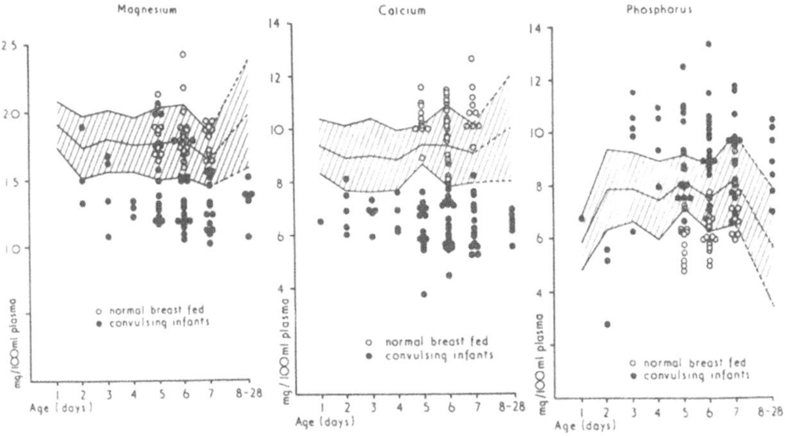

Fig. 13

cows' milk formula to resemble human milk more closely has partially corrected these abnormalities (Oppé and Redstone, 1968).

Hypocalcemic irritability, like infantile and premature adult cardiovascular diseases, has become more prevalent during this century. Only in the past 10 to 15 years has the dependence of plasma calcium levels in infancy on the magnesium status been accepted. The composite figure 13 (Cockburn et al., 1973) clearly depicts the lesser predilection of bottle-fed infants to convulsions, and the simultaneously low plasma magnesium and calcium and high phosphorus in the convulsing (bottle-fed) infants. The better response of hypocalcemic convulsions to magnesium than to calcium or barbiturate is depicted in Table 11. (Turner et al., 1977).

Infants that are particularly susceptible to falling magnesium levels after birth are those that suffer from IUGR (Tsang and Oh, 1970; Tsang, 1972) and infants of diabetic mothers (Tsang et al., 1972; Tsang and Brown, 1977). Diabetics are subject to magnesium deficiency (Martin, 1969). The nature of feeding these latter infants was not designated, but the mothers being American, formula was probably used.

DISCUSSION

The practice of medicine has changed substantially during the past 40 years, not only because of new diagnostic and therapeutic developments, but because new diseases have emerged or increased in incidence. In a commentary on the change in pediatric practice from the 1930s to the 1950s, Hutchison

Table 11. Pre- and Post-Treatment Plasma Magnesium, Calcium and Phosphorus in Response to Treatment of Neonatal Tetany*

Results of Treatment with Magnesium, Calcium, or Phenobarbitone (Mean ± SD)

	Magnesium Therapy (37)		*Calcium Therapy (34)*		*Barbiturate Therapy (33)*	
	Pre-Treatment	*Post-Treatment*	*Pre-Treatment*	*Post-Treatment*	*Pre-Treatment*	*Post-Treatment*
Plasma magnesium (mEq/L)	1.18 ± 0.34	1.75 ± 0.41	1.21 ± 0.18	1.27 ± 0.22	1.17 ± 0.22	1.28 ± 0.21
Plasma calcium (mg/100 ml)	6.16 ± 0.64	8.19 ± 0.97	5.80 ± 0.72	7.24 ± 1.12	6.11 ± 0.66	7.05 ± 1.06
Plasma phosphorus (mg/100 ml)	9.7 ± 1.05	9.02 ± 1.42	9.94 ± 1.04	8.94 ± 1.26	9.71 ± 1.32	8.53 ± 1.13
Number of seizures	1.86 ± 0.9	(After ℞ started) 3.24 ± 4.23	1.72 ± 0.9	(After ℞ started) 8.36 ± 10.2	1.67 ± 0.8	(After ℞ started) 8.93 ± 9.4
Number of doses required for cure		2.31 ± 0.5		15.63 ± 5.9		12.48 ± 5.8

*Adapted from Turner, Cockburn and Forfar, 1977.

(1955) noted new renal and pancreatic diseases and considered the possibility that measures taken to abolish rickets might have resulted not only in infantile hypercalcemia (then prevalent in Great Britain—see Seelig, 1969b), but in new organic diseases. A variety of pediatric cardiovascular abnormalities has also been increasingly reported during the same era, and has persisted to the present. Direct and inferential evidence has been presented that the changed nutritional patterns since the 1930s might be to blame for a variety of cardiovascular and related or associated abnormalities that might be acquired during gestation and intensified during infancy, or that emerge during infancy or later life. Physicians who care for adults with IHD, atherosclerosis, hyperlipemia and hypertension, and epidemiologists and geneticists seeking explanations for the increased incidence of these disorders are increasingly looking to the infant years for clues as to origins and means of prevention of what has become a major epidemic.

Stress, in this paper, has been on magnesium deficiency—absolute and induced by dietary and other factors—as an important factor in sudden, unexpected cardiac death (during infancy, childhood, and early adult life—especially in men), and in chronic cardiovascular diseases. It is possible that the damage caused by vitamin D excess intensifies that produced by dietary magnesium deficiency, and that the primary lesion might be the cardiovascular necrosis and subsequent fibrosis, that can be produced experimentally by magnesium deficiency alone. Excess vitamin D increases blood pressure, the calcific process, and arterial fatty infiltration. Excess dietary fat further increases the tendency towards atheroma formation. The similarity of some of the cardiac and other defects and growth and mental retardation associated with the fetal alcohol syndrome (Hanson et al., 1976), and with the use of lithium (Weinstein and Goldfield, 1975) or of anticonvulsants (Speidel and Meadow, 1972; Anderson, 1976) to those seen with vitamin D excess suggests that each of these agents might cause the damage by means of a common mechanism. Anticonvulsants interfere with vitamin D metabolism (Christiansen et al., 1975), and cause hypomagnesemia (Christiansen et al., 1974). Alcoholism has long been known to cause magnesium depletion (Flink et al., 1954; Flink, 1980). Lithium alters magnesium metabolism, a subject discussed by Birch (1981) (in this symposium) as possibly related to the fetal cardiovascular damage in infants born to mothers receiving lithium during pregnancy. Thus, there is at least circumstantial evidence that several pharmacologic agents that adversely affect magnesium retention or metabolism can cause cardiac and related congenital diseases.

There is much still to be done before we understand the complete picture of nutritional factors involved in the pathogenesis of cardiovascular diseases. We hope that as investigations progress, nutritional intervention can be modified and new steps taken, so as to prevent some of the diseases that have reached epidemic proportions during the past 40 years.

REFERENCES

Anderson, R.C. Cardiac defects in children of mothers receiving anticonvulsant therapy during pregnancy. *J. Ped.* 89, 318-319 (1976).

Anderson, T. A new view of heart disease. *New Scient.* 9, 374-376 (1978).

Anderson, T.W. The changing pattern of ischemic heart disease. *Can. Med. Assoc. J.* 108, 1500-1508 (1973).

Anderson, W.R., Edland, J.F., and Schenk, E.A. Conducting system changes in the sudden death syndrome. *Am. J. Path.* 59, 35a (1970).

Ashe, J.R., Schofield, F.A., and Gram, M.R. The retention of calcium, iron, phosphorus, and magnesium during pregnancy: the adequacy of prenatal diets with and without supplementation. *Am. J. Clin. Nutr.* 32, 286-291 (1979).

Beuren, A.J., Apitz, J., Stoermer, J., Kaiser, B., Schlanger, H.V., Berg, W., and Jorgensen, G. Vitamin D-hypercalcemische Herz und Gefasserkrankung. *Mschr. Kinderh.* 114, 457-470 (1966).

Beuren, A.J., Schulze, C., Eberle, P., Harmanj, D., and Apitz, J. The syndrome of supravalvular aortic stenosis, peripheral pulmonary stenosis, mental retardation, and similar facial appearance. *Am. J. Card.* 13, 471-483 (1964).

Birch, N.J. The role of magnesium in the pharmacology of lithium and in development of fetal cardiovascular defects, in Proceedings of Symposium, American College of Nutrition, University of Minnesota, Minneapolis, 1978. SP Medical & Scientific Books, Jamaica, N.Y. (1982), pp. 295-300.

Blanc, W.A., Franciosi, R.A., and Cadotte, H. L'infarctus et la fibrose du myocarde en pathologie foetale et infantile. *Med. Hyg.* 24, 216-220 (1966).

Blumberg, R.W., and Lyon, R.A. Endocardial sclerosis. *Am. J. Dis. Child.* 84, 291-308 (1952).

Bogert, L.J., and Trail, R.K. Studies in inorganic metabolism. *J. Biol. Chem.* 54, 753-761 (1922).

Brehm, W. Potential dangers of viosterol during pregnancy with observations of calcification of placentae. *Ohio State Med. J.* 33, 990-993 (1937).

Bryan, C.S., and Oppenheimer, E.H. Ventricular endocardial fibroelastosis. Basis for its presence or absence in cases of pulmonic and aortic atresia. *Arch. Path.* 87, 82-86 (1969).

Burch, G.E., and Giles, T.D. The importance of magnesium deficiency in cardiovascular disease. *Am. Heart J.* 94, 649-657 (1977).

Byrne, P.A., and Cadell, J.L. The magnesium load test. I. Correlation of the clinical and laboratory data in neonates. *Clin. Ped.* 14, 460-465 (1975).

Caddell, J.L. The magnesium load test. I. A design for infants. *Clin. Ped.* 14, 449-459, 518-519 (1975).

Caddell, J.L., Byrne, P.A., Triska, R.A., and McElfresh, A.E. The magnesium load test. III. Correlation of clinical and laboratory data in infants from one to six months of age. *Clin. Ped.* 14, 478-484 (1975a).

Caddell, J.L., Saier, F.L., and Thomasen, C.A. Parenteral magnesium load tests in post-partum American women. *Am. J. Clin. Nut.* 28, 1099-1104 (1975b).

Charbon, G.A., and Hoekstra, M.H. On the competition between calcium and magnesium. *Acta Physiol. Pharm. Neerland.* 11, 141-150 (1962).

Christiansen, C., Nielsen, S.P., and Rodbro, P. Anticonvulsant hypomagnesemia. *Br. Med. J.* 1, 198-199 (1974).

Christiansen, C., Rodbro, P., Munck, O., and Minck, O. Actions of vitamins D_2 and 25-OH-D_3 in anticonvulsant osteomalacia. *Br. Med. J.* 2, 363-365 (1975).

Chu, H.I., Liu, S.H., Hsu, H.C., Choa, H.C., and Cheu, S.H. Calcium, phosphorus, nitrogen, and magnesium metabolism in normal young Chinese adults. *Chin. Med. J.* 59, 1-33 (1941).

Cockburn, F., Brown, J.K., Belton, N.R., and Forfar, J.O. Neonatal convulsions associated with primary disturbance of calcium, phosphorus and magnesium. *Arch. Dis. Childh.* 48, 99-108 (1973).

Coleman, E.N. Infantile hypercalcemia and cardiovascular lesions. Evidence, hypothesis and speculation. *Arch. Dis. Childh.* 40, 535-540 (1965).

Committee on Nutrition, American Academy of Pediatrics. The prophylactic requirement and the toxicity of vitamin D. *Pediatrics* 31, 512 (1963).

Coons, C.M., Schiefelbusch, A., Marshall, G.B., and Coons, R. Studies in metabolism during pregnancy. *Oklahoma Agric. Exp. Stat. Bull.* 223 (1935).

Craig, J.M. Congenital endocardial sclerosis. *Bull. Int. A.M. Mus.* 30, 15-67 (1949).

Danilevicus, Z. When does CHD start? *JAMA* 230, 1565-1566 (1974).

Dancis, J., Springer, D., and Cohlan, S.Q. Fetal homeostasis in maternal malnutrition. II. Magnesium malnutrition. *Pediat. Res.* 5, 131-136 (1971).

Davies, J.N.P., and Coles, R.M. Some considerations regarding obscure disease affecting the mural endocardium. *Am. Heart J.* 59, 600-631 (1960).

Dock, W. The predilection of atherosclerosis for the coronary arteries. *JAMA* 131, 875-878 (1946).

Elliott, G.B., and Elliott, J.D.A. Myocardial component in fibroelastoses scar. *Arch. Path.* 95, 321-324 (1973).

Esterly, J.R., and Oppenheimer, E.H. Some aspects of cardiac pathology in infancy and childhood. IV. Myocardial and coronary lesions in cardiac malformations. *Pediatrics* 39, 896-903 (1967).

Fanconi, G. Variations in sensitivity to vitamin D, in *Bone Structure and Metabolism*. G. Wolstenholme and C. O'Connor, eds. Little, Brown, Boston (1956), pp. 187-205.

Fangman, R.J., and Hellwig, C.A. Histology of coronary arteries in newborn infants. *Am. J. Path.* 23, 901-902, 1947.

Finola, G.C., Trump, R.A., and Crimson, M. Bone changes in the fetus following administration of dicalcium-phosphate and viosterol to the pregnant mother. *Am. J. Obst. Gyn.* 34, 955-958 (1937).

Flink, E.B. Clinical manifestations of acute magnesium deficiency in man, in *Magnesium in Health and Disease,* Proceedings of the Second International Symposium on Magnesium, American College of Nutrition; Society for Development of Research in Magnesium, University of Montreal, Montreal, Canada. M. Cantin and M.S. Seelig, eds. SP Medical & Scientific Books, Jamaica, N.Y. (1980), pp. 865-882.

Flink, E.B., Stutzman, F.L., Anderson, A.R., Konig, T., and Fraser, R. Magnesium deficiency after prolonged parenteral fluid administration and after alcoholism complicated by delirium tremens. *J. Lab. Clin. Med.* 43, 169-183 (1954).

Flowers, C.E., Jr. Magnesium sulfate in obstetrics. *Am. J. Obst. Gyn.* 91, 763-776 (1965).

Flowers, C.E., Jr., Easterling, W.E., Jr., White, F.D., Jung, J.M., and Fox, J.T., Jr. Magnesium sulfate in toxemia of pregnancy. *Obst. Gyn.* 19, 315-327 (1962).

Food and Nutrition Board, National Research Council, National Academy of Sciences. *Recommended Dietary Allowances: Mineral Elements,* 9th ed. U.S. Government Printing Office, Washington, D.C. (1980).

Franciosi, R.A., and Blanc, W.A. Myocardial infarcts in infants and children. I. A necropsy study in congenital heart disease. *J. Ped.* 73, 309-319 (1968).

Freeman, R.M., and Pearson, E. Hypomagnesemia of unknown etiology. *Am. J. Med.* 41, 645–656 (1966).
Friedman, W.F., and Roberts, W.C. Vitamin D and the supravalvular aortic stenosis syndrome. The transplacental effects of vitamin D on the aorta of the rabbit. *Circulation* 34, 77–86 (1966).
Friend, B. Nutrients in the United States food supply. A review of trends. *Am. J. Clin. Nutr.* 20, 907–914 (1967).
Gross, P. Concept of fetal endocarditis. *Arch. Path.* 31, 163–177 (1941).
Gruenwald, P. Necrosis in the coronary arteries of newborn infants. *Am. Heart J.* 38, 889–897 (1949).
Haddy, F.J., and Seelig, M.S. Magnesium and the arteries, in *Magnesium in Health and Disease.* Proceedings of the Second International Symposium on Magnesium, American College of Nutrition, Society for Development of Research in Magnesium, University of Montreal, Montreal, Canada, 1976. M. Cantin and M.S. Seelig, eds. SP Medical & Scientific Books, Jamaica, N.Y. (1980), pp. 639–657.
Hall, D.C. Serum magnesium in pregnancy. *Obst. Gyn.* 9, 158–162 (1957).
Hanson, J.W., Jones, K.L., and Smith, D.W. Fetal alcohol syndrome. Experience with 41 patients. *JAMA* 235, 1458–1460 (1976).
Harbert, G.M., Claiborne, H.A., McGaughy, H.S., Wilson, L.A., and Thornton, W.N. Convulsive toxemia. A report of 168 cases managed conservatively. *Am. J. Obst. Gyn.* 100, 336–342 (1968).
Harris, I., and Wilkinson, A.W. Magnesium depletion in children. *Lancet* 2, 735–736 (1971).
Hogg, G.R. Cardiac lesions in hemolytic disease of the newborn. *J. Ped.* 60, 352–360 (1962).
Horley, J.F. Foetal fibroelastosis. *Br. Med. J.* 1, 765–768 (1955).
Hummel, F.C., Sternberger, H.R., Hunscher, H.A., and Macy, I.G. Metabolism of women during the reproductive cycle. IV. Utilization of inorganic elements. (A continuous case study of a multipara). *J. Nutr.* 11, 235–255 (1936).
Hummel, F.C., Hunscher, H.A., Bates, M.F., Bonner, P., and Macy, I.G. A consideration of the nutritive state in the metabolism of women during pregnancy. *J. Nutr.* 13, 263–278 (1937).
Hurley, L.S. Magnesium deficiency in pregnancy and its effects on the offspring, in *Proceedings of the First International Symposium on Magnesium* I, Vittel, France, 1971. J. Durlach, ed. (1971), pp. 481–492.
Hutchinson, H.T., Nichols, M.M., Kuhn, C.R., and Vasicka, A. Effects of magnesium sulfate on uterine contractility, intrauterine fetus, and infant. *Am. J. Obst. Gyn.* 88, 747–758 (1963).
Hutchison, J.H. Some new diseases in pediatrics. *Br. Med. J.* 2, 339–342 (1955).
Johnson, F.R. Anoxia as a cause of endocardial fibroelastosis in infancy. *Arch. Path.* 54, 237–247 (1952).
Johnson, N.E., and Philipps, C.A. Magnesium contents of diets of pregnant women, in *Magnesium in Health and Disease.* Proceedings of the Second International Symposium on Magnesium, American College of Nutrition, Society for Development of Research in Magnesium, University of Montreal, Montreal, Canada, 1976. M. Cantin and M.S. Seelig, eds. SP Medical & Scientific Books, Jamaica, N.Y. (1980), pp. 827–831.
Kastor, J.A. Electrical disorders of the heart. *JAMA* 224, 1031–1033 (1973).
Kelly, J., and Andersen, D.H. Congenital endocardial fibroelastosis. *Pediatrics* 18, 539–555 (1956).

Kontopoulos, V., Seelig, M.S., Dolan, J., Berger, A.R., and Ross, R.S. Influence of parenteral administration of magnesium sulfate to normal pregnant and to preeclamptic women, in *Magnesium in Health and Disease.* Proceedings of the Second International Symposium on Magnesium, American College of Nutrition, Society for Development of Research in Magnesium, University of Montreal, Montreal, Canada, 1976. M. Cantin and M.S. Seelig, eds. SP Medical & Scientific Books, Jamaica, N.Y. (1980), pp. 839–848.

Lehr, D. The role of certain electrolytes and hormones in disseminated myocardial necrosis, in *Electrolytes and Cardiovascular Disease. I. Fundamental Aspects.* E. Bajusz, ed. Williams and Wilkins, New York (1965), pp. 248–273. [S. Karger, Basel, 1965].

Lehr, D., and Krukowski, M. About the mechanism of myocardial necrosis induced by sodium phosphate and adrenal corticoid overdosage. *Ann. N.Y. Acad. Sci.* 105, 135–182 (1963).

Lev, M., Croenen, J., and Lambert, E.C. Infantile coronary sclerosis with atrioventricular block. *J. Ped.* 70, 87–94 (1967).

Leverton, R.M., Leichsenring, J.M., Linkswiler, H., Fox, H., and Meyer, F.L. The metabolic response of young women to a standardized diet. *Home Economics Res. Report No. 16.* U.S. Department of Agriculture, Washington, D.C. (1962).

Lim, P., Jacob, E., Dong, S., and Khoo, O.T. Values for tissue magnesium as a guide in detecting magnesium deficiency. *J. Clin. Path.* 22, 417–421 (1969).

Linden, V. Correlations of vitamin D intake to ischemic heart disease, hypercholesterolemia and renal calcinosis, in *Nutritional Imbalance in Infant and Adult Disease.* Proceedings of the Annual Meeting of the American College of Nutrition, New York, 1975. M.S. Seelig, ed. SP Medical & Scientific Books, Jamaica, N.Y. (1977), pp. 23–42.

McGanity, W.J. Discussion of Flowers, C.E. *Am. J. Obst. Gyn.* 71, 775 (1965).

Martin, H.E. Clinical magnesium deficiency. *Ann. N.Y. Acad. Sci.* 162, 891–900 (1969).

Miller, R.A., Mehta, A.B., Rodriquez-Coronel, A., and Lev, M. Congenital atrioventricular block with multiple ectopic pacemakers. Electrocardiographic and conduction system correlation. *Am. J. Card.* 30, 554–558 (1972).

Mischel, W. Die anoganische Bestanteile der Placenta. *Arch. Gynaek.* 8, 11, 228, 384, 638 (1957).

Moller, J.H., Lucas, R.V., Jr., Adams, P., Jr., Anderson, R.C., Jorgens, J., and Edwards, J.E. Endocardial fibroelastosis. A clinical and anatomic study of 47 patients with emphasis on its relationship to mitral insufficiency. *Circulation* 30, 759–782 (1964).

Muller, P. La therapeutique magnésienne moderne en gynecologie et en obstetrique. *Strasbourg Med.* 19, 117–132 (1968).

Muller, P., Dellenbach, P., and Frenot, M. Deficit magnésique en pathologie gyneco-obstetricale, in *Proceedings of the First International Symposium on Magnesium II,* Vittel, France, 1971. J. Durlach, ed. (1971), pp. 459–480.

Naeye, R.L., Messmer, J. III, Specht, T., and Merrett, T.A. Sudden infant death syndrome temperament before death. *J. Ped.* 88, 511–515 (1976).

Neufeld, H.N., and Vlodaver, Z. Structural changes in the coronary arteries of infants. *Bull. Assoc. Card. Ped. Eur.* 4, 35–39 (1968).

Neufeld, H.N., and Vlodaver, Z. Structural changes of coronary arteries in young age groups. *Intl. Card.* 2, 56–78 (1971).

Oppé, T.E., and Redstone, D. Calcium and phosphorus levels in healthy newborn infants given various types of milk. *Lancet* 1, 1045–1048 (1968).

Oppenheimer, E.H., and Esterly, J.R. Cardiac lesions in hypertensive infants and children. *Arch. Path.* 84, 318–325 (1967).

Ornoy, A., Menczel, J., and Nebel, L. Alterations in the mineral composition and metabolism of rat fetuses and their placentas as induced by maternal hypervitaminosis D_2. *Isr. J. Med. Sci.* 4, 827–832 (1968).

Pincus, J.B., Gittleman, I.F., Sobel, A.E., and Schmerzler, E. Effects of vitamin D on the serum calcium and phosphorus levels in infants during the first week of life. *Pediatrics* 13, 178–185 (1954).

Potvliege, P.R. Hypervitaminosis D_2 in gravid rats. Study of its influence on fetal parathyroid glands and a report of hitherto undescribed placental alterations. *Arch. Path.* 73, 371–382 (1962).

Pritchard, J.A. The use of the magnesium ion in the management of eclamptogenic toxemias. *Surg. Gyn. Obst.* 100, 131–140 (1955).

Robertson, J.H. The significance of intimal thickening in the arteries of the newborn. *Arch. Dis. Child.* 35, 588–590 (1960).

Sabiston, D.C., Jr., Pelargonia, S., and Taussig, H.B. Myocardial infarction in infancy. The surgical management of a complication of congenital origin of the left coronary artery from the pulmonary artery. *J. Thor. Cardiovasc. Surg.* 40, 321–336 (1960).

Schornagel, H.E. Intimal thickening in the coronary arteries in infants. *Arch. Path.* 62, 427–432 (1956).

Scott, K.E., and Usher, R. Fetal malnutrition: its incidence, causes and effects. *Am. J. Obst. Gyn.* 94, 951–963 (1966).

Scoular, F.I., Pace, J.K., and Davis, A.M. The calcium, phosphorus, and magnesium balances of young college women consuming self-selected diets. *J. Nutr.* 62, 489–501 (1957).

Seelig, M.S. The requirement of magnesium by the normal adult. Summary and analysis of published data. *Am. J. Clin. Nutr.* 14, 342–390 (1964).

Seelig, M.S. Electrocardiographic patterns of magnesium depletion appearing in alcoholic heart disease. *Ann. N.Y. Acad. Sci.* 162, 906–917 (1969a).

Seelig, M.S. Vitamin D and cardiovascular, renal, and brain damage in infancy and childhood. *Ann. N.Y. Acad. Sci.* 147, 537–582 (1969b).

Seelig, M.S. Are American children still getting an excess of vitamin D? Hyperreactive children at risk. *Clin. Ped.* 9, 380–383 (1970).

Seelig, M.S. Human requirements of magnesium; factors that increase needs, in *Proceedings of the First International Symposium on Magnesium I,* Vittel, France, 1971. J. Durlach, ed. (1971), pp. 10–38.

Seelig, M.S. Myocardial loss of functional magnesium. II. In cardiomyopathies of diverse etiology, in *Recent Advances in Studies on Cardiac Structure and Metabolism. I. Myocardiology.* E. Bajusz and G. Rona, eds. University Park Press, Baltimore (1972), pp. 626–638.

Seelig, M.S. Magnesium deficiency with phosphate and vitamin D excesses. Possible role in pediatric cardiovascular disease. *Cardiovasc. Med.* 3, 637–650 (1978).

Seelig, M.S. *Magnesium Deficiency in the Pathogenesis of Disease.* L.V. Avioli, ed. Plenum Medical Book Co., New York (1980).

Seelig, M.S., and Bunce, G.E. Contribution of magnesium deficit to human disease, in *Magnesium in the Environment.* Proceedings of Symposium at Fort Valley State College, Georgia (1972), pp. 61–106.

Seelig, M.S., and Haddy, F.J. Magnesium and the arteries. I. Effects of magnesium on arteries and on the retention of sodium, potassium, and calcium, in *Magnesium in Health and Disease.* Proceedings of the Second International Symposium on Magnesium, American College of Nutrition, Society for Development of Research in Magnesium, University of Montreal, Montreal, Canada, 1976. M. Cantin and M.S. Seelig, eds. SP Medical & Scientific Books, Jamaica, N.Y. (1980), pp. 605-638.

Seelig, M.S., and Heggtveit, H.A. Magnesium interrelationships in ischemic heart disease: A review. *Am. J. Clin. Nutr.* 27, 59-79 (1974).

Selye, H. *The Chemical Prevention of Cardiac Necrosis.* Ronald Press, New York, (1958).

Sos, J. An investigation into the nutritional factors of experimental cardiopathy, in *Electrolytes and Cardiovascular Diseases. I. Fundamental Aspects.* E. Bajusz, ed. Williams and Wilkins Co., New York (1965), pp. 161-180. [S. Karger, Basel, Switzerland (1965)].

Speidel, B.D., and Meadow, S.R. Maternal epilepsy and abnormalities of the fetus and newborn. *Lancet* 2, 839-843 (1972).

Taussig, H.B. On the evolution of our knowledge of congenital malformations of the heart. *Circulation* 31, 768-777 (1965).

Taussig, H.B. Possible injury to the cardiovascular system from vitamin D. *Ann. Int. Med.* 65, 1195-1200 (1966).

Tsang, R.C. Neonatal magnesium disturbances. *Am. J. Dis. Child.* 124, 282-293 (1972).

Tsang, R.C., and Brown, D.R. Calcium and magnesium in premature infants and infants of diabetic mothers, in *Nutritional Imbalances in Infants and Adults.* M.S. Seelig, ed. SP Medical & Scientific Books, Jamaica, N.Y. (1977), pp. 141-152.

Tsang, R.C., and Oh, W. Serum magnesium levels in low birth weight infants. *Am. J. Dis. Child.* 120, 44-48 (1970).

Tsang, R.C., Kleinman, L.I., Sutherland, J.M., and Light, I.J. Hypocalcemia in infants of diabetic mothers. *J. Ped.* 80, 384-395 (1972).

Turner, T.L., Cockburn, F., and Forfar, J.O. Magnesium therapy in neonatal tetany. *Lancet* 1, 283-284 (1977).

Walker, M.A., and Page, L. Nutritive content of college meals. III. Mineral elements. *J. Am. Dietet. Assoc.* 70, 260-266 (1977).

Warkany, J., Monroe, B.B., and Sutherland, B.S. Intrauterine growth retardation. *J. Dis. Child.* 102, 249-279 (1961).

Weaver, K. A possible anticoagulant effect of magnesium in pre-eclampsia, in *Magnesium in Health and Disease.* Proceedings of the Second International Symposium on Magnesium, American College of Nutrition, Society for Development of Research in Magnesium, University of Montreal, Montreal, Canada. M. Cantin and M.S. Seelig, eds. SP Medical & Scientific Books, Jamaica, N.Y. (1980), pp. 833-838.

Weinstein, M.R., and Goldfield, M.D. Cardiovascular malformations with lithium use during pregnancy. *Am. J. Psychiat.* 132, 529-531 (1975).

Widdowson, E.M., and Dickerson, J.W.T. Chemical composition of the body, in *Mineral Metabolism 2* (Part A). C.L. Comar and F. Bronner, eds. Academic Press, New York (1962), pp. 2-247.

Widdowson, E.M., McCance, R.A., and Spray, C.M. Chemical composition of the body. *Clin. Sci.* 10, 113-125 (1951).

Wigglesworth, J.S.L. Foetal growth retardation. *Br. Med. Bull.* 22, 13-15 (1966).

Witzleben, C.L. Idiopathic infantile arterial calcification–A misnomer? *Am. J. Card.* 26, 305-309, 1970.

4

Ischemic Heart Disease: Updating the Zinc/Copper Hypothesis

LESLIE M. KLEVAY

INTRODUCTION

It is hypothesized that "a metabolic imbalance in regard to zinc and copper is a major factor in the etiology of coronary or ischemic heart disease. This imbalance is either "relative or absolute deficiency of copper characterized by a high ratio of zinc to copper" (Klevay, 1975, 1977c). The hypothesis is called the *zinc/copper hypothesis;* it is based on the production of hypercholesterolemia in animals and on the association of altered copper and zinc metabolism with many apparently dissimilar observations on the epidemiology of ischemic heart disease and the metabolism of cholesterol in people. Some of these observations are summarized in Tables 1 and 2 (Klevay, 1977a).

ZINC/COPPER CHOLESTEROLEMIA

Hypercholesterolemia can be produced in rats and mice by a high ratio of zinc to copper or by copper deficiency (Klevay, 1973; Jacob et al., 1977; Allen and Klevay, 1978 a, b, c, 1980; Lei, 1977, 1978). Hypocholesterolemia can be produced in pigs and rats by zinc deficiency (Burch et al., 1975; Patel et al., 1975).

In copper-deficient rats, the concentration of copper in liver correlated negatively with both the concentration of cholesterol in plasma (Allen and Klevay, 1978b) and the incorporation of radioactivity from mevalonic acid into plasma cholesterol (Allen and Klevay, 1978c). Apparently the copper in

Table 1. Epidemiology of Ischemic Heart Disease[a]

Environmental Characteristic	*IHD Risk*[b]	*Possible Explanation*
Diets low in fat and sucrose and high in vegetable fiber	<	Have low Zn/Cu, or contain phytate, a protective chelate
Nursing of infants	<	Human milk has low Zn/Cu ratio
Cirrhosis of the liver	<	Increased loss of Zn
Exercise	<	Zn/Cu of sweat = 16, or synthesis of muscle and bone traps Zn
Chronic kidney disease	>	Bone loss releases Zn, or Zn infused during treatment
Availability of hard water	<	Decreased absorption of Zn

[a]These concepts are excerpted from an article (Klevay, 1975) in which data from many references were found to be consonant with the zinc/copper hypothesis. This table was published in *Perspectives in Biology and Medicine.* 1977a. All observations pertain to humans, except that concerning the decreased absorption of zinc in response to the calcium of hard water.
[b]< = decreased; > = increased.

Table 2. Metabolism of Cholesterol[a]

Agent or Physiological State	*Serum Cholesterol*[b]	*Possible Explanation*
Calcium	<	Decreased absorption of Zn
Ethylenediaminetetraacetate	<	Increased loss of Zn
Pregnancy	>	Increased loss of Cu
Bread	<	Decreased absorption of Zn
Nephrotic syndrome	>	Increased loss of Cu
Acute viral hepatitis	<	Increased loss of Zn
Sandfly fever	<	Decreased loss of Cu

[a]See Table 1. All of these data were obtained from studies of humans.
[b]<= decreased, >= increased.

liver microsomes is important in this process as microsomal copper and plasma cholesterol were correlated negatively (Jacob et al., 1978) in another experiment in which rats were fed adequate, but not luxuriant amounts of copper. Liver is the major site of synthesis and catabolism of cholesterol (Dietschy and Wilson, 1970).

Copper deficiency does not increase cholesterol concentration in liver (Allen and Klevay, 1978c). Bile acid excretion increases, but the increase is not great enough to eliminate the hypercholesterolemia (Allen and Klevay, 1978b, c). The increase in serum total cholesterol concentration is reflected as an increase in low-density lipoprotein cholesterol, but a decrease in high-density lipoprotein cholesterol as a percent of total cholesterol (Allen and Klevay, 1980). From these findings one can conclude that synthesis and clearance of cholesterol into the plasma pool is more rapid in copper deficiency.

PREDICTIONS BASED ON THE ZINC/COPPER HYPOTHESIS

Frieden (1978) outlined ten steps in metal metabolism in mammals. The steps are (1) dietary availability; (2) absorption; (3) transport; (4) storage; (5) mobilization to target tissue; (6) metalloprotein biosynthesis; (7) metalloenzyme role; (8) metalloprotein catabolism; (9) recycling, etc.; and (10) excretion. These steps of metal metabolism also may be steps where metallic elements interact, or where interactions with nonmetallic dietary components occur. Only a few of the steps can be implicated now in the zinc/copper phenomenon.

The original experiments on the effect of zinc/copper on cholesterol metabolism (Klevay, 1973) were done using a diet deficient in copper and zinc with supplements of copper and zinc salts in the drinking solutions given to the animals. These experiments may correspond to Frieden's step 1. Greger et al. (1978) may have identified an interaction between copper and zinc at the second step. They found that increased fecal loss of copper in adolescent girls was achieved by increasing the dietary zinc intake from 11 mg to 15 mg. The increased zinc consumption was through the intake of lemonade containing zinc sulfate.

The effects of ascorbic and phytic acids on cholesterol metabolism and the effect of extra dietary zinc in acrodermatitis may be examples of interactions in step 2, absorption. As ascorbic acid seems to inhibit the absorption of copper from the intestinal tract of animals (Evans, 1973), one might expect excessive consumption to produce adverse affects. Ascorbic acid fed to rats produced hypercholesterolemia (Klevay, 1976a). The amount fed (150 mg/kg of diet) corresponds to between 82 and 630 mg of ascorbic acid over normal adult dietary amounts, depending on the method used to calculate the dose for an adult human from the dose fed to the rats. With the current fashion, many people probably are ingesting greater amounts of ascorbic acid.

Phytic acid is a naturally occurring chelating agent of vegetable origin. Because of studies in vitro and in vivo (for references see Klevay, 1977b) it was suggested (Klevay, 1973, 1975) that phytic acid may be a protective material in fibrous diets which are associated with low risk of ischemic heart disease (for references see Klevay, 1976b). Sodium phytate fed to rats (Klevay, 1977b) resulted in hypocholesterolemia and a decreased ratio of zinc to copper in the hair of the animals. This latter observation is consonant with the belief that the change in cholesterol was produced by a change in the metabolism of copper and zinc (Klevay, 1978).

Patients with acrodermatitis chronica enteropathica, a chronic, often fatal disease which can be treated with zinc sulfate, have low concentrations of cholesterol in plasma (for references see Klevay, 1977c). It was suggested (Klevay, 1977c) that this finding may be related to the hypocholesterolemia of zinc deficiency found in animals. Data on the concentration of cholesterol in serum before and after treatment with zinc are now available; in three out of four patients the concentration of cholesterol increased with zinc therapy (Hambidge et al., 1978).

One of the primary stimuli to my work on trace elements and ischemic heart disease has been the association between low risk of disease and the availability of hard drinking water. It was suggested (Klevay, 1973, 1975, 1977c) that calcium, the major constituent of hard water, would produce a lower ratio of zinc to copper in liver. Romasz et al. (1977) confirmed the suggestion by feeding rats a wide range of dietary calcium. As dietary calcium increased, the concentration of cholesterol in serum decreased, and the concentrations of copper and zinc in liver increased and decreased, respectively. This finding may represent an example of Frieden's step 4, storage.

OTHER OBSERVATIONS CONSONANT WITH THE ZINC/COPPER HYPOTHESIS

Carroll (1966) found that the risk of death due to non-rheumatic heart diseases was proportional to the concentration of zinc in the air over 28 cities in the United States. Valentine and Chambers (1976) found the risk of death due to arteriosclerotic heart disease to be proportional to the concentration of zinc in reservoirs storing water for nine study areas in Houston. Considering the very small amounts of zinc in air and water compared to dietary amounts, perhaps these findings are representative of other environmental characteristics that influence risk of death. The association of the ratio of zinc to copper of milk available in 47 cities of the United States with mortality due to coronary heart disease in the cities (Klevay, 1974) is more likely to involve a nutritional mechanism.

It was noted (Klevay, 1977c) that most analyses of diets in the United States done since 1966 have shown daily amounts of copper substantially less than the 2 mg thought to be required by adults according to the Food and Nutrition Board of the National Academy of Sciences (1974). Other data on diets low in copper (Brown et al., 1977; van Berge Henegouwen et al., 1977; Greger et al., 1978; Klevay et al., 1979; Holden et al., 1979; Milne et al., 1980) have been found. A mean daily intake of more than 3 mg of copper (Walker and Page, 1977) stands almost alone. Diets low in copper have been found in eight States and the District of Columbia. Similarly low diets have been found in Finland (Koivistoinen et al., 1970) and New Zealand (Guthrie and Robinson, 1977), two other countries in which risk of ischemic heart disease is high. Some of the diets have ratios of zinc to copper greater than that which produced hypercholesterolemia in rats.

Hair analysis seems to have promise in the assessment of copper and zinc nutriture (Klevay, 1978). Copper in the hair of rats correlates with copper liver (Jacob et al., 1978). If this finding is confirmed in humans, hair analysis will provide a means of examining a relatively inaccessible part of the body (i.e., liver) that is an important site of lipid metabolism.

Animals deficient in copper die suddenly (Coulson and Carnes, 1963; Davis, 1976; Allen and Klevay, 1978a) with various pathologic changes in the anatomy of the heart and arteries (Shields et al., 1962; Coulson and Carnes, 1963; Kelly et al., 1974; Davis, 1976; Allen and Klevay, 1978a). In hearts of various species of animals that were made copper deficient, myocardial degeneration, focal necrosis, fatty change, infarction, subendocardial fibroplasia, and aneurysms have been found with ruptures, hemopericardium, and hemothorax. In arteries, these findings have been noted: decreased, distorted, and fragmented elastic tissue, including the internal elastic lamina, accumulation of amorphous material, dissecting hemorrhages, medial fissuring and necrosis, and increased collagen.

The hearts of people who have died of myocardial infarction are low in copper (Wester, 1965; Anderson et al., 1975; Chipperfield and Chipperfield, 1978). Uninfarcted myocardium from infarction victims was compared with myocardial samples from accident victims and others who died of causes unrelated to ischemic heart disease.

CONCLUSIONS

The zinc/copper hypothesis on the etiology of ischemic heart disease has been broadened since its proposal (Klevay, 1973, 1975) in a series of theoretical and experimental papers. It is consonant with more aspects of the epidemiology of ischemic heart disease and the metabolism of cholesterol than any other hypothesis. With the exception of ethanol, copper and zinc are the only dietary components associated with risk of death due to ischemic heart disease in an epidemiologic study in the continental United States. Relative or absolute deficiency of copper is the only nutritional insult which can produce direct, unfavorable alterations in lipid metabolism and the anatomy of arteries and hearts.

REFERENCES

Allen, K.G.D., and Klevay, L.M. Cholesterol metabolism in copper deficient rats. *Life Sci.* 22, 1691–1698 (1978a).

Allen, K.G.D., and Klevay, L.M. Cholesterolemia and cardiovascular abnormalities in rats caused by copper deficiency. *Atherosclerosis* 29, 81–93 (1978b).

Allen, K.G.D., and Klevay, L.M. Copper deficiency and cholesterol metabolism in the rat. *Atherosclerosis* 31, 259–271 (1978c).

Allen, K.G.D., and Klevay, L.M. Hyperlipoproteinemia in rats due to copper deficiency. *Nutr. Rep. Int.* 22, 295–299 (1980).

Anderson, T.W., Neri, L.C., Schreiber, G.B., Talbot, F.D.F., and Zdrojewski, A. Ischemic heart disease, water hardness, and myocardial magnesium. *Can. Med. Assoc. J.* 113, 199–203 (1975).

Brown, E.D., Howard, M.P., and Smith, J.C., Jr. The copper content of regular, vegetarian and renal diets. *Fed. Proc.* 36, 1122 (1977).

Burch, R.E., Williams, R.V., Hahn, H.K.J., Jetton, M.M., and Sullivan, J.F. Serum and tissue enzyme activity and trace-element content in response to zinc deficiency in the pig. *Clin. Chem.* 21, 568–577 (1975).

Carroll, R.E. The relationship of cadmium in the air to cardiovascular disease death rates. *JAMA* 198, 177–179 (1966).

Chipperfield, B., and Chipperfield, J.R. Differences in metal content of the heart muscle in death from ischemic heart disease. *Am. Heart J.* 95, 732–737 (1978).

Coulson, W.F., and Carnes, W.H. Cardiovascular studies on copper-deficient swine. V. The histogenesis of the coronary artery lesions. *Am. J. Path.* 43, 945–954 (1963).

Davis, G.K. Copper and cardiac integrity, in *The Biomedical Role of Trace Elements in Aging.* J.M. Hsu, R.L. Davis, and R.W. Neithamer, eds. Eckerd College Gerontology Center, St. Petersburg, Florida (1976), pp. 81–90.

Dietschy, J.M., and Wilson, J.D. Regulation of cholesterol metabolism. *New Eng. J. Med.* 282, 1128–1138, 1179–1183, 1241–1249 (1970).

Evans, G.W. Copper homeostasis in the mammalian system. *Physiol. Rev.* 53, 535–570 (1973).

Frieden, E. Modes of metal metabolism in mammals, in *Trace Element Metabolism in Man and Animals, vol. 3.* M. Kirchgessner, ed. Institut für Ernährungsphysiologie, Freising, W. Germany (1978), pp. 8–14.

Greger, J.L., Zaikis, S.C., Abernathy, R.P., Bennett, O.A., and Huffman, J. Zinc, nitrogen, copper, iron, and manganese balance in adolescent females fed two levels of zinc. *J. Nut.* 108, 1449–1456 (1978).

Guthrie, B.E., and Robinson, M.F. Daily intakes of manganese, copper, zinc, and cadmium. *Br. J. Nut.* 38, 55–63 (1977).

Hambidge, K.M., Nelder, K.H., Walravens, P.A., Weston, W.L., Silverman, A., Sabol, J.L., and Brown, R.M. Zinc and acrodermatitis enteropathica, in *Zinc and Copper in Clinical Medicine.* K.M. Hambidge and B.L. Nichols, Jr., eds. SP Medical & Scientific Books, Jamaica, N.Y. (1978), pp. 81–98.

Jacob, R.A., Baesler, L.G., Klevay, L.M., Lee, D.E., and Wherry, P.L. Hypercholesterolemia in mice with meat anemia. *Nut. Rep. Int.* 16, 73–79 (1977).

Jacob, R.A., Klevay, L.M., and Logan, G.M., Jr. Hair as a biopsy material. V. Hair metal as an index of hepatic metal in rats: copper and zinc. *Am. J. Clin. Nut.* 31, 477–480 (1978).

Kelly, W.A., Kesterson, J.W., and Carlton, W.W. Myocardial lesions in the offspring of female rats fed a copper deficient diet. *Exp. Mol. Path.* 20, 40–56 (1974).

Klevay, L.M. Hypercholesterolemia in rats produced by an increase in the ratio of zinc to copper ingested. *Am. J. Clin. Nut.* 26, 1060–1068 (1973).

Klevay, L.M. The ratio of zinc to copper in milk and mortality due to coronary heart disease: An association, in *Trace Substances in Environmental Health VIII.* D.D. Hemphill, ed. University of Missouri Press, Columbia (1974), pp. 9–14.

Klevay, L.M. Coronary heart disease: The zinc/copper hypothesis. *Am. J. Clin. Nut.* 28, 764–774 (1975).

Klevay, L.M. Hypercholesterolemia due to ascorbic acid. *Proc. Soc. Exp. Biol. Med.* 151, 579–582 (1976a).

Klevay, L.M. Ischemic heart disease: The fiber hypothesis. Proceedings of the Miles Symposium 1976 on "Dietary Fibre," presented by the Nutrition Society of Canada. Halifax (1976b), pp. 33–39.

Klevay, L.M. Elements of ischemic heart disease. *Perspect. Biol. Med.* 20, 186–192 (1977a).

Klevay, L.M. Hypocholesterolemia due to sodium phytate. *Nut. Rep. Int.* 15, 587–595 (1977b).

Klevay, L.M. The role of copper and zinc in cholesterol metabolism, in *Advances in Nutritional Research, vol. I.* H.H. Draper, ed. Plenum Press, New York (1977c), pp. 227–252.

Klevay, L.M. Hair as a biopsy material. Progress and prospects. *Arch. Int. Med.* 138, 1127–1128 (1978).

Klevay, L.M., Reck, S., and Barcome, D.F. Evidence of dietary copper and zinc deficiencies. *JAMA* 241, 1916–1918 (1979).

Koivistoinen, P., Ahlström, A., Nissinen, H., Pekkarinen, M., and Roine, P. Mineral element compositions of Finnish diets. Part 1: Fe, Cu, Mn, Zn, Mg, Na, K, Ca, and P. *Suomen Kemistilehti* B 43, 426–430 (1970).

Lei, K.Y. Cholesterol metabolism in copper-deficient rats. *Nut. Rep. Int.* 15, 597–605 (1977).

Lei, K.Y. Oxidation, excretion, and tissue distribution of [26-^{14}C] cholesterol in copper-deficient rats. *J. Nut.* 108, 232–237 (1978).

Milne, D.B., Schnakenberg, D.D., Johnson, H.L., and Kuhl, G.L. Trace mineral intake of enlisted military personnel. *J. Amer. Dietet. Assoc.* 76, 41–45 (1980).

Patel, P.B., Chung, R.A., and Lu, J.Y. Effect of zinc deficiency on serum and liver cholesterol in the female rat. *Nut. Rep. Int.* 12, 205–210 (1975).

Recommended Dietary Allowances. Food and Nutrition Board, National Research Council, National Academy of Sciences, Washington, D.C. (1974), pp. 95–96.

Romasz, R.S., Lemmo, E.A., and Evans, J.L. Diet calcium, sex and age influences on tissue mineralization and cholesterol in rats, in *Trace Substances in Environmental Health XI.* D.D. Hemphill, ed. University of Missouri Press, Columbia (1977), pp. 289–296.

Shields, G.S., Coulson, W.F., Kimball, D.A., Carnes, W.H., Cartwright, G.E., and Wintrobe, M.M. Studies on copper metabolism. XXXII. Cardiovascular lesions in copper-deficient swine. *Am. J. Path.* 41, 603–621 (1962).

Valentine, J.L., and Chambers, L.A. Distribution of trace elements in the Houston environment: Relationship to mortality from arteriosclerotic heart disease. *Texas Rep. Biol. Med.* 34, 331–339 (1976).

van Berge Henegouwen, G.P., Tangedahl, T.N., Hofmann, A.F., Northfield, T.C., LaRusso, N.F., and McCall, J.T. Biliary secretion of copper in healthy man. *Gastroenterology* 72, 1228–1231 (1977).

Walker, M.A., and Page, L. Nutritive content of college meals. *J. Am. Diet. Assoc.* 70, 260–266 (1977).

Wester, P.O. Trace elements in human myocardial infarction determined by neutron activation analysis. *Acta Med. Scand.* 178, 765–788 (1965).

Holden, J.M., Wolf, W.R., and Mertz, W. Zinc and copper in self-selected diets. *J. Amer. Dietet. Assoc.* 75, 23–28 (1979).

5

A Public Health Approach to Nutrition, Mass Hyperlipidemia, and Atherosclerotic Diseases

HENRY BLACKBURN

INTRODUCTION

Atherosclerotic coronary heart disease (CHD) is a public health phenomenon of affluent cultures. Population comparisons suggest that *mass* hyperlipidemia is a prime requisite for *mass* atherosclerosis. On the basis of available evidence, the habitual diet of a culture is, in turn, the chief factor leading to *mass* hyperlipidemia. Specific components of the habitual diet are principal contributors to population levels of blood lipids, in contrast to the predominant influence of nondietary factors on an individual's usual lipid level. Changes in population levels of blood lipids are generally predictable and safely attainable from changes in habitual diet.

Mass hyperlipidemia is also influenced by mass caloric overconsumption and obesity. Similarly, the mass frequency of adult hypertension, a primary risk characteristic for CHD, is related to the nutritional factors of obesity, alcohol consumption, and habitually excessive salt intake in entire populations. Thus, diet composition and energy balance appear to be central to the public health issue of mass hyperlipidemia and to the public health burden of atherosclerotic diseases. Change in the national eating pattern probably requires multiple strategies within a long-term national plan and policy. Changes in the mass levels of certain blood lipoproteins requires a public health objective, a preventive approach to health education, and changes in the production, marketing, availability, and consumption of appropriate foods.

These ideas represent the major public health considerations about nutrition and CHD and reflect a public health view of the issues. These ideas, derived from population studies, in no way diminish the importance of individual variation or of continued basic research on specific mechanisms relating nutrition to atherosclerosis. Neither do they deprecate the effect on blood lipid levels of dietary factors other than fatty acids and cholesterol, as so effectively presented in Chapters 1 and 12 of Naito, 10 of Kritchevsky, and 11 of Davignon and Lussier-Cacan of this volume. Finally, these ideas do not deny, but rather attempt to place in public health perspective, the effect of nondietary factors so central to lipid regulation in the individual. This public health approach attempts to bring ideas together to provide a rational basis for preventive strategies in the whole population, while accounting for specific needs of individuals and special groups in the population.

THE NEED FOR PRIMARY PREVENTION OF ATHEROSCLEROSIS

The immense social and personal burden of the atherosclerotic diseases, manifest as premature cardiovascular disability and death, compels scientific interest and public health concern. The nature of atherosclerosis, illustrated by a few salient facts, necessitates a preventive strategy: There is a high rate of sudden coronary death outside the hospital, and insidious development of arterial damage, an absence of any effective cure, and a permanent excess risk among survivors of heart attack or stroke (Inter-Society Commission on Heart Disease Resources Report, 1970; Blackburn, 1974).

THE POTENTIAL FOR PRIMARY PREVENTION OF ATHEROSCLEROSIS

The potential for a primary preventive approach to atherosclerosis is similarly contained in a few cogent facts: men in Mediterranean and Oriental cultures have little atherosclerotic CHD during the middle years of life (Keys, 1970); coronary risk factors demonstrated within populations "explain" about one-half the variability in disease rates between populations (Keys et al., 1972); congruence of evidence from population studies and from clinical and experimental disciplines suggests strongly that the primary risk factors of habitual diet, elevated blood lipid levels, elevated blood pressure, and cigarette smoking are truly causal factors. The evidence suggests that a necessary factor for mass atherosclerosis is mass hyperlipidemia, an elevation of particular blood lipoproteins, caused in turn by a population diet high in calories, saturated fats, and cholesterol (Inter-Society Commission on Heart Disease Resources Report, 1970).

The apparent causes of large population differences in heart and vascular disease attack rates are characteristics greatly influenced by environment, cultural patterns, and health-related behavior. But natural as well as manmade experiments suggest that population changes can and do occur, both in health behavior and in risk factor levels, and that these changes may be paralleled by changes in disease rates (National Diet-Heart Study Research Group, 1968; Walker, 1977).

These are central factors to the public health view about need and potential for primary prevention of atherosclerotic diseases, which point, in turn, to appropriate tactics for a successful preventive strategy.

THE PUBLIC HEALTH ISSUE AND NUTRITION

If the public health concern is with mass atherosclerosis and its widespread, prematurely disabling, and fatal consequences in affluent societies, then the public health goal is primary prevention of atherosclerosis in the masses. If the public health demonstration is that the habitual diet of a population is an essential factor in mass hyperlipidemia and a mass social burden of atherosclerosis, then the public health aim must be to reduce mass hyperlipidemia. To be effective, the preventive strategy probably requires a combination of forces among the health professions, voluntary health agencies, and the health care system, as well as between agriculture and the food industry, the mass media and community leadership, and the consuming public and its representative government. Public health tactics for primary prevention include health education, public and professional, and community organization to disseminate a message effecting modifications in cultural values and in the environment, in national dietary goals, and in personal patterns of eating and health behavior. Individual and family change in eating patterns and health behavior require new efforts in education, along with sociocultural supports of the new behavior. Significant change in the national diet requires practical changes in the food supply, greater availability, acceptability, and habitual use of foods conducive to reducing mass hyperlipidemia. Finally, significant change in the national diet and nutrition-related health issues would probably benefit from a national plan and policy.

THE CONTRIBUTION OF POPULATION STUDIES

The population evidence shows clearly that there are vast population differences in the frequency of adult, complicated atherosclerotic plaques and their clinical counterparts of coronary disease, stroke, and peripheral arterial disease (McGill, 1968; Inter-Society Commission on Heart Disease Resources Report, 1970; Keys, 1970; Gordon et al., 1974). Sound epidemiologic studies among large heterogenous populations, using systematic methods of observation, reveal strong correlations among atherosclerotic disease inci-

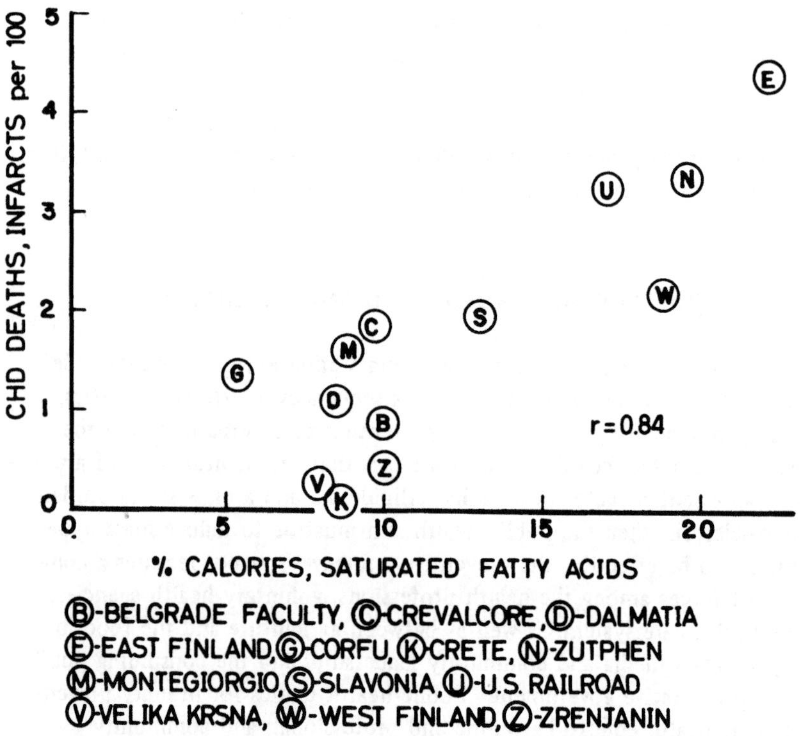

Fig. 1. Diet-heart associations. B, Belgrade faculty; C, Crevalcore; D, Dalmatia; E, East Finland; G, Corfu; K, Crete; N, Zutphen; M, Montegiorgio; S, Slavonia; U, United States railroads; V, Velika Krsna; W, West Finland; Z, Zrenjanin. (From Keys, 1970.)

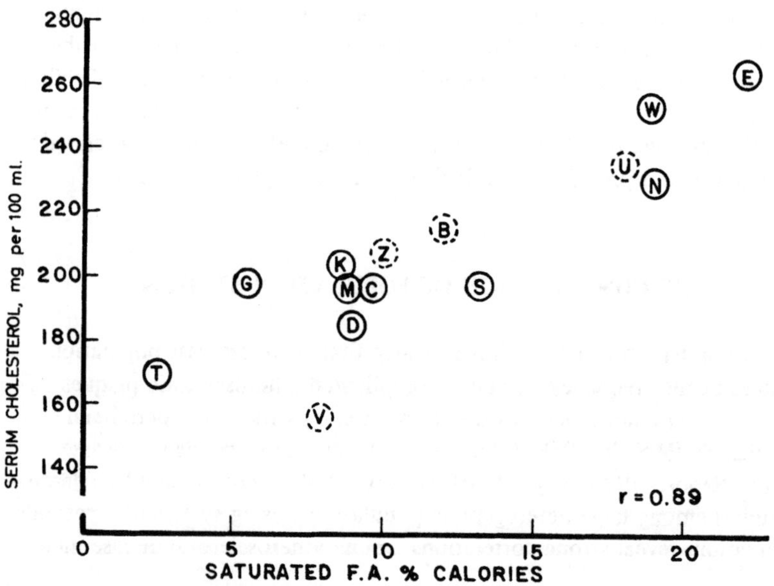

Fig. 2. Association between average serum cholesterol levels among populations and habitual diet. (From Keys, 1970.)

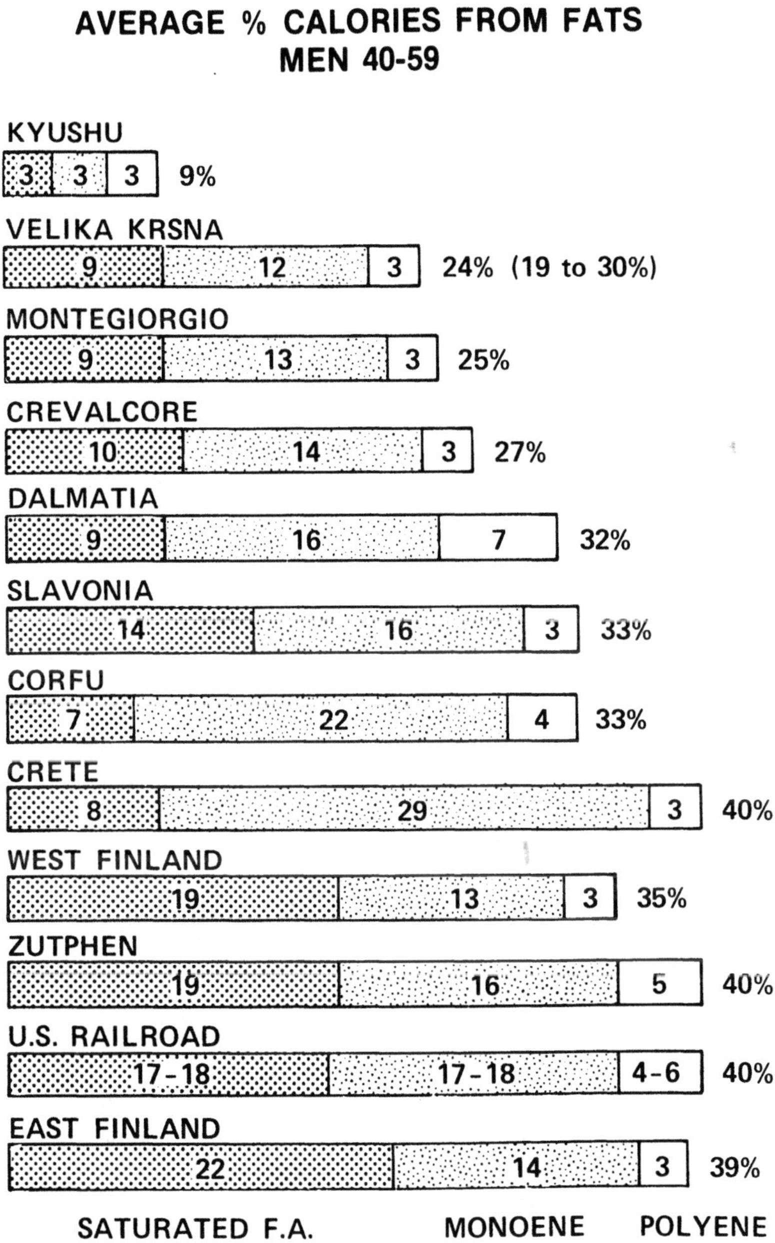

Fig. 3. Average percentage of calories from fats in men aged 40 to 59 years. (From Keys, 1970.)

dence, mass hyperlipidemia, especially average total serum cholesterol levels, and habitual diet of the population. The diets in high-risk cultures are characterized by relatively high amounts of saturated fats and dietary cholesterol and relatively low amounts of complex carbohydrates. In populations of the Seven Countries Study, CHD incidence was assessed in standardized fashion by trained teams, diets were chemically analyzed from sampled households during all four seasons of the year, and blood lipids were measured in a standard way in one central laboratory (Keys, 1970). Much of the difference in CHD (Keys, 1970) incidence could be attributed to habitual diet differences in saturated fat *if* the diet-heart associations are causal (Fig. 1) (Keys, 1970). Similarly, most of the difference in average serum cholesterol levels among those populations could be explained by differences in habitual diet; there is direct evidence that this association in populations is causal (Fig. 2). Populations characterized by high average cholesterol levels and high atherosclerotic disease rates have diets in the realm of 15 percent or more of saturated fat calories. Those characterized by low frequencies of coronary disease and low average serum cholesterol levels have diets on the order of 10 percent or less of saturated fat calories. There is no consistent relationship between the monosaturated and polysaturated fat consumption and either the values for blood lipids or the incidence rates for atherosclerotic disease (Fig. 3; Keys, 1970).

Figure 4 illustrates that hyperlipidemia is a mass phenomenon that is poorly defined by use of normal statistical or clinical distributions and criteria. It indicates that the mean and entire distributions of total serum cholesterol values in a culture may be high relative to that in other populations. These dramatic curves show little overlap between the highest cholesterol values among men in southern Japan (Ushibuka, Kyushu) (Kimura, 1967) and the lowest values among East Finns (Karelia) (Karvonen et al., 1967). Similarly, Fig. 5 indicates that a whole population may be obese relative to others, in this case, sedentary United States rail workers compared to active Serbian farmers (Djordjevic et al., 1967). These graphs illustrate the basis for a public health concern to find preventive approaches to mass hyperlipidemia, mass obesity, mass atherosclerosis, and CHD.

In the scientific public health model (in contrast to the individual case in which nondietary factors may be predominant influences), the population evidence is interpreted to mean that habitual diet and hyperlipidemia are central factors in the mass burden of atherosclerosis and its complications. In other words, without the habitual population diet high in calories, saturated fat, and dietary cholesterol, a mass problem of adult atherosclerosis and coronary disease simply does not exist—even in the presence of strong smoking. The classic natural experiment to illustrate this phenomenon is Japan, where mass hypertension, in the presence of excessive salt intake involves

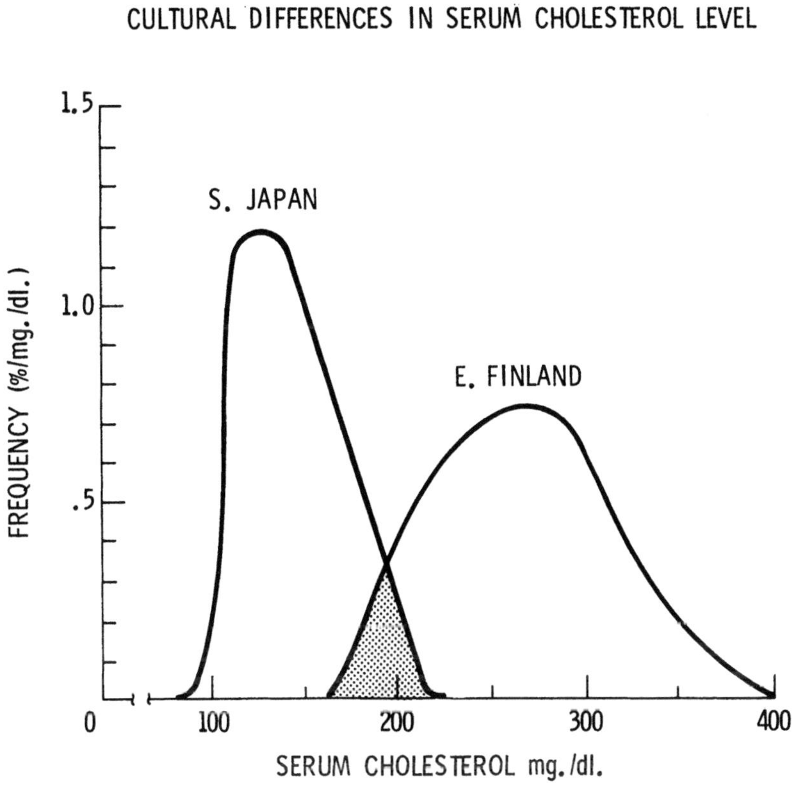

Fig. 4. Cultural differences in serum cholesterol levels. (From Karvonen et al., 1967; Kimura, 1967.)

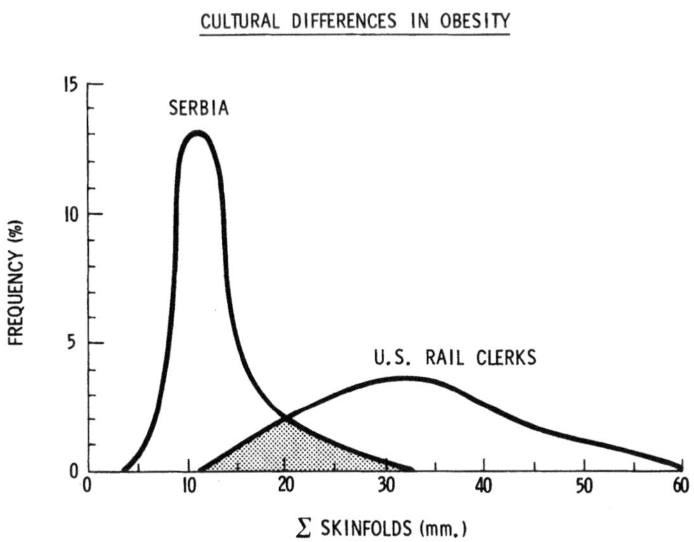

Fig. 5. Cultural differences in obesity. (From Djordjevic et al., 1967; Keys et al., 1967.)

20 to 30 percent of the adult population, and in a culture of heavy cigarette smokers. This combination has resulted in little mass burden of CHD, at least until the late 1960s. However, Japan is the industrial nation having the highest habitual carbohydrate intake (±75 percent of calories) and the lowest habitual total fat (±10 percent) and saturated fat intake (±3 percent) (Keys, 1970). These findings confirm (but do not establish) a public health view.

At the opposite end of the scale of habitual saturated fat consumption from Japan is the natural experiment of the eastern region of Finland, where the diet is about 22 percent saturated fat calories and the distribution of blood pressure and cigarette smoking is not significantly different from that in central and southern Europe. Mass hyperlipidemia is the most striking finding in eastern Finland, with serum cholesterol average levels around 275 mg/dl. In fact, the Finns have among the higher atherosclerotic disease rates of any culture in which the rates have been measured directly and systematically (Keys, 1970).

Such a simple interpretation makes inadequate allowance for many questions, for example, the different functional and predictive roles of the lipid fractions. But the public health view assumes that effective applications may not require knowledge of detailed atherogenic mechanisms at the cellular level, nor the operation of other unknown and awaited "X-factors" of risk. The public health and pragmatic model accepts the fact that total serum or plasma cholesterol is a marker highly influenced by habitual diet and either directly or indirectly related to the atherosclerotic process. It accepts the possibility that more research findings, for example, of the different functional roles of the lipid fractions, as well as dietary and other influences, are desirable in order to refine and elucidate causal mechanisms and to enhance the potential for prevention. But the public health argument also maintains that these and other mechanisms of atherosclerosis, as presently understood, are not expected to invalidate the conclusions that (1) a habitual population diet high in saturated fat and cholesterol is a primary and necessary factor in mass hyperlipidemia and results in a large social burden of atherosclerosis; and (2) a habitual national diet lower in saturated fat and cholesterol is probably a necessary component of the public health solution to CHD.

DIETARY VERSUS NONDIETARY CONTRIBUTIONS TO SERUM CHOLESTEROL LEVEL

Two simple models in Tables 1 and 2 are used to illustrate the dietary and nondietary contributions to serum cholesterol levels. These models ignore some details, including the different functional roles of lipid fractions. They involve many assumptions. Nevertheless, they portray the great importance

Table 1. A Model of Individual Diet-Serum Cholesterol Relationships with Individual Examples[a]

Minimum Genetic Value[b] *(mg/dl)*	*Mean Diet Effect (mg/dl)*[c] *0*	*+25*	*+75*	*+100*
75	75	100	150	175
150	150	175	225	250
300	300	325	375	400

a

bA pure assumption.
cBased on the cholesterol-raising properties of diets tested in Minnesota experiments.

Table 2. Model of Population Diet-Serum Cholesterol Relationships with Population Examples[a,b]

	Mean Serum Cholesterol (mg/dl)				
Mean Diet-Cholesterol Effect[c]	*Japan* *0*	*Greece* *+25*	*Italy* *+50*	*U.S.* *+75*	*Finland* *+100*
Population mean	150	175	200	225	250
Lower limit (2.5%)	75	100	125	150	175
Upper limit (97.5%)	225	250	275	300	325

a

bThe table assumes an estimated universal mean genetic serum cholesterol level of 150 mg/dl and an estimated total serum cholesterol SD ± 37.5 mg/dl.
cSeven Countries Study approximations of the cholesterol-raising properties of the national habitual diet, based on 2S-P or Keys Minnesota equation.

of the nondietary, presumably genetic, contributions to serum lipid regulation in the *individual.* In contrast, they illustrate the apparent overriding importance of the contribution of habitual diet composition to different means and distributions of blood lipids between *populations.* The models illustrate both the individual problem and the public health concern. They provide the basis for a public health view of nutrition and atherosclerosis.

THE INDIVIDUAL MODEL

Table 1 shows the relative effect of habitual diet and of the nondietary effect, here called the "minimum genetic value," on individual total cholesterol levels. The model assumes that each individual is born with, or early develops, a particular intrinsic regulatory capacity for serum lipids. Superimposed on this capacity is the average cholesterol-raising effect of various habitual diets, as shown in controlled metabolic experiments. This depicts why individuals on the same diet exhibit different average serum cholesterol levels; that is, the nondietary factor is a large contributor to interindividual differences in blood cholesterol levels. Similarly depicted is why individuals on different diets may have the same serum cholesterol level, also due predominantly to intrinsic blood lipid metabolism.

THE POPULATION MODEL

In contrast, the population model in Table 2 assumes an equal distribution among large, heterogenous population groups of the intrinsic factors that regulate serum lipid levels. Obviously, departures from this model exist due to different gene distributions among small cultural isolates. If it is assumed for large populations that the distribution of nondietary influences contributes to a theoretical universal population mean serum cholesterol level of 150 mg/dl, then the overwhelming effect of dietary differences on the population means and distributions of serum cholesterol becomes apparent.

VALIDATION OF THE MODELS

These models are not entirely theoretical. They were retrospectively developed and based on (1) knowledge of variability in serum cholesterol and its measurement as made in samples of general populations; and (2) the cholesterol-raising effects observed in controlled feeding experiments in humans. In fact, the means and upper and lower 2.5 percent limits of serum cholesterol in these models fit the experience observed in systematic population comparisons carried out by Ancel Keys in this laboratory, and by colleagues internationally (Keys et al., 1967; Keys, 1970). The Japanese diet would be cholesterol-lowering by American dietary standards; here, however, for simplicity, it is assumed to be non-cholesterol-raising. This results in an estimated average cholesterol level for the Japanese identical to the genetically (or nondietary) determined cholesterol level, which is assumed for all populations to be 150 mg/dl with an appropriate standard deviation of ±37.5 mg/dl. Estimates are not far from the observed mean levels in a Japanese population (Keys et al., 1967; Kimura, 1967). Similarly, the cholesterol-raising properties of the habitual diet of the East Finns would anticipate an effect sufficient to yield a mean value of 250 mg/dl and a distribution around the mean as depicted. This estimate is not far from the cholesterol values observed in the Finnish population (Karvonen et al., 1967; Keys et al., 1967).

These crude models of the relative intrinsic and dietary influences on serum cholesterol are further confirmed by the experience comparing Japanese

Table 3. Prevalence of Hypercholesterolemia in Japanese Men[a]

Age-Adjusted Prevalence Rate per 1,000 of Serum Cholesterol ⩾260 mg/dl		
Japan	*Hawaii*	*California*
N = 2,138	*N* = 7,961	*N* = 1,816
31.6	124.0	162.5

[a]Modified from Marmot et al., 1975.

populations on the mainland and in Hawaii and California, as shown in Table 3. In these Japanese populations, there is little likelihood that selective immigration (in regard to genes) to Hawaii or California could account for the considerable difference in the frequency of hypercholesteremia. In fact, there is evidence that the genetic composition of these Japanese families is similar in regard to common genetic markers. The difference in the observed frequency of elevated cholesterol values among these Japanese immigrants suggests an overwhelming contribution to mass hyperlipidemia of sociocultural factors, which are predominantly dietary (Marmot et al., 1975).

On these facts, assumptions, and models rests the case for the primary prevention of atherosclerosis, in part through mass dietary change. Powerful sociocultural influences that affect these levels of blood lipids in populations are, in the public health view, major issues of nutrition and public health. These forces, and important recent changes in their strength and direction, are considered in detail elsewhere (Blackburn, 1979).

REFERENCES

Blackburn, H. Progress in the epidemiology and prevention of coronary heart disease, in *Progress in Cardiology.* P. Yu and J. Goodwin, eds. Lee and Febiger, Philadelphia (1974), pp. 1–36.

Blackburn, H. Diet and mass hyperlipidemia: A public health view, in *Nutrition, Lipids, and Coronary Heart Disease.* R. Levy, B. Rifkind, B. Dennis, and N. Ernst, eds. Raven Press, New York (1979), pp. 309–347.

Djordjevic, B.S., Josipovic, V., Nedelkovic, S.I., Strasser, T., Slavkovic, V., Simic, B., Keys, A., and Blackburn, H. Men in Velika Krsma, a Serbian village. *Acta Med. Scand.* 460S, 267–277 (1967).

Gordon, T., Garcia-Palmieri, M.R., Kagan, A., Kannel, W.B., and Schiffman, J. Differences in coronary heart disease mortality in Framingham, Honolulu and Puerto Rico. *J. Chron. Dis.* 27, 329–344 (1974).

Inter-Society Commission on Heart Disease Resources Report. The primary prevention of atherosclerosis. *Circulation* 42, A-55 (1970).

Karvonen, M.J., Blomquist, G., Kallio, V., Orma, E., Punsar, S., Rautaharju, P., Takkunen, J.I., and Keys, A. Men in rural east and west Finland. *Acta Med. Scand.* 460S, 169–190 (1967).

Keys, A. (ed). Coronary heart disease in seven countries. *Circulation* 41S, 211 (1970).

Keys, A., Aravanis, C., Blackburn, H., van Buchem, F.S.P., Buzina, R., Djordjevic, B.S., Dontas, A.S., Fidanza, F., Karvonen, M.J., Kimura, H., Lekos, D., Monti, M., Puddu, V., and Taylor, H.L. Epidemiological studies related to coronary heart disease: Characteristics of men aged 40–59 in seven countries. *Acta Med. Scand.* 460S, 8–392 (1967).

Keys, A., Aravanis, C., Blackburn, H., van Buchem, F.S.P., Buzina, R., Djordjevic, B.S., Fidanza, F., Karvonen, M.J., Menotti, A., Puddu, V., and Taylor, H.L. The probability of middle-aged men developing coronary heart disease in five years. *Circulation* 45, 815–828 (1972).

Kimura, N. A farming and a fishing village in Japan: Tanushimaru and Ushibuka. *Acta Med. Scand.* 460S, 231–249 (1967).

McGill, H.D., Jr., ed. *Geographic Pathology of Atherosclerosis.* Williams and Wilkins, Baltimore (1968).

Marmot, M.G., Syme, S.L., Kato, H., Cohen, J.B., and Belsky, J. Epidemiologic studies of coronary heart disease and stroke in Japanese men living in Japan, Hawaii, and California. Prevalence of coronary disease and hypertensive heart disease and associated risk factors. *Am. J. Epidem.* 102, 514–525 (1975).

National Diet-Heart Study Research Group. The national diet-heart study final report. *Circulation* 38, suppl. 1, 428 (1968).

Walker, W.J. Changing U.S. life-style and declining vascular mortality: Cause or coincidence. *New Eng. J. Med.* 297, 163–165 (1977).

6

Epidemiology of Sudden Cardiac Death: Minerals and the "Water Story"

L.C. NERI
J.R. MARIER

Ever since Kobayashi, in 1957, noted a parallel between the geographical distribution of the acidity of water in Japanese rivers and the distribution of apoplexy (what was then one of the major causes of mortality in Japan), an increasing number of investigators all over the world have attempted to elucidate and confirm a geographical relationship between quality of drinking water and mortality, particularly from cardiovascular causes (Neri and Johansen, 1978). The now voluminous literature in this field has been subject to several comprehensive reviews most of which have been discussed in a 1979 monograph by Marier, Neri, and Anderson.

As remarkable as the geographic diversity of these studies is there has been a great diversity of the hypotheses favored by different investigators, both with regards to the identity of the water-borne factor to which they impute as good or bad influence, and with regards the nature of the disease or pathological process induced. Recently, we expressed regret at the lack of any emerging consensus among those who have contributed to the literature over the last 20 years, and at the failure of most studies to yield evidence capable of discriminating among any of 64 major classes of hypotheses that need to be considered (Neri, Hewitt and Schiber, 1974). Kobayashi (1957) did not refer to any category other than apoplexy but ecological studies, from 1960 on (Schroder, 1960), have usually tried several cause-specific death rates as dependent variables.

If the series of investigations by the various researchers from the various countries on the association between water hardness and cardiovascular disease

Table 1. Surveys of the Dietary Magnesium Intake in Various Regions of the World[a]

Reference	Country	Subjects Studied	Mg Requirement[b] mg day^{-1}	Mg Requirement[b] mg kg^{-1} day^{-1}	Average Mg Intake mg day^{-1}	Average Mg Intake mg kg^{-1} day^{-1}	Intake Requirement (%)
Leverton et al. (1961)	U.S.A.	30 Young women	320	5.3	279	4.7	87
		Lowest value	–	–	174	–	54
Fodor et al. (1978)	Newfoundland (Canada)	83 Males	–	5.0	189	2.7	55
		105 Females	–	5.0	143	2.4	48
Holtmeier and Kuhn (1972)	West Germany	Dietary survey of 1852 persons	360	5.1	235	3.5	65
Greger (1977)	U.S.A.	34 Elderly women	300	5.0	283	4.2	94
		31 Elderly men	350	5.0	251	3.5	72

[a]In balance studies, Selling (1964) had recommended a daily Mg intake of 6 mg kg^{-1}, that is, 360 or 420 mg for persons weighing 60 or 70 kg, respectively. In adult patients relying exclusively on parenteral nutrition, Freeman and Wittine (1977) found that the daily magnesium requirement averaged 400 mg.
[b]As cited by the authors in the above table.

had not followed, one wonders in which possible ways investigators could have arrived at the theory that a mineral deficiency (namely Mg) may be responsible for the increased mortality rate which is found in some geographical areas. What we propose to do in this chapter is to start at the present-day point in the water story and to see if the findings make any sense when viewed in retrospect. Let us begin, therefore, with the proposition that, in North America, the intake of magnesium is below what it should be.

A review of available studies on total intake of magnesium is summarized in Table 1, which shows that the average intake is from 6 to 35 percent lower than the daily recommended allowance (Leverton et al. 1961; Fodor, 1978; Holtmeier and Kuhn, 1972; Greger, 1977). (Note also the individual distribution of intakes ranging down to 46 percent lower than the adult daily minimum requirement.)

Moreover, this Mg deficiency—as we will see later—appears to vary on a regional basis, so that it is conceivably influenced by environmental factors,

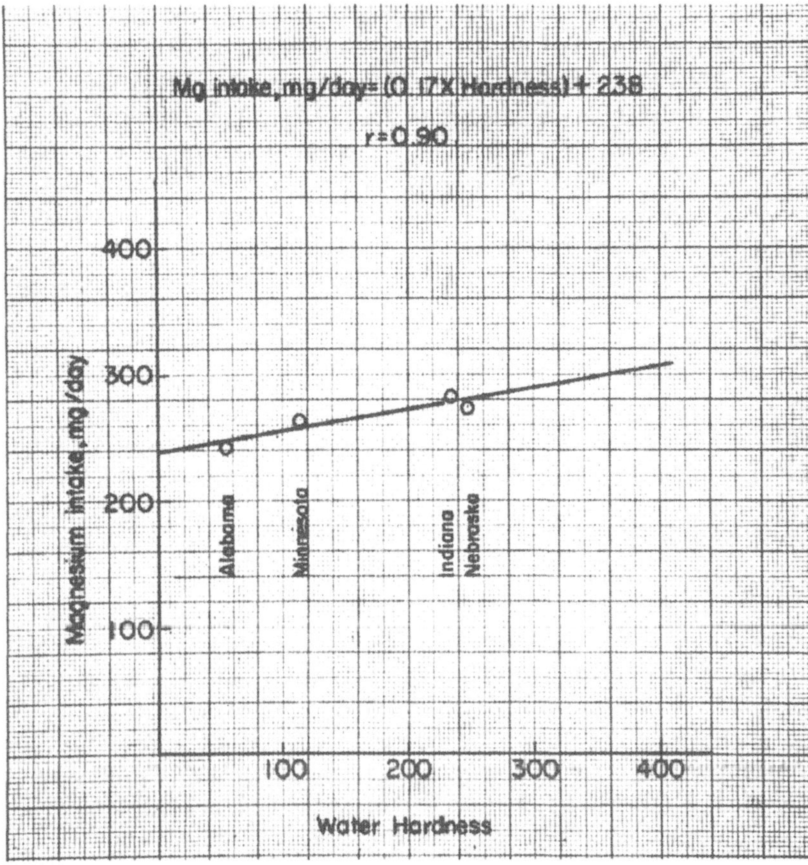

Fig. 1 From Marier (1968).

such as sociocultural factors (i.e., local eating habits) and low supplementation of Mg in local food products, etc.

When confronted by this evidence of mg deficiency, we would probably have started thinking about which of the environmental factors is most likely to affect the magnesium intake. And, by systematically exploring the various possibilities, we would sooner or later have arrived at the idea of looking at the intake of magnesium from sources other than foods, and this in turn would probably had led us to explore whether or not the local drinking waters might be the factor that would explain the geographical variations in magnesium intake.

Figure 1 shows the trend obtained by plotting magnesium intake as measured in comparable studies conducted in four geographical areas of the United States, in relation to the hardness of waters in those localities. The association appears striking. If, then, there is a great likelihood that the magnesium intake in North America is below what it should be, then there are likely to be health consequences which leads to increased mortality and morbidity. We do not really know what health effects to expect from this situation. Clinical descriptions of effects of rather severe states of magnesium deficiency do exist; however, these acute short-term manifestations are not what we are looking for. Instead, it is preferable to attempt to assess what a marginal or subclinical magnesium deficiency might mean in terms of affecting the longevity of a middle-aged (and possibly overweight) population chronically exposed to a moderate degree of magnesium deficiency.

The ideal way to investigate this problem would be a large-scale dietary survey, with follow-up studies to determine the health consequences associated with different levels of magnesium intake. The second best way, in our opinion, would be a retrospective study to reconstruct the magnesium intake of individuals with relatively better and worse health. The third best method is the one based on ecological correlations, and Table 1 has shown us the direction that such an ecological study would take: It would take the form of comparing mortality rates in soft- and hard-water areas.

However, this graph (Figure 1) also indicates that such studies, based on community averages, would be likely to underestimate the effect of magnesium deficiency. If it is true that the recommended daily requirement of magnesium is 300 to 360 mg (for normal adults), then an adequate intake occurs in only a few localities. And even when this ideal situation occurs, it would still be based on the average intake of individuals. This would mean that one half of the population in such places could be below the desirable level of magnesium intake. A quantitative appraisal of this situation would be possible if we had detailed data on the variation between individuals. The standard deviations (S.D.) of the relevant variables vary from 10 percent of the mean value in our tissue studies (about which more will be said later) to 22 percent of the mean value in the surveys of magnesium intake conducted by Leverton et al. (1961). In terms of the correlation we have shown, this would mean that reliance on averages would fall somewhat short of indicating the total protection obtainable by remedying the magnesium insufficiency in *all* individuals.

Since we were not in a position to conduct a full-scale dietary survey, nor to do a retrospective study of magnesium intake status among individuals, we were left with the option of comparing the tissue concentrations of selected elements in people who died violent deaths in two selected areas (one region with soft- and one region with hard-water), and comparing these results with the tissue concentrations of these elements in people who died from natural causes in the same two areas, with special emphasis on the possible influence of different magnesium intakes in the two types of region.

Table 2. Elimination on Tissue Analysis Grounds (Seven Candidate Elements)[a]

Heart Muscle Dry Weight Concentration of Zinc and Chromium (Males Only) (ppm)

	Soft-water areas	
	Zn	*Cr (X 100)*
Cardiovascular cases	100.9 ± 19.0	7.1 ± 11.1
Accident cases	100.5 ± 13.3	13.2 ± 15.2
P	N.S.[b]	N.S.
	Accident cases	
	Zn	*Cr (X 100)*
Hard-water areas	101.1 ± 17.9	19.8 ± 21.9
Soft-water areas	100.5 ± 13.3	13.2 ± 15.2
P	N.S.	N.S.

[a]Do not differ between healthy and cardiovascular subjects.
[b]N.S. = not significant.

We will present what we found in Canada, in terms of what we call "progressive eliminations" of various possible coexisting elements, that is to say, systematic exclusion of the less likely minerals and zeroing-in on the more promising ones. Although, for the purposes of this chapter, we have pretended to begin with foreknowledge of the magnesium deficiency situation, we—in fact—arrived at this conclusion only *after* ecological correlation studies of the "water factor," thus following Schroeder's steps (1960).

The design of our tissue studies, conducted in collaboration with Dr. T.W. Anderson of the University of Toronto, provides for the comparison of the metal content of the heart and of control muscles in residents of hard- and soft-water areas, and specifically those dying from myocardial infarction and from accidents (Anderson et al., 1973, 1975; Neri et al., 1975). This last group is taken as being representative of healthy subjects. For the purposes of this study, we established the following criteria so as to enable us to decide which of the various elements might be implicated as the suspected element:

1. The tissue concentration must differ between cardiac deaths and accidental deaths.
2. The difference in tissue concentration must be consistent with the postulated biological effect of a particular element.
3. The difference in concentration among control patients from each type of area must be consistent with the mineral content of the water consumed.

On this overall basis, we were able to eliminate zinc and chromium, because the concentrations of these two elements are not different in healthy and cardiac subjects (see Table 2). In Table 3, the reader can see that we

Table 3. Elimination on Tissue Analysis Grounds (Seven Candidate Elements)[a]

Heart Muscle Dry Weight Concentration of Pb (Males Only) (ppm)

	Soft-water areas		*Accident cases*
Cardiovascular	0.01 ± 0.04	Hard water	0.26 ± 0.85
Accident	0.18 ± 0.43	Soft water	0.18 ± 0.43
P	N.S.[b]	*P*	N.S.

[a]Is not consistent with the postulated effect.
[b]N.S. = not significant.

Table 4. Elimination on Tissue Analysis Grounds (Seven Candidate Elements)[a]

Heart Muscle Dry Weight Concentration of Metals (Males Only) (ppm)

	Accident cases	
	Ca	*Cd*
Hard-water areas	230.7 ± 50.1	0.21 ± 0.15
Soft-water areas	214.6 ± 38.1	0.18 ± 0.12
P	N.S.[b]	N.S.
	Soft-water areas	
	Ca	*Cd*
Cardiovascular cases	293.3 ± 124.0	0.30 ± 0.37
Accident cases	214.6 ± 38.1	0.18 ± 0.12
P	<.001	N.S.

[a]Lack of consistent difference among healthy residents in soft- and hard-water areas.
[b]N.S. = not significant.

also eliminated lead, because the results were not consistent with its postulated toxicologic effect.

Similarly, Table 4, shows that we eliminated calcium and cadmium, which were found in increasing concentrations in the hearts of subjects dying from myocardial infarct as compared with accident cases, and because the concentration of these elements does not differ among healthy residents in soft- and hard-water areas.

We are, thus, left with two possible elements, copper and magnesium.

Copper (see Table 5) is found to be decreased by a significant amount in the hearts of myocardial infarction cases, but is also found to decrease in healthy residents of soft-water areas. Here, there is a paradox, because the concentration of copper in soft waters tended to be about two-fold greater than that in hard waters, and one would expect the tissue copper concentrations to be *higher,* rather than lower.

Magnesium showed the greatest difference between the subjects dying from myocardial infarction and accident cases, a difference that is present in both hard- and soft-water areas. Moreover, the hearts of healthy residents

Table 5. Elimination on Tissue Analysis Grounds (Seven Candidate Elements)

Heart Muscle Dry Weight Concentration of Cu (Males Only) (ppm)			
	Soft-water areas		*Accident cases*
Cardiovascular	12.7 ± 3.8	Hard water	16.7 ± 2.5
Accident	15.8 ± 2.2	Soft water	15.8 ± 2.2
P	<.001	*P*	N.S.[a]
Heart Muscle Dry Weight Concentration of Mg (Males Only) (ppm)			
	Soft-water areas		*Accident cases*
Cardiovascular	685.3 ± 153.6	Hard water	994.9 ± 139.9
Accident	925.7 ± 113.4	Soft water	925.7 ± 113.4
P	<.001	*P*	<.02

[a]N.S. = not significant.

Table 6. Elimination on Water Analysis Grounds (15 Candidate Elements)[a]

Elements	*No. of Loc. Tested*	*Percentage Found*	*Limit of Detection (ppb)*	*Method of Analysis*
Ag	239	0.1	001–005	N.A.[b]
Mo	239	0.1	050–200	N.A.
Se	239	0.8	001–008	N.A.
Sb	239	6.3	004	N.A.

[a]Detectable in less than 10% of water tested.
[b]N.A. = neutron activation.

in hard-water areas also contained more magnesium than those in soft-water areas.

As we have said previously, the third best option for studies of this type is based on ecological correlations (i.e., studies of water and mortality averages). To obtain baseline data on the hardness and elemental content of drinking waters, we examined randomly selected tapwaters obtained in more than 500 localities across Canada, each of them having a communal water supply. A list of 15 candidate elements was selected, on the basis of suggestions that had been proposed by previous investigators.

Again, we went through a sequence of progressive eliminations, based on fixed criteria, in a fashion similar to the one used in the tissue studies, that is:

1. The suspected element must be found in the waters consumed.
2. The trend seen with a particular element must be compatible with the geographical distribution of hardness, that is, if the element is protective, it must be present in larger quantities in hard waters; if the element is toxic, it must be found in larger amounts in soft waters.

Table 7. Elimination on Water Analysis Grounds (15 Candidate Elements)[a]

Mean Concentration	Water Hardness Ranges (ppm) 0–14	15–29	30–59	60–99	100–149	150–249	250+	No. of Localities
Ni (ppb)	2.9	4.9	5.2	6.4	4.3	3.5	7.2	233
Pb (ppb)	42.9	16.9	10.7	7.3	9.0	10.7	8.7	234
Zn (ppm)	0.2	0.2	0.3	0.3	0.3	0.3	0.3	510
Cd (ppb)	1.0	0.3	0.1	0.4	0.4	0.3	0.9	510

Element	Daily Requirement	Daily Intake from Average Diet	Estimated Intake from 2 Liters of Water per Day: Soft-water Areas <30 ppm	Hard-water Areas >150 ppm
Ni (μg)	?	400	7.8	10.7
Pb (μg)	Toxic	130	59.8	19.4
Zn (mg)	16–27	12–15	0.4	0.6
Cd (μg)	Toxic	215	1.3	1.2

[a]Not appropriately related to hardness vs. softness.

Table 8. Elimination on Water Analysis Grounds (15 Candidate Elements)[a]

Element	Daily Requirement	Daily Intake from Average Diet	Estimated Intake from 2 Liters of Water per Day: Soft-water Areas (<30 ppm)	Hard-water Areas (>150 ppm)
Ca (mg)	800–1000	1000	8.9	144.0
Co (μg)	1	300	0.5	1.6

Mean Concentration	Water Hardness Ranges (ppm) 0–14	15–29	30–59	60–99	100–149	150–249	250+	No. of Localities
Ca (ppm)	2.4	6.5	12.6	22.8	35.8	50.6	93.2	501
Co (ppb)	0.2	0.3	0.4	0.4	0.7	0.8	0.8	239

[a]Intake from water too small, relative to other sources.

3. A particular element must be present in sufficient quantities in the waters consumed so as to make an appreciable contribution to total dietary intake.

On this basis (see Table 6) we could eliminate silver, selenium molybdenum, and antimony—all supposedly protective elements—because they were detected in less than 10 percent of the waters that we tested.

We also eliminated (see Table 7) nickel, lead, zinc, and cadmium, because they were not consistently related to the hardness-softness gradient.

Table 9. Short List[a,b]

Element	Daily Requirement	Daily Intake from Average Diet	Estimated Intake from 2 Liters of Water per Day: Soft-water Areas	Hard-water Areas
Hg (μg)	Toxic	20	19.2	4.1
Cu (mg)	2.1	2–4	1.2	0.6
Cr (μg)	20–500	5–100	0.6	4.1

Mean Concentration	Water Hardness Ranges (ppm): 0–14	15–29	30–59	60–99	100–149	150–249	250+	No. of Localities
Hg (ppb)	11.1	8.1	10.9	7.6	3.1	2.1	2.0	239
Cu (ppm)	0.7	0.5	0.4	0.2	0.2	0.3	0.3	510
Cr (ppb)	0.0	0.6	0.7	0.3	1.1	1.7	2.4	239

Correlation Coefficient Between Male Mortality Rates and Certain Water Quality (Age Standardized 35–64; Combined Years 1950–52 and 1960–1962)

Cause	Hg	Cu	Cr
Coronary Mortality	– 0.01	.02	– 0.16
All Causes	– 0.01	.04	– 0.09
N	129.0	510.0	39.0

[a]No positive evidence.
[b]Excluding less than the limit of detection.

Table 10. Short List[a]

Element	Daily Requirement	Daily Intake from Average Diet	Estimated Intake from 2 Liters of Water per Day: Soft-water Areas	Hard-water Areas
Mg (mg)	300–500	250–300	2.3	52.1
Li	?	1 mg	0.1	1.3

Mean Concentration	Water Hardness Ranges (ppm): 0–14	15–29	30–59	60–99	100–149	150–249	250+	No. of Localities
Mg (ppm)	0.8	1.5	2.8	5.8	8.4	17.3	34.1	509
Li (ppm)	0.0	0.1	0.2	0.2	0.3	0.4	0.9	509

[a]With positive evidence.

In addition (see Table 8) we eliminated calcium and cobalt, because intake of these elements from drinking water was too small in comparison with intake from other sources.

Among the remaining five elements, there are three (see Table 9), that is, mercury, chromium, and copper, that also merit exclusion because of the lack of consistant supporting evidence from studies in Canada and elsewhere. In fact, mercury, found in 60 percent of the sampled waters, has a gradient

Table 11. Statistically Significant Correlation Coefficient Between Male Mortality Rates and Certain Water Quality Age Standardized 35–64 (Combined Years 1950–52 and 1960–62)[a,b]

	Li	*Ca*	*Mg*	*Hardness*	*Ni*
N	*522*	*522*	*522*	*522*	*239*
Canada					
ASHD[c] (420 + 422)	– .09*	– .07	– .10**	– .09*	– .12*
All causes	– .09*	– .11**	– .18***	– .13**	– .17**
N	*159*	*159*	*159*	*159*	–
Ontario					
ASHD (420 + 422)	– .24**	– .11**	– .27**	– .28***	–
All causes	– .16**	– .16*	– .25***	– .21**	–

[a]Tested but found not significant: Cu, Zn, pH, Pb, Cr, Cd, Co, Hg, Sb, and Mg.
[b]Adapted from Neri et al. (1975).
[c]ASHD = atheroschlerotic heart disease.

of decreasing concentration with increasing hardness. This could fit the hypothesis of a toxic element, contained in soft waters, that provides an average of 10 μg of mercury per day (i.e., five times the amount received from hard waters). However, in the correlation studies, mercury does not correlate significantly with mortality; in the few instances in which it does, it has a negative sign indicating a protective effect. Chromium, found in 16 percent of the sampled waters, is found in its highest values in hard waters. If the form of chromium found in water is optimal for absorption, this could account for a large proportion of the daily chromium intake in some hard-water areas; however, mortality correlations in most countries do not provide any conclusive evidence of a water-borne chromium effect. Copper also deserves more attention. It is found in decreasing amounts with increasing hardness, and its highest values are found in the softest groups of water. However, copper concentration is not significantly associated with mortality on the list of suspect elements.

This leaves magnesium and lithium (see Table 10).

Magnesium is the strongest correlate in our correlation matrix (see Table 11), that is, stronger than either calcium or hardness, with lithium ranking fourth. Of course, it must be stated that all of these factors are highly intercorrelated. The daily requirement of magnesium, as we have seen, is considered to be 300 to 360 mg, and may be as high as 400 mg. (Seelig, 1964; Freeman and Wittine, 1977). Diet alone rarely provides a reassuring margin of safety; thus, the amount of magnesium that is obtained from water could become critical, especially on a long-term basis.

At this point in our presentation, it is time to connect our anachronistic narrative to the actual historical sequence in which events really happened. First of all, let us try to validate Table 1 (i.e., the table concerned with dietary magnesium intakes).

In Table 12, it can be seen, first, that by using a calculation based on the regression equation shown in the earlier graph (first two columns), and, second, by using a calculation based on the contribution of water-borne magnesium to total hardness, we obtain very similar estimates of total magnesium intake per day, including the amount contributed by water. We must emphasize that these estimated intakes include the use of water for food and beverage preparation.

Table 13 illustrates how much magnesium is contributed by hard waters of various types. There are some rather meaningful differences revealed in this table. In particular, we wish to draw attention to the bottom line. We really do not see any easy way to account for all the geographical differences in mortality rates associated with water hardness in Britain, certainly not on the basis of variations in water-borne magnesium. This is something that most probably will have to be explained on the basis of *total* daily intake of magnesium. Such data, as well as geochemical data regarding the distribution of magnesium-depleted areas in the U.K., are sorely lacking.

There are a number of ways in which one may try to characterize the risk of mortality that is associated with soft-water residence. The use of the International Classification of Disease to categorize death is not a particularly rewarding one, for various reasons. One shortcoming is that the traditional reliance on the cardiovascular or noncardiovascular designation does not really isolate the water effect in Canada or in other countries. Witness to this are the findings of correlations with a bronchitis effect, or an infancy mortality effect, and, particularly in Canada, an effect on mortality from all causes.

The implications of the preceding findings give rise to two possibilities: (1) either the effects extend *outside* the cardiovascular area; or (2) we are in the very complicated situation of finding that water has a real effect on cardiovascular diseases, along with discovering that there is an altogether different reason for the increase found in noncardiovascular mortality.

Another approach has been tried, and perhaps it is the only one that has been tried thoroughly: it is the distinction between sudden and nonsudden deaths. Currently, this distinction has been done only on a portion of the all causes mortality pattern, that is, the cardiac-related segment. In this regard, the results of studies done in Ontario were somewhat encouraging; but unfortunately, these were not confirmed for the remainder of Canada, nor in the State of Washington. Perhaps, the most recent attempt to investigate the sudden death subject is the one recently published by

Table 12. Comparison of Two Calculations for Estimation of Daily Magnesium Intake, Including the Contribution by Water-borne Mg

Calculation Based on Water Composition

Total hardness of water	*Estimated Mg intake, mg day^{-1}* [a]	*Total hardness × 0.33 = Mg hardness*	*Mg hardness × 0.24 = Mg (ppm)*	*Mg intake from 2.4 liters water day^{-1} (mg)* [b]	*Total daily Mg intake (water + baseline) (mg)*
0	238	–	–	0	238
100	255	33	8.0	19 (= 7.4%)	257
200	272	66	16.0	38 (= 13.9%)	276
300	289	99	24.0	57 (= 19.6%)	295
400	306	133	32.0	76 (= 24.5%)	314

[a] Mg intake, mg day^{-1} = (0.17 × hardness) + 238.
[b] A daily water intake of 2.4 liters (in all forms) is in agreement with the findings of ICRP (1975), Spencer et al. (1970), and Schroeder et al. (1969).

Table 13. Compositional Diversity of Waters from Different Regions[a]

Authors	*Locale*	*Total Hardness*	*Ca (mg $liter^{-1}$)*	*Mg (mg $liter^{-1}$)*	*Mg Intake From 2.0 Liters Water (mg day^{-1})*
Schroeder (1960)	163 U.S. metropolitan areas	118	31.1	9.75	19.5
Schroeder (1960)	25 U.S. cities with lowest death rates from coronary disease	125	22.5	16.50	33.0
Anderson et al. (1975)	Five Ontario soft waters	33	8.9	2.80	5.6
	Three Ontario hard waters	421	119.4	29.40	58.8
Crawford et al. (1968)	Nine British soft waters	31	8.5	2.50	5.0
	Six British hard waters	293	102.0	9.25	18.5

[a] Adapted from Marier (1968).

Table 14. Death Rates from IHD and Percentage of Sudden Deaths (Males 30–59)[a]

Rates for Ischemic Heart Disease (IHD)	*6 Soft-water Towns*	*6 Hard-water Towns*	*Difference*
Rates per 10^5	251	151	90
Percentage of definite sudden deaths	41.9	35.0	6.9
Rate of sudden deaths	105	55	49
Rate of nonsudden deaths	146	105	41

[a]Adapted from Crawford, Shaper et al. (1977).

Crawford et al. (1977). The authors themselves state that "the results do not constitute firm evidence that the proportion of ischemic heart disease (IHD) deaths which are sudden is higher in soft- than in hard-water towns." And (in fact) our own analysis of their data shows (see Table 14) that the distinction is indeed not clear but implies that the effect of water hardness is an almost equally strong effect in sudden and nonsudden cardiac deaths. It would seem, therefore, that the separation between sudden and nonsudden deaths, although encouraging, does not define what the conditions for the occurrence of disease are, nor what are the causes of death that are found in excess in areas where the water is soft. Within the category of cardiovascular disease, however, sudden-death findings are consistent for us to consider them a better approximation to what specifically relates to soft-water mortality. One of the difficulties may be that the deaths classified as "sudden" may not be sudden at all, in the sense that we are concerned with: for example, deaths following a series of episodes of ischemic attacks.

A distinction based on unexpected premature deaths could conceivably turn out to be a better criterion of the water hardness effect. But, even then, this may not explain the entire story, especially if the search is confined to the traditional subject of exploration: the cardiovascular area.

The above epidemiologic considerations, when viewed together with the clinical and experimental work conducted in the area of stress (we refer here to stress imposed on the cardiac function), suggests an hypothesis capable of tying together most of the findings. This is the concept of the unstable, vulnerable heart, which–possibly because of some metabolic deficiency (likely related to magnesium deficiency)–is capable of responding to a sudden upsurge of functional demand. This can conceivably happen in several situations in which the cause of death would not be classified as cardiac on the medical certificate of death, particularly in cases such as chronic bronchitis and maybe even some of the cancers. The selective magnesium depletion found in the myocardia of our tissue studies, in the study by Behr and Burton (1973) in England, and by various other studies in experimental animals, is in line with this theory. One cannot expect that the epidemiologic evidence collected up to now would be able to confirm an hypothesis such as this.

Studies will have to be designed to test the specific hypothesis, and the ultimate answer will hopefully emerge during a magnesium intervention trial.

We would, at this point, ask you to set aside the water story in order to examine the available clinical and experimental data that would support the proposed theory. The place to begin is with the evidence stemming from clinical observations. Data recently became available indicating the importance of magnesium as a therapeutic agent in various syndromes, whether or not these can be considered as being primarily cardiac-related syndromes. For instance, Chadda's (1972) work has shown that magnesium supplements are very effective in stabilizing arrhythmia in patients admitted to cardiac intensive care units; in comparison, potassium supplements were ineffective by themselves. A similar situation has also been seen at the University of Montreal, where magnesium supplements have prevented adrenalin-induced cardiopathy; here again, potassium supplements were ineffective (Savoie, 1972). Magnesium supplements can prevent histamine shock during the "sudden unexpected infant death" syndrome (Caddell, 1972) and can also enhance thiamin utilization in undernourished individuals (Ziere, 1975). In addition, it has been found that magnesium supplementation has a vasodilator effect in hypertensive patients, and increases the cardiac output in most types of patients (Mroczek et al., 1977).

A review by Burch and Giles (1977) illustrates how an inadequate magnesium status in the body can cause noticeable aberrations in electrocardiographic patterns, and another review by Marier (1978) has emphasized that all these recent studies on human beings indicate the beneficial role that magnesium can have, particularly at the cardiac site. These observations may relate to some noncardiac syndromes in a multitude of metabolic situations in which magnesium has been demonstrated to be very helpful.

To turn to the experimental evidence, many publications which have dealt with experimental work on animals also indicates that magnesium protects against various types of stress. For instance, contrasting with the effect of acute magnesium deficiencies, subacute deficiencies, such as the one possible in soft-water areas, can produce a significant fall in heart tissue magnesium content in experimental animals, a fall that is not accompanied by a similar response in other muscles, and which has been found to cause selective myocardial calcifications. Such studies have shown magnesium supplementation to be demonstrably protective against cardiotoxic substances and against stress.

Because of the long-recognized crucial importance of magnesium as a vital cofactor for various enzymatic and metabolic processes, a myocardium that is deficient in magnesium is likely to be particularly vulnerable to a variety of stressful situations. In fact, myocardial magnesium depletion can be regarded as the "sensitizer" in Hans Selye's "sensitizer-challenger" concept in which the "challenger" is most probably a sudden surge of stimulus at the cardiac site (Selye, 1968). What will then be our conclusion? If the myocardium can (1) become selectively depleted in magnesium, and (2) can thereby become impaired in its responses to a sudden demand for increased cardiac output, we have the prerequisites for an increased likelihood of fatalities, probably sudden fatalities, whether or not they will be ultimately ascribed to the cardiac domain.

In terms of the Canadian experience, such an hypothesis is fully applicable to the so-called Water Story. It can also be related to the inadequate intake of magnesium from dietary source, sometimes referred to as "empty-calorie diets" in the modern-day world.

REFERENCES

Anderson, T.W., Le Riche, W.H., and MacKay, J.S. Sudden death and ischemic heart disease–correlation with hardness of local water supply. *New Engl. J. Med.* 280, 805–807 (1969).

Anderson, T.W., Hewitt, D., Neri, L.C., Schreiber, G., and Talbot, F. Water hardness and magnesium in heart muscle. *Lancet,* Dec. 15, 1973, p. 1390.

Anderson, T.W., Neri, L.C., Schreiber, G., Talbot, F.D.F., and Zdrejewski, A. Ischemic heart disease, water hardness, and myocardial magnesium. *Can. Med. Assoc. J.* 113, 199–203 (1975).

Behr, G., and Burton, P. Heart muscle magnesium. *Lancet,* Aug. 25, 1973, p. 450.

Burch, G.E., and Giles, T.D. The importance of magnesium deficiency in cardiovascular disease. *Amer. Heart J.* 94, 649–657 (1977).

Caddell, J.L. Magnesium deprivation in sudden unexpected infant death. *Lancet,* Aug. 5, 1972, pp. 258–262.

Chadda, K.D., Gupta, P.K., and Lichstein, E. Magnesium in cardiac arrhythmia. *New Engl. J. Med.* 287, 1102 (1972).

Crawford, M.D., Clayton, D.G., Stanley, F., and Shaper, A.G. An epidemiological study of sudden death in hard- and soft-water areas. *J. Chron. Dis.* 30, 69–80 (1977).

Crawford, M.D., Gardner, M.J., and Morris, J.N. Mortality and hardness of local water supplies. *Lancet,* Apr. 20, 1968, pp. 827–831.

Greger, J.L., Marhefka, S., Huffman, J., Baligar, P., Peterson, T., Zaikis, S., and Sickles, V. Comparison of analysed and calculated nitrogen, zinc, magnesium, phosphorus, and iron content of diets. *Nutr. Rep. Internat.* 18, 345–352 (1978).

Holtmeier, H.J., and Kuhn, M. Zinc and magnesium mangel beim menschen. *Therapiewoche* 22, 4536–4646 (1972).

Kobayashi, J. Geographical relation between the chemical nature of river water and death-rate from apoplexy. *Ber. Ohara Inst. Landwirtsch. Biol.,* Okayama Univ. 11, 12–21 (1957).

Marier, J.R. Cardio-protective contribution of hard waters to magnesium intake. *Rev. Canad. Biol.* 37, 115–125 (1978).

Marier, J.R., Neri, L.C., and Anderson, T.W. *Water Hardness, Human Health and the Importance of Magnesium.* National Research Council of Canada Publication, NRCC No. 17581 (1979).

Mroczek, W.J., Lee, W.R., and Davidov, M.E. Effect of magnesium sulfate on cardiovascular hemodynamics. *Angiology* 28, 720–724 (1977).

Neri, L.C., Hewitt, D., and Mandel, J.S. Risk of sudden death in soft-water areas. *Amer. J. Epidemiol.* 94, 101-104 (1971).

Neri, L.C. and Hewitt, D. Review and implications of ongoing and projected research outside the European Communities (1975). (See reference to "CEC 1975", pp. 443–466).

Neri, L.C., Hewitt, D., Schreiver, G.B., Anderson, T.W., Mandel, J.S., and Zdrojewsky, A. Health aspects of hard and soft waters. *J. Amer. Water Works Assoc.* 67(8), 403–409 (1975).

Neri, L.C. and Johansen, H.L. Water hardness and cardiovascular mortality. *Ann. N.Y. Acad. Sci.* 304, 203–219 (1978).

Peterson, D.R., Thompson, D.J., and Nam, J.M. Water hardness, arteriosclerotic heart disease, and sudden death. *Amer. J. Epidemiol.* 92, 90–93 (1970).

Schroeder, H.A. Relation between mortality from cardiovascular disease and treated water supplies. *J. Amer. Med. Assoc.* 172, 98/1902–104/1908 (1960).

Schroeder, H.A. Municipal drinking-water and cardiovascular death rates. *J. Amer. Med. Assoc.* 195, 81/125–85/129 (1966).

Selye, H. *Anaphylactoid Edema.* St. Louis, Missouri: W.H. Green, Inc. (1968).

Zieve, L. Role of co-factors in the treatment of malnutrition, as exemplified by magnesium. *Yale J. Biol. Med.* 48, 229–237 (1975).

7

Dietary Studies of Ten-year-old Children in the Bogalusa Heart Study

GAIL C. FRANK
LARRY S. WEBBER
GERALD S. BERENSON

INTRODUCTION

One of the major questions concerning the pathogenesis of atherosclerosis and hypertension is, "What environmental factors influence the development of these major cardiovascular diseases?" Of the environmental factors, nutrition plays a major role. The Bogalusa Heart Study, a large epidemiologic program of the Specialized Center of Research–Arteriosclerosis (SCOR-A) at the Louisiana State University Medical Center, is conducting research on the early natural history of arteriosclerosis (a term used here to encompass both atherosclerosis and hypertension). Risk factor variables, similar to those that have been described in adults, are being studied in Bogalusa, Louisiana, as a total community study of children in a biracial population. Since risk factors in adults have been shown to be predictive of the development of morbid events complicating coronary artery disease and hypertension (American Heart Association, 1973), it is important to observe the early onset and progression of the risk factors.

We now know that coronary artery disease and very likely essential hypertension begin in childhood, progressing silently over several decades until clinical disease is expressed. When focusing attention on children it is appropriate to begin by studying the onset of obesity, hypertension, and hyperlipoproteinemia and to look at the interrelationship of these and other risk factor variables, as shown in Fig. 1. In children we can describe the levels of blood pressure, height, weight, and serum lipids, but obviously at this point we cannot define them as precise factors placing the child at risk. Unfortunately, little information heretofore has elucidated risk factor variables

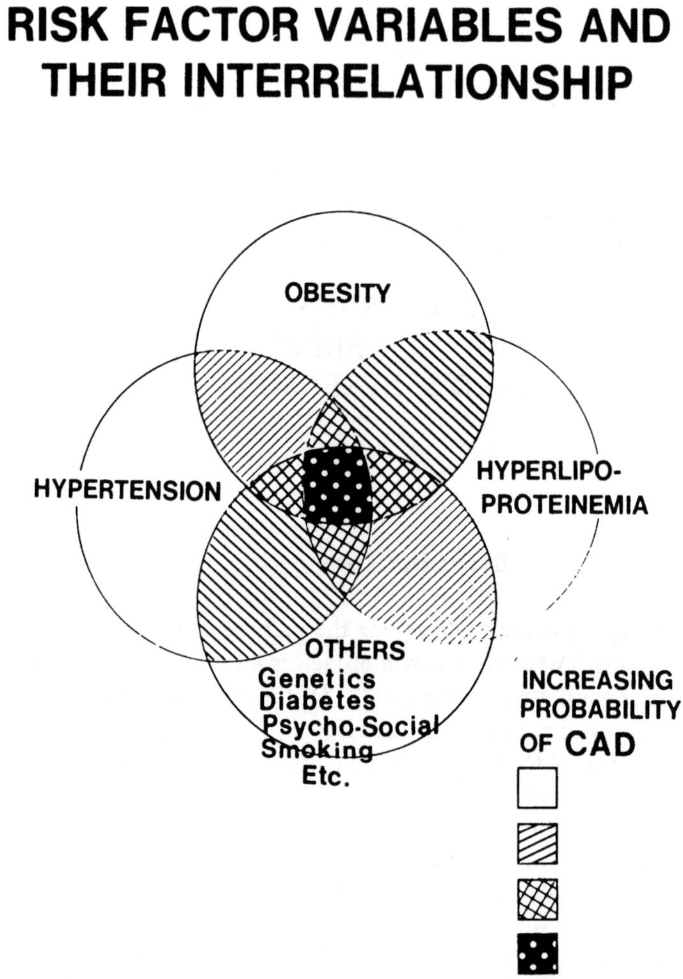

Fig. 1. Risk factor variables and their interrelationship. An interrelationship of multiple risk factors occurs. In children these cannot be defined for risk at the present time, but the variables obviously interrelate as they do in adults.

in children, their occurrence, their interrelationship, or their changes over time. The LSU SCOR-A has posed four basic questions with regard to these risk factor variables in children: (1) What are their distribution and prevalence?; (2) What are their interrelationships?; (3) What is their course over time?; and (4) What are their determinants (genetic versus environmental)?

Information to help answer the first two questions has now been published for the Bogalusa children (Foster et al., 1977; Frerichs et al., 1976;

Srinivasan et al., 1976b; Voors et al., 1976). The present discussion primarily concerns the fourth question which pertains to the environmental determinants of risk factor variables in children, specifically diet. Identification of dietary practices in children that might relate to the development of risk factors would be important in understanding how to prevent arteriosclerosis.

EXAMINATION OF SCHOOL CHILDREN

In 1973–74 the distribution of serum lipid and blood pressure levels and indices of obesity were characterized in 93 percent of Bogalusa's pediatric population, aged 5 to 15 years, totaling 3524 children. Each child rotated through a carefully planned 3½-hour examination where trained physicians and nurses, adhering to established protocols, obtained measurements of risk factor variables and other information. To balance the research studies with service to the children, a physical examination was also conducted.

DIETARY STUDIES

Because of technical limitations in obtaining reliable and quantitative dietary data, only a subsample of the children could be involved in the dietary studies. During the first year of the cross-sectional study, dietary data were collected on a subsample of ten-year-olds. Although data have been obtained from other age cohorts to encompass changes from birth to adulthood, this presentation will focus on the dietary data of the ten-year-old children.

Two major objectives of the dietary study of ten-year-olds were (1) to determine what a subsample of the pediatric population was consuming; and (2) to observe the diet-risk factor variable interrelationships. Careful consideration was given to selecting both the sample of children and the methods for dietary assessment. Most techniques demand cooperation and time from the participants, and diminish chances of randomizing and examining large samples. Several methods (Young et al., 1952; Rose and Blackburn, 1968; Emmons and Hayes, 1973) used for precise assessment of dietary intakes were also considered but were not found feasible for field studies of children. Even though the 24-hour dietary recall is known to have limitations (Young and Trulson, 1960), we chose this method to identify the most recent food intakes of a group of normal, free-living children. The 24-hour recall allows the child to serve as his or her own respondent even though it relies upon the child's memory. The method is relatively short, not overtaxing, and is primarily acceptable for group characterization. In addition, quality controls can be incorporated to improve its accuracy.

Several methods and quality controls for improvement of the recall method were tested on 68 students, 10 to 16 years old, in a pilot study in Franklinton, Louisiana, 20 miles from Bogalusa (Frank et al., 1977a,b).

1. A *detailed protocol* was developed to cover all areas of dietary data collection and calculation, including a dialogue for an interview and verbal probes to identify and document the foods eaten.

2. *Graduated food models,* similar to those employed in the Ten-State Nutrition Survey (Moore et al., 1967), were used. They do not depict any one food item but are coded for equivalents which can be used to convert foods to grams.

3. A *product identification notebook* (Frank et al., 1977a) was developed to aid in careful characterization of snack foods consumed by children. This notebook pictorially categorizes snacks into five groups based on texture and content, such as "crunchy crumbles," "baked bits," "sugary sweets," and "soft surprises."

4. *School lunch measurement.* On the day before the recall, school staff selected three representative lunch trays from the serving line. The foods were weighed for an average portion size and one-cup weights were obtained to establish one-eighth cup equivalents used for the graduated food models. School lunch recipes were computerized prior to analysis of a child's food intake.

5. *Verification by parent.* Type of fat used in cooking, salting habits, preparation techniques, and home recipes were verified by telephone contact with parents.

6. *Collection feedback mechanism.* Each nutritionist completed the recalls she collected, while another nutritionist checked her observations and provided an immediate feedback of calculation errors.

7. *Duplicate recalls.* Intermittent duplicate recalls were inserted during the collection period to indicate the repeatability and standardization of data collection. To obtain a duplicate, two nutritionists independently interviewed the same child within an hour. A third interviewer compared and recorded any differences that might warrant further training of the interviewers. The computed mean intakes of selected nutrients were compared by a paired *t*-test. All of the comparisons have shown no significant differences between interviewers.

8. *Retraining sessions.* In an attempt to minimize interviewer traits that would bias the responses of the children, retraining sessions of the interviewers were interspersed throughout the collection period.

9. *Computerized food composition data bank.* We used a computerized food composition table, the "Extended Table of Nutrient Values" (ETNV)

Table 1. Risk Factor Variable Levels of Ten-year-olds[a]

Variable	*Mean Level* Boys $N = 96$	Girls $N = 89$
Skinfold average (mm)	11	13
Weight (kg)	34	34
Height (cm)	139	141
Serum cholesterol (mg%)	164	168
Serum triglyceride (mg%)	65	69
Systolic blood pressure (mm Hg)	98	99
Diastolic blood pressure (mm Hg)	61	61

[a] $N = 185$.

(Moore et al., 1971), to analyze our data; the ETNV is a collaborative data bank with over 2000 food items. Analysis for 58 dietary components is currently available per food item.

The improved 24-hour dietary recall was then employed in Bogalusa to describe the dietary intakes and meal patterns and to explore the risk factor variable-diet relationship of a random sample of children from the ten-year-old age group. The sample totaled 185 children, which was half of the students ten years of age, 35 percent black and 65 percent white, with 89 girls and 96 boys. These students would serve only indirectly to reflect the dietary intakes of all children of school age. Table 1 shows the levels of risk factor variables for this sample.

Each child responded to a 30- to 40-minute interview regarding what he or she ate during the previous 24-hour period. Three sets of ten children were interviewed in duplicate, and 15 children were interviewed four times during the screening year to note any seasonal variation.

RESULTS AND DISCUSSION

As shown in Table 2, the mean energy intake for the Bogalusa children was 2141 calories. Of the total calories, 13 percent were from protein and 49 percent from carbohydrate. Fat provided 38 percent of the total calories with twice the percentage from animal as vegetable fat. This high animal fat intake resulted in a polyunsaturated/saturated fatty acid ratio (P/S) of 0.3. The children consumed twice as much protein from animal sources as vegetable sources, and both the black and white boys ingested roughly 10 g more protein than their female counterparts. Average carbohydrate consumed was 262 g, with an equal proportion of sucrose to starch.

Cholesterol intake averaged 324 mg, an intake of about 10 mg/kg of body weight. When these data were compared to Framingham, Massachusetts adults

Table 2. Mean Intake and Percentage of Total Calories from Dietary Components in 24-Hour Recalls of Ten-year-olds[a]

Dietary Component	*Mean Intake*	*Percentage of Total Calories*
Energy (kcal)	2141	–
Protein (g)[b]	69	13
Animal	47	9
Vegetable	22	4
Carbohydrate (g)[c]	262	49
Starch	88	17
Sugar[d]	144	27
Sucrose	98	18
Fat (g)	93	38
Animal	59	25
Vegetable	25	10
P/S ratio[e]	0.3	–
Cholesterol (mg)	324	–
Sodium (g)	3.3	–

[a]$N = 185$.
[b]Protein = sum of amino acid values.
[c]Carbohydrate = sum of starch, fructose, glucose, lactose, maltose, sucrose, pectic substances, other known, and unknown.
[d]Sugar = sum of fructose, glucose, lactose, maltose, and sucrose.
[e]Polyunsaturated/saturated = sum of linoleic, linolenic, arachidonic divided by the total saturated fatty acids.

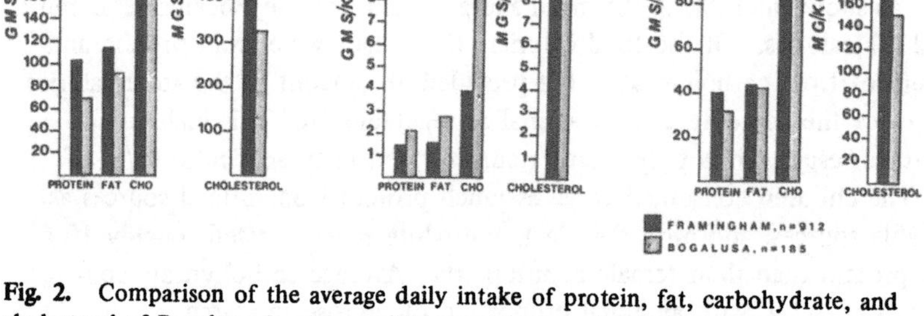

Fig. 2. Comparison of the average daily intake of protein, fat, carbohydrate, and cholesterol of Bogalusa, Louisiana children with that of Framingham, Massachusetts adults.

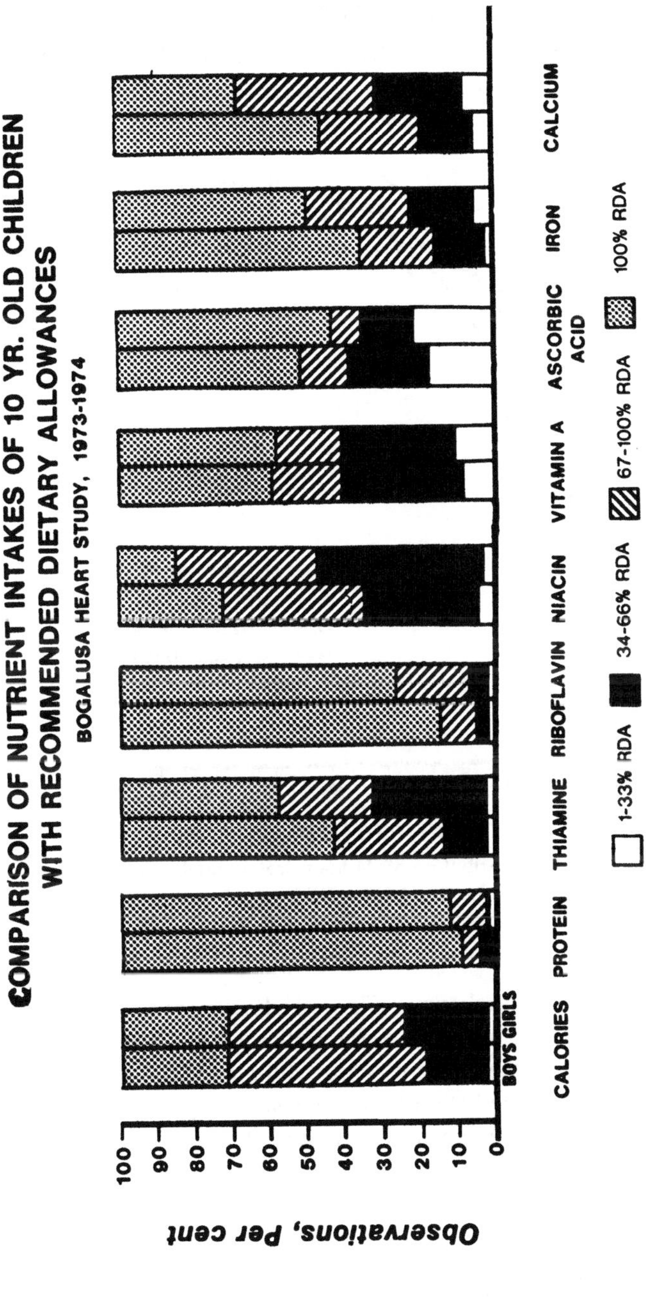

Fig. 3. Comparison of the nutrient intakes of ten-year-old children with recommended dietary allowances. Bogalusa Heart Study, 1973–74. The percentages of children consuming various percentages of RDAs are shown.

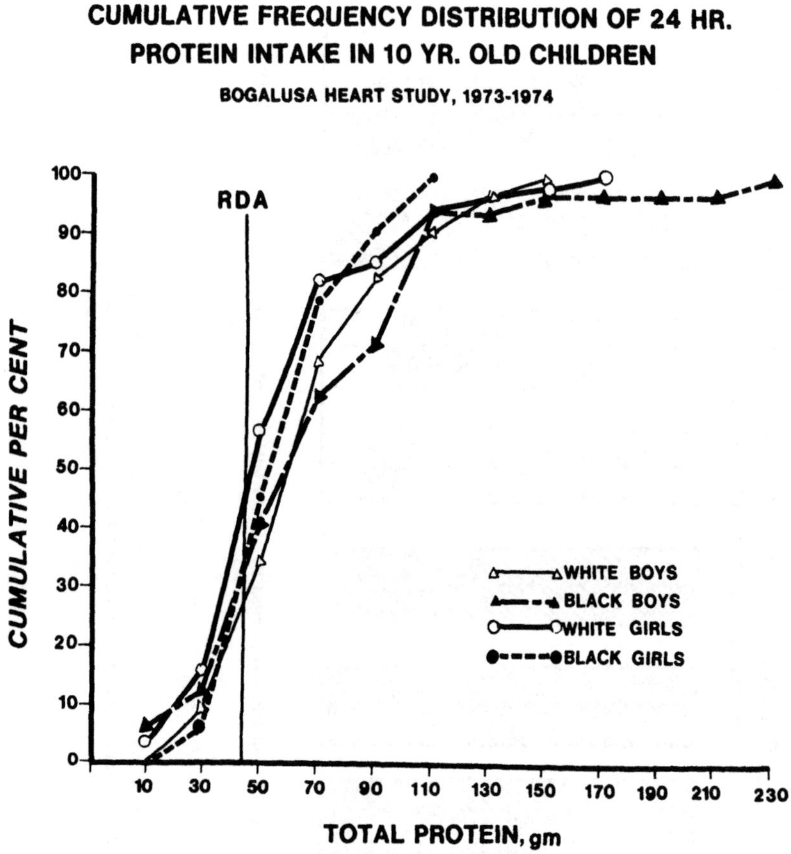

Fig. 4. Cumulative frequency distribution of 24-hour protein intake in ten-year-old children with a vertical line inserted at the protein RDA for 11-year-old children (44 g). Bogalusa Heart Study, 1973–74.

(Kannel and Gordon, 1976), as shown in Fig. 2, adults averaged only 8.5 mg/kg. The childrens' diets reflected a greater concentration of cholesterol, even though the mean intake of the adults was over 700 mg. Although the Framingham data were gathered almost ten years ago, they serve as a reference for individuals observed in a similar cardiovascular survey.

A general description of meal patterns showed that most children ate lunch and snacks. Fewer blacks than whites ate breakfast, which provided 17 percent of the total calories for the children. Lunch provided roughly one-fourth and snacks one-third of the total calories.

A comparison of the total daily nutrient intake with Recommended Dietary Allowances (RDA) (Food and Nutrition Board, 1974) showed that boys achieved higher recommended levels of most nutrients than did girls, as illustrated in Fig. 3. At least 45 percent of the girls did not meet two-thirds the recommended levels for vitamin A, ascorbic acid, calcium, thiamin, niacin, and iron. Of particular interest was the more than adequate protein intake with 92 percent of the boys and 88 percent of the girls achieving greater than 100 percent of their RDA for protein. Figure 4 illustrates this point even when the RDA for eleven-year-olds is inserted.

Taken from other observations on the children, the mean hemoglobin level was 12.9 g/100 ml which ranked 9.7 percent of the blacks and 3.5 percent of the whites as low using a level of 10–11.4 g/dl. However, no significant correlations were noted between iron intakes and hemoglobin levels in the Bogalusa children.

Comparing the mean energy and nutrient intakes of the Bogalusa sample with children the same age interviewed in the Ten-State Nutrition Survey (U.S. Department of Health, Education, and Welfare, 1968–70) and a 1965 U.S. Department of Agriculture Survey (U.S. Department of Agriculture, 1969) we find that energy and iron intakes were similar, but protein and calcium intakes appeared somewhat lower for our population.

The 185 Bogalusa children were divided into three groups according to the number of hours between the first and last foods eaten in the 24-hour period (eating spans): 19 children ate within ten hours; 95 children ate within 10 to 13 hours; and 71 children had eating spans exceeding 13 hours.

The three groups were then compared for mean intakes of diet components (see Table 3). The children with the longest eating span had significantly greater intakes of energy, fat, cholesterol, carbohydrate, and sodium. Serum cholesterol was the only risk factor variable that showed significant differences among the eating span groups. As discussed below, even though studies within populations do not clearly reflect a relationship of dietary intake to serum lipids, (Keys et al., 1956; Kannel et al., 1971; Anderson et al., 1976); interestingly, as shown in the table, these children with greater eating spans had higher levels of serum cholesterol.

Table 3. Influence of Eating Span on Dietary Components in Ten-year-old Children[a,b]

	<10 hours	*10 to 13 hours*	*>13 hours*
Energy (kcal)	1708	2011	2431**
Protein (g)	58	66	76*
Fat (g)	72	89	105*
Carbohydrate (g)	209	242	301***
Sodium (g)	2.7	3.1	3.8**
Serum cholesterol (mg%)	157	163	174*

[a] $N = 185$.
[b] $p = < 0.05$ (*); < 0.01 (**); < 0.001 (***).

Table 4. Pearson Correlation Coefficients[a] for Risk Factor Variables and Dietary Components as Expressed per se and per 1000 Calories for 185 Bogalusa Ten-year-old Children

	Risk Factor Variable							
				Cholesterol				
Dietary component per se	*Total cholesterol*	*Triglyceride*	*Systolic blood pressure (Baum)*	*β-LP*	*Pre-β LP*	*α-LP*	*Wt/ht²*	*Skinfold*
Vegetable fat	—[b]	−.159[c]	—	—	—	—	—	—
Arachidonic acid	.154[c]	—	—	.176[c]	—	—	—	—
Cholesterol	—	—	—	.171[c]	—	—	—	—
Dietary component/1000 kcal								
Protein	—	—	—	—	—	—	.145[c]	—
Fat	.151[c]	—	—	—	—	—	.146[c]	—
Vegetable	—	−.194[d]	—	—	—	—	—	—
Polyunsaturated fatty acids	—	−.156[c]	—	—	—	—	—	—
Saturated fatty acids	—	—	—	—	—	—	—	.154[c]
Arachidonic acid	—	—	—	.152[c]	—	—	−.143[c]	—
Linoleic acid	—	−.160[c]	—	—	—	—	—	—
Carbohydrate	−.151[c]	—	—	—	—	—	−.176[c]	—
Starch	—	—	—	—	—	.149[c]	—	—
Sucrose	−.165[c]	.148[c]	—	—	—	−.189[c]	—	—
Sodium	—	—	.143[c]	—	—	—	—	—

[a]Only statistically significant correlation coefficients shown.
[b]— designates not significant.
[c]$p < .05$.
[d]$p < .01$.

Major food groups supplying carbohydrate were bread and starches, 26 percent of total carbohydrate; desserts, 14 percent; beverages, 14 percent; candy, 13 percent; and milk, 10 percent. As a food group, breads and starches were also the major source of sodium, 31 percent; then vegetables, 17 percent, which according to Southern custom includes seasoned meats in preparation; beef, 7 percent, and milk, 7 percent.

No significant differences were noted between the four sex-race groups for cholesterol or fat intakes, although significant differences were noted for starch and sodium. Both the white boys and the black girls had significantly greater intakes of starch than the white girls ($p < .01$). The black girls had a significantly greater mean sodium intake (4.0 g) than white girls (3.0 g) ($p < .01$), and both black (3.2 g) and white boys (3.3 g) ($p < .05$).

As an approach to examining the interrelationship of the dietary information with the risk factor variables, the correlation matrix in Table 4 indicates a few weak correlations between dietary components and some of the other observations. Even though on an individual basis there is a close relationship between diet and serum lipids, within a given population the range of dietary cholesterol or fat intake is relatively narrow and the individual variability of serum cholesterol levels is so great that correlations of this type cannot be observed.

Knowing this, we then grouped our sample according to high- or low-risk factor variable level, for example, below the twenty-fifth percentile, between the twenty-fifth and seventy-fifth percentiles, and equal to or greater than the seventy-fifth percentile. The mean intakes of 22 dietary components expressed as actual intake and per 1000 kcal were compared for the three groups for each risk factor variable. Table 5 shows the comparison of mean intakes for children grouped according to serum cholesterol level. When various fat components were expressed per 1000 kcal, the mean fat intakes of children of the middle and upper serum cholesterol groups were significantly greater than the mean fat intakes of the lowest serum cholesterol group. The reverse relation was true for carbohydrate and sucrose intakes but no difference was found for exogenous cholesterol and serum cholesterol.

These observations are noteworthy in that grouping the children according to levels of the risk factor variable, serum cholesterol, did give us a clue to the influence of diet on serum lipids in our population sample. Other studies point out the difficulty of relating diet to serum lipids and imply that there is no association. Obviously, environmental influences on the genetic response and metabolic makeup of an individual are expressed but difficult to detect. Our studies are leads to show that dietary components do have an effect on lipids, which can be detected by careful investigation. Other SCOR-A studies involving nonhuman primates are in concert with

Table 5. Mean Intake of Dietary Components for Children Grouped According to Serum Cholesterol Level Percentile[a]

Dietary Component	*Serum Cholesterol Level Percentile* Group 1 (<25th) N = 49	Group 2 (25th ⩽ x < 75th) N = 81	Group 3 (⩾75th) N = 49
		g	
Total fat	75.3	100.6[c]	101.4[c]
TF/1000 kcal	38.1	44.8[d]	44.3[d]
Animal fat (AF)	44.9	65.6[b]	65.5[b]
AF/1000 kcal	23.1	29.4[b]	28.5[b]
Saturated fatty acid (SFA)	30.7	41.0[b]	42.3[b]
SFA/1000 kcal	15.6	18.4[d]	18.5[b]
Unsaturated fatty acid (USFA)	40.1	53.4[b]	52.4[b]
USFA/1000 kcal	20.2	23.6[c]	22.9[b]
Carbohydrate/1000 kcal	133.3[f]	119.5	120.2
Sucrose/1000 kcal	53.1[e]	43.5	43.1
Iron/1000 kcal	6.6[g]	5.8	5.3
Sodium	2.9	3.5[b]	3.6[b]

[a]Other variables compared but not found significant.
[b]Mean greater than mean for Group 1 ($p < .05$).
[c]Mean greater than mean for Group 1 ($p < .01$).
[d]Mean greater than mean for Group 1 ($p < .001$).
[e]Mean greater than mean for Group 2 ($p < .05$) and Group 3 ($p < .05$).
[f]Mean greater than mean for Group 2 ($p < .01$) and Group 3 ($p < .01$).
[g]Mean greater than mean for Group 3 ($p < .05$).

these findings (Srinivasan et al., 1974; Srinivasan et al., 1976a; Srinivasan et al., 1977), and these along with our clinical studies provide directions for future research.

SUMMARY

Dietary data were collected on a random sample of 50 percent of the ten-year-old children participating in a cardiovascular survey for risk factor variables for early atherosclerosis and hypertension. An improved 24-hour dietary recall method was used to obtain reliable information on the food intake of the children and to provide clues to the diet-risk factor variable interaction.

The children's food patterns reflected a high consumption of total fat and saturated fat, low P/S ratio, and an equal proportion of sucrose to starch. A marked difference in eating span was observed; as eating spans increased, so did serum cholesterol, total kcal, and major dietary components. By grouping children according to risk factor variable percentiles, significant differences were noted in fat and saturated fat, which were less in children with the lowest levels of serum cholesterol. Significant sex-race differences were noted for carbohydrate and sodium intakes; in particular, the black girls consumed significantly more sodium than the other children.
than the other children.

Population studies are helpful in determining the role of food as an environmental determinant of risk factors for cardiovascular disease and in complementing observations of metabolic studies of individual subjects and experimental animals.

ACKNOWLEDGMENTS

Supported by funds from the National Heart, Lung, and Blood Institute of the United States Public Health Service, Specialized Center of Research–Arteriosclerosis (SCOR-A), HL15103.

REFERENCES

Anderson, J.D., Grande, F., and Keys, A. Independence of the effects of cholesterol and degree of saturation of the fat in the diet on the serum cholesterol in man. *Am. J. Clin. Nut.* 29, 1184 (1976).

Committee on Reduction of Risk of Heart Attack and Stroke of the American Heart Association. *Coronary Risk Handbook.* American Heart Association, New York (1973).

Emmons, L., and Hayes, M. Accuracy of 24-hr. recalls of young children. *J. Am. Diet. Assoc.* 62, 409 (1973).

Food and Nutrition Board. *Recommended Dietary Allowances.* Eighth revised edition. National Academy of Science, Washington, D.C. (1974).

Foster, T.A., Voors, A.W., Webber, L.S., Frerichs, R.R., and Berenson, G.S. Anthropometric and maturation measurements of children, ages 5–14 years, in a biracial community–The Bogalusa Heart Study. *Am. J. Clin. Nut.* 30, 582–591 (1977).

Frank, G.C., Berenson, G.S., Schilling, P.E., and Moore, M.C. Adapting the 24-hr. recall for epidemiologic studies of school children. *J. Am. Diet. Assoc.* 71, 26 (1977a).

Frank, G.C., Voors, A.W., Schilling, P.E., and Berenson, G.S. Dietary studies of rural school children in a cardiovascular survey. *J. Am. Diet. Assoc.* 71, 31 (1977b).

Frerichs, R.R., Srinivasan, S.R., Webber, L.S., and Berenson, G.S. Serum cholesterol and triglyceride levels in 3,446 children from a biracial community–The Bogalusa Heart Study. *Circulation* 54, 302–309 (1976).

Kannel, W.B., and Gordon, T., eds. *The Framingham Study: An Epidemiological Investigation of Cardiovascular Disease, Section 24–The Framingham Diet Study: Diet and the Regulation of Serum Cholesterol.* U.S. Department of Health, Education, and Welfare–National Institute of Health, Washington, D.C. (1976).

Kannel, W.B., Garcia, M.J., McNamara, P.M., and Pearson, G. Serum lipid precursors of coronary heart disease. *Hum. Path.* 2, 129–151 (1971).

Keys, A., Anderson, J.D., Mickelsen, O., Adelson, S.F., and Fidanza, F. Diet and serum cholesterol in man: lack of effect of dietary cholesterol. *J. Nut.* 59, 39–56 (1956).

Moore, M.C., Goodloe, M.H., and Schilling, P.E. Extended table of nutrient values. Louisiana State University Medical Center, New Orleans (1971).

Moore, M.C., Judlin, B.C., and Kennemur, P.M. Using graduated food models in taking dietary histories. *J. Am. Diet. Assoc.* 51, 447–450 (1967).

Rose, G.A., and Blackburn, H. *Cardiovascular Survey Methods.* World Health Organization, Geneva, Switzerland (1968).

Srinivasan, S.R., McBride, J.R., Jr., Radhakrishnamurthy, B., and Berenson, G.S. Comparative studies on serum lipoprotein and lipid profiles in subhuman primates. *Comp. Biochem. Phys.* 47B, 711–716 (1974).

Srinivasan, S.R., Radhakrishnamurthy, B., Smith, C.C., Wolf, R.H., and Berenson, G.S. Serum lipid and lipoprotein responses of six nonhuman primate species to dietary changes in cholesterol levels. *J. Nut.* 106, 1757–1767 (1976a).

Srinivasan, S.R., Frerichs, R.R., Webber, L.S., and Berenson, G.S. Serum lipoprotein profile in children from a biracial community–The Bogalusa Heart Study. *Circulation* 54, 309–318 (1976b).

Srinivasan, S.R., Radhakrishnamurthy, B., Dalferes, E.R., Jr., Webber, L.S., and Berenson, G.S. Serum lipoprotein responses to exogenous cholesterol in spider monkeys: Effect of levels of dietary protein. *Proc. Exp. Biol. Med.* 154, 102–106 (1977).

Voors, A.W., Foster, T.A., Frerichs, R.R., Webber, L.S., and Berenson, G.S. Studies of blood pressure in children, ages 5–14 years in a total biracial community–The Bogalusa Heart Study. *Circulation* 54, 319–327 (1976).

Young, C.M., and Trulson, M.F. Methodology for dietary studies in epidemiological surveys. II. Strengths and weaknesses of existing methods. *Am. J. Pub. Health* 50, 803–814 (1960).

Young, C.M., Hagan, G.C., Tucker, R.E., and Foster, W.D. A comparison of dietary study methods. 2. Dietary history vs. seven-day record vs. 24-hr. recall. *J. Am. Diet. Assoc.* 28, 218–221 (1952).

U.S. Department of Agriculture. *Food Intake and Nutritive Value of Diets of Men, Women, and Children in the United States.* Washington, D.C. ARS-62-18 (March 1969).

U.S. Department of Health, Education, and Welfare. *Ten State Nutrition Survey.* U.S. Government Printing Office, Washington, D.C. Department of Health, Education, and Welfare Publication No. (HSM) 72-8133, V.101 (1968–70).

8

Aortic Fatty Streaking and Alterations of Serum Cholesterol, Amino Acids, and Copper in Miniature Pigs Fed Atherogenic Diet

MUSHTAQ A. KHAN
JENG M. HSU
FRANCIS L. EARL
FELIX P. HEALD

INTRODUCTION

The pig has been used as a model for studies of atherogenesis because it is similar to humans in blood vessel wall structure (French et al., 1965), response to high-fat-high-cholesterol diets (Florentin et al., 1968) and to the development of atherosclerosis (Ratcliffe and Luginbuhl, 1971). Serum cholesterol levels are increased in pigs when they are fed diets containing butter (Bragdon et al., 1957) or beef tallow (Pfeifer and Lundberg, 1958; Barnes et al., 1959a, b). Diets low in protein have also been known to cause hypercholesterolemia (Elvehjem, 1956). While the metabolic interconversion of fat, carbohydrate, and protein has been well established (Conn and Stumpf, 1972), the effects of atherogenic diets on serum free amino acids have received less attention. Among the essential microminerals, manganese, a known cofactor in the biosynthesis of squalene, has been shown to be directly related to serum cholesterol levels in humans and chickens (Doisy, 1972). Schroeder et al. (1971) have shown that chromium deficiency is associated with hypercholesterolemia in rats. An inverse relationship has been reported between serum copper and cholesterol levels in the rat (Murthy and Petering, 1976; Petering et al., 1977), and a high zinc/copper ratio has been implicated in hyperlipidemia (Klevay, 1973) and ischemic heart disease (Chapter 4 of the present volume).

Endocrine secretions have been shown to have an important influence on serum cholesterol levels of experimental animals. It has been reported that testosterone lowers serum cholesterol levels in male and female rabbits, while estradiol causes hypercholesterolemia (Fillios and Mann, 1956). How

Table 1. Composition of Diets (Percentage by Weight)

Ingredients	*Stock (USDA-SR-3)*[a]	*Atherogenic (LEY) Diet*
Cornmeal	73.9	
Soybean meal	17.3	
Alfalfa meal	5.0	(USDA SR-3) 33.65
Iodized salt	0.5	
Limestone flour	0.8	
Dicalcium phosphate	2.3	
Vitamin premix (swine)	0.1	0.07
Mineral premix (swine)	0.1	0.07
Dry powder egg yolk	–	16.25
Lard	–	20.0
Dry skin milk powder	–	30.0
Protein	16.0	21.5
Carbohydrate	75.0	41.2
Fat	2.86	29.5
Caloric density (kcal/g)	3.90	5.3
Cholesterol (from egg yolk only)	–	0.22

[a]SR-3 = Swine Ration No. 3 of the USDA at Beltsville, Md. which is a standard pig stock ration.

male sex hormones predispose to fatty streaking and atherosclerosis is still obscure, but several investigators have suggested a possible association of altered testicular function with evolution of fatty streaking in the pubertal years (Holman et al., 1958; Dalldorf, 1961). Castrated pigs have been shown to have higher serum cholesterol concentration and increased fatty streaking of the aorta (Khan et al., 1977).

We have studied the effects of early castration of male miniature pigs on the concentrations of serum cholesterol, trace elements, and free amino acids of pigs fed control and atherogenic diets; the association of these biochemical parameters to the development of aortic fatty streaking was also studied.

MATERIALS AND METHODS

Male miniature Hormel piglets (maintained by the Special Pharmacological Animal Laboratory of the Food and Drug Administration, Beltsville, Maryland) were used. Littermate piglets were randomly castrated by removal of testes or sham-operated at two weeks of age. Isocaloric feeding of the piglets with stock or atherogenic diet (LEY, Lard, egg yolk) (Table 1) was started at nine weeks of age and maintained throughout the one-year study. Daily feed intake for each animal was adjusted every week based on the previous week's body weight and caloric density of the two diets as described previously (Khan et al., 1977). This was done to achieve a uniform intake of calories. The protein content of the atherogenic diet was increased by the addition of dry skim milk powder to ensure similar protein intake. With increasing age and body weight, measures were taken when the diet offered was not fully consumed by reducing the amount of food presented to each animal in order to achieve full consumption of the diet. Water was freely available. The pigs were housed individually in heated pens (during winter) with ample indoor and outdoor runs.

At 52 weeks of age, the animals were fasted for 18 hours and blood was drawn from the anterior vena cava. The serum was separated from the blood cells and stored in a freezer at –25°C, or deproteinized with an equal volume of 9 percent sulfosalicylic acid for 16 hours at 4°C. The treated serum was centrifuged and filtered through a glass sintered Buchner-type fine filter. The clear filtrate was transferred to a Kimble ampule, sealed under a nitrogen atmosphere and hydrolyzed for two hours at 110°C. Free amino acids in the hydrolysate were analyzed by ion-exchange chromatography on a 140 X 0.06 cm single column with a Technicon amino acid analyzer. Gradient elution was carried out with sodium citrate buffers (1) pH 2.88 (0.2 N for Na^+), and (2) pH 4.75 (0.8 N for Na^+), prepared as described in Technicon Monograph No. 1, 1966. Norleucine (0.25 μm) was always included as an internal standard, and a commercially prepared amino acid standard was analyzed periodically. Concentrations of trace elements were determined by atomic absorption spectroscopy. The extent of aortic fatty streaking was assessed as previously described (Khan et al., 1977). Serum cholesterol was determined according to the enzymatic method of Allain et al. (1974). All results were expressed as the mean ± SEM, and were compared statistically by means of Student's *t*-test. Differences were considered significant when the value of p was $\leqslant 0.05$.

RESULTS

The castrated pigs had a significantly higher level of serum cholesterol concentration within five weeks after feeding on the stock diet when compared to the sham-operated pigs. This difference was sustained throughout the experiment. Hypercholesterolemia was more pronounced in castrated and sham-operated pigs fed the LEY diet than in castrated and sham-operated pigs fed the stock diet, respectively. Castrated pigs fed the atherogenic diet had significantly higher serum cholesterol levels. The hypercholesterolemia was associated with increased fatty streaking of the aorta in the castrated pigs (Khan et al., 1977).

Table 2. Concentrations of Serum-free Amino Acids (μmol/1000 ml)

Amino Acid	*Sham* Stock (6)[a]	LEY diet (5)	*Castrate* Stock (6)	LEY diet (7)
Taurine	32.0 ± 2.8[b]	25.2 ± 3.1	32.9 ± 4.5	27.2 ± 0.9
L-aspartic acid	48.3 ± 2.5[c,*]	38.1 ± 2.5[c]	46.3 ± 4.5[d]	32.7 ± 2.7[d]
L-threonine	30.2 ± 1.0[e]	23.1 ± 0.9[e]	27.9 ± 1.6	22.8 ± 2.0
L-serine	18.3 ± 0.7	15.4 ± 0.8	20.9 ± 1.3	17.4 ± 1.5
L-glutamic acid	53.7 ± 3.4	64.9 ± 2.5[f]	49.1 ± 4.2	45.8 ± 4.2[f]
Glycine	123.8 ± 7.7[g,h]	101.6 ± 4.6[h]	87.8 ± 4.0[g]	84.0 ± 5.1[h]
L-alanine	74.8 ± 1.4	67.6 ± 4.7	71.9 ± 3.4	68.2 ± 4.0
L-valine	82.1 ± 3.9[i]	67.3 ± 2.5[i]	57.5 ± 4.7[i]	47.4 ± 1.8[i]
L-methionine	6.7 ± 0.4	5.1 ± 0.9	6.5 ± 0.6	5.8 ± 0.8
L-isoleucine	28.9 ± 1.2[j]	23.7 ± 1.3[k]	14.5 ± 1.1[j]	15.3 ± 0.8[k]
L-leucine	42.6 ± 3.0[l]	35.3 ± 1.6[m]	29.5 ± 2.3[l]	26.5 ± 1.8[m]
L-tyrosine	16.6 ± 1.2	15.8 ± 1.4	14.3 ± 0.6	11.9 ± 1.0
L-phenylalanine	20.8 ± 2.0[n]	19.6 ± 1.4[o]	16.0 ± 0.6[n]	13.5 ± 0.7[o]
Ornithine	15.1 ± 0.5	15.1 ± 1.3	15.4 ± 1.0	17.9 ± 1.5
L-lysine	35.3 ± 3.6	32.0 ± 2.6	34.3 ± 1.9	30.8 ± 2.3
L-histidine	12.7 ± 1.5	12.5 ± 1.1	12.9 ± 1.1	13.0 ± 0.8
L-arginine	27.6 ± 3.1	21.5 ± 1.6	23.6 ± 2.5	16.9 ± 1.6
Alpha-amino-*n*-butyric acid	19.8 ± 1.8[p]	20.1 ± 3.5[q]	4.0 ± 0.3[p]	2.8 ± 0.2[q]

[a]Figures in parentheses represent the number of pigs used in the study.
[b–q]Mean ± SEM.
[r]Values with the same superscripts are significantly different from each other when compared, using the student's t-test ($P \leq 0.05$).

Pigs fed the atherogenic diet had significantly decreased levels of aspartic acid, threonine, serine, glutamic acid, glycine, and valine (Table 2). Castrated pigs fed the stock diet also had lower levels of glycine, valine, isoleucine, leucine, and phenylalanine than did the sham-operated stock-fed group. The most striking difference following castration was a drastic decrease in the level of alpha-amino-*n*-butyric acid: it was about one-fifth that observed in the sham-operated pigs. The feeding of the LEY diet to castrated pigs reduced serum levels of glutamic acid, glycine, valine, isoleucine, leucine, phenylalanine, and alpha-amino-*n*-buytric acid more than similar feeding did in sham-operated pigs.

The LEY diet reduced Cu levels of both the sham-operated and castrated pigs (see Table 3). Serum Zn levels and ratio of Zn:Cu were unaffected by atherogenic diet or castration. Serum Mg was lower in the sham-operated pigs on the LEY diet, but not in the castrated pigs.

Table 3. Serum Concentrations of Zinc, Copper, and Magnesium

	Sham-operated		*Castrated*	
	Stock diet	*LEY diet*	*Stock diet*	*LEY diet*
Zinc (μg/100 ml)	98.9 ± 3.2[a] (9)[b]	93.0 ± 3.4 (5)	106.7 ± 10.6 (6)	95.0 ± 5.7 (5)
Copper (μg/100 ml)	194.4 ± 5.3[c] (9)	164.8 ± 12.6[c] (5)	204.3 ± 10.8[d] (6)	168.8 ± 10.6[d] (5)
Zinc/copper ratio	0.509	0.564	0.522	0.563
Magnesium (mg/100 ml)	3.4 ± 0.4 (5)	2.4 ± 0.2 (5)	2.8 ± 0.1 (4)	2.9 ± 0.4 (5)

[a]Mean ± SEM.
[b]Figures in parentheses indicate number of pigs.
[c]Values with the same superscripts are significantly different from each other ($p \leqslant 0.05$).
[d]

DISCUSSION

This study shows that either an atherogenic diet or castration causes increased serum cholesterol of growing pigs, as has been observed in other animal species (Luden, 1916; Blinoff, 1930; Teilum, 1937). The hyper-cholesterolemia is associated with aortic fatty streaking in the castrated pigs.

Studies with radioactively labeled amino acids have shown that amino acids are convertible to carbohydrates and fat (Conn and Stumpf, 1972). Feeding a high-fat–high-cholesterol but low-carbohydrate diet can enhance gluconeogenesis from amino acids, the decreased concentration of which (Table 2) might result from an increase of transamination reaction. Our results differ from those of Swendseid et al. (1967), who reported an increase in plasma valine, leucine, and isoleucine and a decrease of alanine levels in subjects six days after consumption of a high-fat diet. These discrepancies might be due to differences in animal species, amount and nature of the diet, and duration of the experiment. There were decreases in concentrations of two essential amino acids: threonine and valine, and three nonessential amino acids: aspartic acid, serine, and glycine in pigs fed the LEY diet. Castration reduced the concentration of four essential amino acids: the three branch-chain amino acids valine, isoleucine, leucine, and phenylalanine.

Kochakian (1965) has shown that castration decreases the RNA and polysome concentrations with concomitant changes in the rate of amino acid incorporation into protein, a response reflected by the synergistic effect of castration and high-fat diet on serum amino acid levels observed in this study. Among the four groups, castrated pigs on atherogenic diet had lower concentrations of serum aspartic acid, threonine, glutamic acid, glycine, valine, leucine, tyrosine, phenylalanine, lysine, arginine, and α-amino-*n*-butyric acid.

Acetyl CoA, formed from fatty acid metabolism, enters the citric acid cycle and is converted to alpha-ketoglutarate and oxalacetate which undergo transamination to form glutamate and aspartate, respectively. The relationship between fat metabolism and amino acids is also exemplified in the fatty liver disorder produced by an imbalance or deficiency of essential amino acids. Fatty livers in rats have been attributed to dietary imbalances involving lysine, tryptophan, and threonine (Dent, 1947; Harper, 1958) or in fat transport from liver in threonine deficiency (Yoshida and Harper, 1960). Similarly, rats reared on diets which completely lacked tryptophan (Adamstone and Spector, 1950), isoleucine (Lyman et al., 1964), methionine (Dick et al., 1952), and histidine or threonine (Singal et al., 1953) also developed fatty livers.

Many factors affect the concentration of amino acids in the blood. Among them are the degree of absorption at the intestinal wall, the rate of amino acid metabolism in the liver, the ability of various tissues to incorporate amino acid, etc. It is difficult to assign a definite significance to the amino acid patterns observed in this study. It is to be expected, however, that the variations in the concentration of free amino acids cause imbalance in the pool of free amino acids and this, in turn, could affect the rate of protein synthesis.

Our studies show that serum amino acids are also affected not only by high-fat–high-cholesterol (LEY) diet, but by castration. The decline in levels of alpha-amino-*n*-butyric acid of castrated pigs is provocative. This amino acid is a metabolite of threonine or methionine (catalyzed by threonine dehydrase and amino transferase). Deficiency of either enzyme could result in a decrease of alpha-amino-*n*-butyric acid. Cystathionine, an intermediate amino acid from demethylation of methionine, is cleaved to cystine and alpha-ketobutyric acid; the latter is aminated to form alpha-amino-*n*-butyric acid. Further evidence of such conversion is the increase of alpha-amino-*n*-butyric acid in the urine of humans who have ingested methionine (Dent, 1947). It seems reasonable that the castrated animals may have impaired methionine and/or threonine metabolism. Testosterone administration to elderly individuals has been shown to restore the normal concentrations of plasma serine, isoleucine, and lysine (Ackerman and Kheim, 1964). Whether the abnormalities observed in hypercholesterolemic pigs are reversible by the administration of testosterone remains to be studied. Results of the present study showing the decreased serum threonine levels of pigs fed the LEY diet provide additional evidence of a possible relationship between serum threonine levels and fat metabolism.

It may be postulated that the decline in the levels of amino acids (especially the branch-chain amino acids) in castrated animals may reflect amino acid catabolism resulting in enhanced synthesis of adipose tissue and cholesterol, which in turn causes fatty streaking of the aorta. These studies also suggest that male sex hormones, in the pig at least, protect against development of hypercholesterolemia and fatty streaking—a finding in contrast to current beliefs in humans.

The decline in serum concentration of copper in the group fed the atherogenic diet may be significant because of the reported inverse relationship between serum copper and cholesterol levels (Klevay, 1973; Petering et al., 1977). Although the precise mechanism of this decline in levels of copper cannot be ascertained in our study, the inverse relationship between cholesterolemia and copper levels is apparent.

ACKNOWLEDGMENTS

The authors express their deepest gratitude to Miss Eileen Marks and Messrs. Vernon Smith and Roger Mathews for their help during these studies.

Supported by National Institute of Health grant NS 06779-08, Medical Research Service of the Veterans Administration, and the Frank G. Bressler Research Fund.

REFERENCES

Ackermann, P.G., and Kheim, T. The effect of testosterone on plasma amino acid levels in elderly individuals. *J. Geront.* 19, 207–210 (1964).

Adamstone, F.B., and Spector, H. Tryptophan deficiency in the rat. *Arch. Path.* 49, 173–184 (1950).

Allain, C.C., Poon, L.S., Chan, C.S.G., Richmond, W., and Fu, P.C. Enzymatic determination of total serum cholesterol. *Clin. Chem.* 20, 470–475 (1974).

Barnes, R.H., Kwong, E., Fiala, G., Rechcigl, M., Jr., Lutz, R.M., and Loosli, J.K. Dietary fat and protein and serum cholesterol. I. Adult swine. *J. Nut.* 69, 261–268 (1959a).

Barnes, R.H., Kwong, E., Pond, W., Lowry, R., and Loosli, J.K. Dietary fat and protein and serum cholesterol. II. Young swine. *J. Nut.* 69, 269–273 (1959b).

Blinoff, A. Cholesterinemie chez le chien. Influence de l' hyperthyroidie et de la castration. *Comp. Rend. Soc. Biol.* 10, 188–189 (1930).

Bragdon, J.H., Zeller, J.H., and Stevenson, J.W. Swine and experimental atherosclerosis. *Proc. Soc. Exp. Biol. Med.* 95, 282–284 (1957).
Conn, E.E., and Stumpf, P.K. *Outlines of Biochemistry,* 3rd ed. Conn and Stumpf, eds. Wiley, New York (1972), pp. 535.
Dalldorf, F.G. Arteriosclerotic vascular disease and testicular fibrosis. *Circulation* 24, 1367–1371 (1961).
Dent, C.E. Methionine metabolism and aminobutyric acid. *Science* 105, 335–336 (1947).
Dick, F., Jr., Hall, W.K., Sydenstricker, V.P., McCollum, W., and Bowles, L.L. Accumulation of fat in the liver with deficiencies of threonine and of lysine. *Arch. Path.* 53, 154–159 (1952).
Doisy, E.A., Jr. Micronutrient controls on biosynthesis of clotting proteins and cholesterol, in *Trace Substances in Environmental Health,* vol. 6. D.D. Hemphill, ed. University of Missouri Press, Columbia (1972), pp. 193–199.
Elvehjem, C.A. Amino acid balance in nutrition. *J. Am. Diet. Assoc.* 32, 305–308 (1956).
Fillios, L.C., and Mann, G.V. Importance of sex in variability of the cholesteremic response of rabbits fed cholesterol. *Circ. Res.* 4, 406–412 (1956).
Florentin, R.A., Nam, S.C., Daoud, A.S., Jones, R., Scott, R.J., Morrison, E.S., Kim, D.N., Lee, K.T., Thomas, W.A., Dodds, W.J., and Miller, K.D. Dietary-induced atherosclerosis in miniature swine. *I-V Exp. Mol. Path.* 8, 263–301 (1968).
French, J.E., Jennings, M.A., and Florey, J.H.W. Morphological studies on atherosclerosis in swine. *Ann. N.Y. Acad. Sci.* 127, 780–799 (1965).
Harper, A.E. Nutritional fatty livers in rats. *Am. J. Clin. Nut.* 6, 242–253 (1958).
Holman, R.L., McGill, H.C., Jr., Strong, J.P., and Greer, H.C. The natural history of atherosclerosis. The early aortic lesions as seen in New Orleans in the middle of the 20th century. *Am. J. Path.* 35, 209–235 (1958).
Khan, M.A., Earl, F.L., Farber, T.M., Miller, E., Husain, M.M., Nelson, E., Gertz, S.D., Forbes, M.S., Rennels, M.L., and Heald, F.P. Elevation of serum cholesterol and increased fatty streaking in egg-yolk: lard-fed castrated miniature pigs. *Exp. Mol. Path.* 26, 63–74 (1977).
Klevay, L.M. Hypercholesterolemia in rats produced by an increase in the ratio of zinc to copper ingested. *Am. J. Clin. Nut.* 26, 1060–1068 (1973).
Klevay, L.M. Ischemic heart disease: Updating the zinc/copper hypothesis, in *Proceedings of the Symposium on Cardiovascular Disease and Nutrition,* Herbert K. Naito, ed. SP Medical & Scientific Books, Jamaica, N.Y. (1981), pp. 000–000.
Kochakian, C.D. Mechanism of anabolic action of androgens, in *Mechanism of Hormone Action,* P. Karlson, ed. Academic Press, New York (1965), pp. 191–196.
Luden, G. Observations on the changes in the cholesterol content of the blood of goats, following cholesterol feeding alone, roentgen treatment alone, and cholesterol feeding combined with roentgen treatment and subsequent castration. *J. Biol. Chem.* 27, 273–297 (1916).
Lyman, R.L., Cook, C.R., and Williams, M.A. Liver lipid accumulation in isoleucine deficient rats. *J. Nut.* 82, 432–438 (1964).
Murthy, L., and Petering, H.G. Effect of dietary zinc and copper interrelationship on blood parameters of the rats. *J. Ag. Food Chem.* 24, 808–811 (1976).
Petering, H.G., Murthy, L., and O'Flaherty, E. Influence of copper ana zinc on rat lipid metabolism. *J. Ag. Food Chem.* 25, 1105–1109 (1977).
Pfeifer, J.J., and Lundberg, W.O. Influence of total calories, fat calories, and fat unsaturation on blood lipids. *Fed. Proc.* 17, 288 (1958).

Ratcliffe, J.L., and Luginbuhl, J. The domestic pig: A model for experimental atherosclerosis. *Atherosclerosis* 13, 133–136 (1971).

Schroeder, H.A., Mitchener, M., and Nason, A.P. Influence of various sugars, chromium, and other trace metals on serum cholesterol and glucose of rats. *J. Nut.* 101, 247–258 (1971).

Singal, S.A., Hazan, S.J., Sydenstricker, V.P., and Littlejohn, J.M. The production of fatty livers in rats on threonine and lysine-deficient diet. *J. Biol. Chem.* 200, 867–874 (1953).

Swendseid, M.E., Yamada, C., Vinyard, E., Figuero, W.G., and Drenick, E.J. Plasma amino acid levels in subjects fed iso-nitrogenous diets containing different proportions of fat and carbohydrate. *Am. J. Clin. Nut.* 20, 52–55 (1967).

Technicon Monograph No. 1, Technicon Corp., Tarrytown, N.Y. (1966).

Teilum, G. Sur l' hypercholesterilemie apres castration chez l' homme. *Comp. Rend. Soc. Biol.* 125, 577–580 (1937).

Yoshida, A., and Harper, A.E. Effect of threonine and choline deficiencies on the metabolism of ^{14}C-labeled acetate and palmitate in the intact rat. *J. Biol. Chem.* 235, 2586–2589 (1960).

9

Quantitation of Lesions During Progression and Regression of Atherosclerosis in Rhesus Monkeys

DRAGOSLAVA VESSELINOVITCH
ROBERT W. WISSLER
THOMAS J. SCHAFFNER

INTRODUCTION

We have recently reported evidence that a highly restrictive, very low fat and essentially cholesterol free diet, as well as a less rigorous prudent diet, either alone or in combination with cholestyramine, will lead to regression of advanced atherosclerosis (Wissler et al., 1975; Vesselinovitch et al., 1976; Wissler and Vesselinovitch, 1976; Vesselinovitch et al., 1977; Wissler and Vesselinovitch, 1977; Vesselinovitch et al., 1978). Current studies confirm and extend previous observations by us and other investigators that substantial reversal of atherosclerotic lesions at various stages of development is possible in rhesus monkeys by diet and/or drug therapy (Armstrong, 1970; Tucker et al., 1971; DePalma, et al., 1972; Stary, 1972; Eggen et al., 1974; Stary, 1974; Wissler et al., 1975; Bond et al., 1976; Bullock et al., 1976; Stary et al., 1976; Vesselinovitch et al., 1976; Wissler and Vesselinovitch, 1976; Strong et al., 1977; Vesselinovitch et al., 1977b; Wissler and Vesselinovitch, 1977; Vesselinovitch et al., 1978).

To quantify changes produced by a prudent diet with or without cholestyramine, or cholestyramine alone, on atherosclerosis in rhesus monkeys, lesion components were measured by point counting. This was done in sections prepared from standardized arterial samples taken at predetermined anatomical sites. One can assume that many pathologic mechanisms contribute to and are reflected in the final makeup of atheromatous lesions of the artery wall. By evaluating the predominant lesion components separately, we hoped to shed some light on the cellularity of lesions, the extent of necrosis and the time course of collagen, elastin and/or glycosaminoglycans (GAGs)

Table 1. Methods of Evaluating Atherosclerotic Lesions

Author	*Methods*
Gore and Tejada (1957) WHO Classification of Atherosclerotic Lesions (1958) Roberts et al. (1959) Daoud et al. (1964) McGill et al. (1968) Massmann and Oestreich (1974) Lee and Downing (1976)	Visual assessment (staining, drawing)
Holman et al. (1960) Eggen et al. (1962) Cranston et al. (1964)	Photoelectric scanning planimetry
Rodriguez and Robbins (1959) Crawford et al. (1961)	Radiopaque-contrast media
Zugibe et al. (1961)	Plastic cast
Mitchell and Cranston (1965)	Point-counting technique "Dunhill method"
Cornhill and Roach (1974)	Projecting of photographs into polar coordinates
Morgan and Adams (1974)	Photo graticule
Insull (1967)	Gross staining
Beadenkopf et al. (1960)	Measurement of wall thickness
Hata et al. (1978)	Xerography

synthesis in lesions. This would help to single out factors that might be used as indicators for assessment of the potential of a lesion to heal or deteriorate. Every component may also be seen as a function of one or more of the various forces by which cells or their products are controlled in this pathogenesis and regression of lesions.

Few data have been reported concerning results of quantitative makeup of lesions during progression and regression of the atherosclerotic process. Although the best data so far are presumably chemical studies, the results are often misleading, depending on the basis of comparison (i.e., tissue, DNA, or tissue protein), and give little or no insight into the potential clinical effect on a given lesion. A survey of reports which deal with the size and type of atheromatous lesions, given in Table 1 (Gore and Tejada; 1957; World Health Organization, 1958; Roberts et al., 1959; Rodriguez and Robbins, 1959; Beadenkopf et al., 1960; Holman et al., 1960; Crawford et al., 1961; Zugibe et al., 1961; Eggen et al., 1962; Cranston et al., 1964; Daoud et al., 1964; Mitchell and Cranston, 1965; Insull, 1967; McGill et al., 1968; Cornhill and Roach, 1974; Massmann and Oestreich, 1974; Morgan and Adams, 1974; Lee and Downing, 1975; Hata, 1978), reveals very few papers that evaluate lesion components.

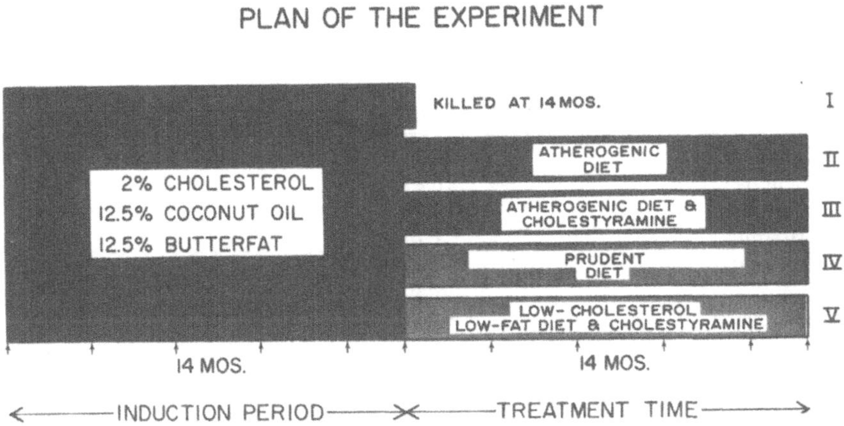

Fig. 1. Plan of the experiment.

A relatively speedy and at the same time accurate and reproducible method which makes it possible to evaluate lesion components without expensive instruments or especially difficult technology is the point-counting technique used and described here. It is relatively simple, inexpensive and reliable. It is based on counts of stainable components per unit area in microscopic sections of known thickness and standard locations. In this study, areas made up predominantly of total, intracellular and extracellular lipid, collagen, elastin, necrosis, glycosaminoglycans, and calcification have been measured. Standard procedures were adapted for this purpose, to ascertain a level of confidence in single measurements of ± 10 percent. In addition, two selected lysosomal enzymes were evaluated histochemically and cholesterol, cholesterol ester, collagen and elastin were analyzed chemically in an anatomically defined sample of aorta.

The main purposes of this study were: (1) to evaluate long-term effects of feeding a prudent diet with or without cholestyramine on regression of advanced, dietarily-induced atherosclerosis in rhesus monkeys; (2) to compare effects on atheromatous lesions of cholestyramine administered along with an atherogenic diet; (3) to evaluate the practical application and usefulness of morphometric methods of measuring lesion regression; and (4) to study and correlate lysosomal enzyme activities with various lesion component changes after progression and regression regimens.

MATERIAL AND METHODS

Plan of the Experiment

Twenty-four male rhesus monkeys were divided on the basis of body weights and serum cholesterol levels into five groups (Fig. 1). During the

Table 2. Diet Preparation[a]
(Expressed as Percentage of Wet Weight)

Ingredients	*Atherogenic diet (%)*	*Prudent diet (%)*
Butter oil	10.87	0.00
Coconut oil	10.87	0.00
Corn oil	0.00	18.00
Cholesterol	1.74	0.05
Vitamin mix	0.87	0.87
Gelatin	1.30	1.30
Monkey chow	61.31	47.61
Orange juice	13.04	13.04
Water	0.00	19.13
Total	100.00 g	100.00 g
Cal/100 g	482	389

[a]Pulverized primate ration with no animal fat added was obtained through the Purina Ralston Company.

14-month induction period, all animals were fed a diet consisting of a specially prepared, low-fat, low-cholesterol ration, which was supplemented with 2 percent cholesterol and 25 percent of a 1:1 mixture of coconut oil and butterfat. Detailed diet information for the atherogenic ration has been published (Vesselinovitch et al., 1976). At the end of the induction period, one group of five animals was autopsied to act as a reference for measurement following therapy (Group I), and two groups were continued on the atherogenic diet, one alone (Group II) and one in combination with 2.5 percent cholestyramine (Group V). Two additional groups were shifted to a prudent diet with (Group IV) or without (Group III) the 2.5 percent of bile acid sequestering agent. The prudent diet was formulated to match recommendations of the American Heart Association for patients with heart disease, to prevent and/or retard atherosclerosis. The prudent diet contained 18 percent corn oil and 0.05 percent cholesterol (Table 2). A constantly formulated pulverized primate ration with the same ingredients for each batch, and without animal fat, was obtained by special arrangement with the Purina Ralston Co. All percentages of diet ingredients are based on net weight. Cholestyramine* a bile acid sequestering agent, was added as 2.5 percent by weight of dry ingredients to the corn-oil-enriched diet or to the atherogenic diet.

*Cholestyramine was purchased in one large batch from Mead Johnson Laboratories, Evansville, Indiana.

Blood and Tissue Chemistry

To determine serum lipid values, fasting animals were bled at the onset of the study and at monthly intervals thereafter. Serum was analyzed for cholesterol (Abell et al., 1952), total lipid (Swahn, 1952), and lipoprotein profile determination (Noble, 1968). Relative serum lipoprotein values were evaluated using agarose gel electrophoresis performed by a modified method of Noble, previously described (Vesselinovitch et al., 1977a).

Tissue Preparation of Histological Studies

The animals were autopsied after exsanguination under Surital anesthesia.† Aortas were removed, cleaned of adventitial fat, opened along the mid-dorsal side, photographed and inspected. Extent of gross aortic disease in each specimen was evaluated and lesions diagramed and estimated independently by two pathologists. Results were averaged for each aorta with the thoracic and abdominal disease estimated separately. Chemical analyses were done on the left half of the aorta while the right half was used for microscopic study. The heart was fixed by pressure perfusion of the coronary arteries using phosphate buffered 2.5 percent glutaraldehyde at a pressure of 90 mm Hg.

Sampling methods have been previously described in detail (Vesselinovitch et al., 1976). Standard sections of aorta and coronary arteries were obtained allowing comparison of identically located portions from individual animals. The sections were stained with hematoxylin and eosin for assessment of necrosis, oil-red-O for lipids, Gomori trichrome aldehyde fuchsin stain, and Van Gieson Sirius red stains for collagen, iron-gallein method for elastin, alcian blue for glycosaminoglycans visualization, and alizarin red to indicate the presence of calcium. For quantitative evaluation of lesion components, an ocular grid or a transparency superimposed on the slide was used. Areas of specifically stained structure and/or components were evaluated by counting the points equally spaced, covering every single type of component. The ocular grid used had a resolution of 400 points and the total magnification was 200X. Points directly on the boundaries were counted as 0.5. As an alternative, transparencies made from graph paper (461610, made by Keuffel and Esser Co.) with letters and numbers as required, were also used. Such transparencies can be temporarily attached to the slide with glycerin. Using a Zeiss projection microscope, the slides were shown on a screen at

†Sodium thiamytal was purchased from Parke-Davis Laboratories, Detroit, Michigan.

$$\text{Number of reticule points required (95\% Confidence limits)} = \left[\frac{200}{\text{Desired accuracy \%}} \times \frac{\text{Standard deviation of 5 to 10 measurments over smallest area}}{\text{Mean number of points from 5 to 10 measurments over the smallest area}} \right]^2$$

Fig. 2. DeHoff formula for reticule point requirements.

appropriate magnification and again points covering individual components were counted.

The most crucial problem in morphometry concerned the sampling procedure. Since we took defined samples, our main concern was to determine the accuracy of single point-counting measurements on individual arteries. The achieved accuracy can be determined by a procedure proposed by DeHoff (Fig. 2). It can be demonstrated that the grid point requirements at a given accuracy and/or confidence level are a function of the square of the standard deviation obtained from several measurements with any test grid (DeHoff, 1968). For our purpose, an ocular 400-point grid was found optimal when two readings were taken for each component in each slide. From these initial counts absolute and percentage values for measured components could easily be calculated and evaluated statistically by one-way analysis of variance. Micrometric determinations of intimal thickness (endothelium, subendothelial space bordering on internal elastic lamina) were made by a filar micrometer at 200X magnification on each section. Lesions were always measured at their thickest points and care was taken to be certain that the transection was consistently perpendicular to the long axis of the vessel. Mean standard deviation and standard error were also calculated. Statistical comparison shown in the accompanying tables was performed using the Behrens-Fisher test for unequal variance. Histochemical determinations and biochemical determination of acid lipase activity were performed as described by Schaffner et al. (1978).

RESULTS

Body Weights, Food Consumption, and Serum Lipids

Monkey weights averaged 3 kg at the onset of the experiment (range: 2.5 to 3.5 kg). At the end of induction (14 mo), average weights had increased to 5.2 kg. At the end of the experiment (28 mo), weights of animals fed the prudent diet with or without cholestyramine averaged 8.2 kg; those of monkeys in groups continued on atherogenic diet with or without cholestyramine averaged 7 and 8.6 kg, respectively.

Table 3. Gross and Microscopic Aortic Lesions

Group	No. of Animals	Treatment	Gross Percentage of Intimal Involvement with Lesions	Microscopic	
				Frequency	Severity
I	5	Atherogenic diet (14 mo)	68 ± 3.9[a]	100	2.3 ± 0.3
II	4	Atherogenic diet (28 mo)	88 ± 4.3	100	2.4 ± 0.3
III	5	Prudent diet	20 ± 8.4[b]	64[b]	0.6 ± 0.3[b]
IV	5	Prudent diet and cholestyramine	7 ± 2.5[b]	52[b]	0.2 ± 0.3[b]
V	5	Atherogenic diet and cholestyramine	43 ± 12.0[b]	88	0.6 ± 0.3[b]

[a]Standard error, p based on Behrens-Fisher Test.
[b]Results different from Groups I and II at $p < 0.05$.

During the induction period animals consumed an average of 200 g of diet per day (963 cal/day). During the regression period food intake varied slightly among the groups, with the highest level (348 g/day) found in monkeys fed a prudent diet and cholestyramine (Group IV).

Serum total lipids and cholesterol levels from all fasted animals at the beginning of the study when they were fed a prudent ration, averaged 491 and 165 mg percent, respectively. At the end of 14 months, just before treatment commenced, the average serum total lipids and cholesterol in all animals increased to 2300 mg percent and 900 mg percent, respectively. Group II, which was fed an atherogenic diet throughout the 28-month experiment, maintained high cholesterol levels. Monkeys fed the prudent diet alone (Group III) or with cholestyramine (Group IV) and animals to which cholestyramine was given with the atherogenic diet (Group V), reduced their cholesterol levels drastically during treatment. This was somewhat more evident in animals fed the prudent ration with cholestyramine (average, 116 mg percent) and less so in animals receiving cholestyramine with an atherogenic diet (average, 299 mg percent).

Details of the levels of serum lipids and lipoproteins have been previously published (Vesselinovitch et al., 1977a).

Gross and Microscopic Findings

Aorta

Table 3 summarizes gross and microscopic observations made on aortas. The percentage of total aortic surface area grossly involved by lesions was high in both groups fed the atherogenic diet for either 14 or 28 months. In

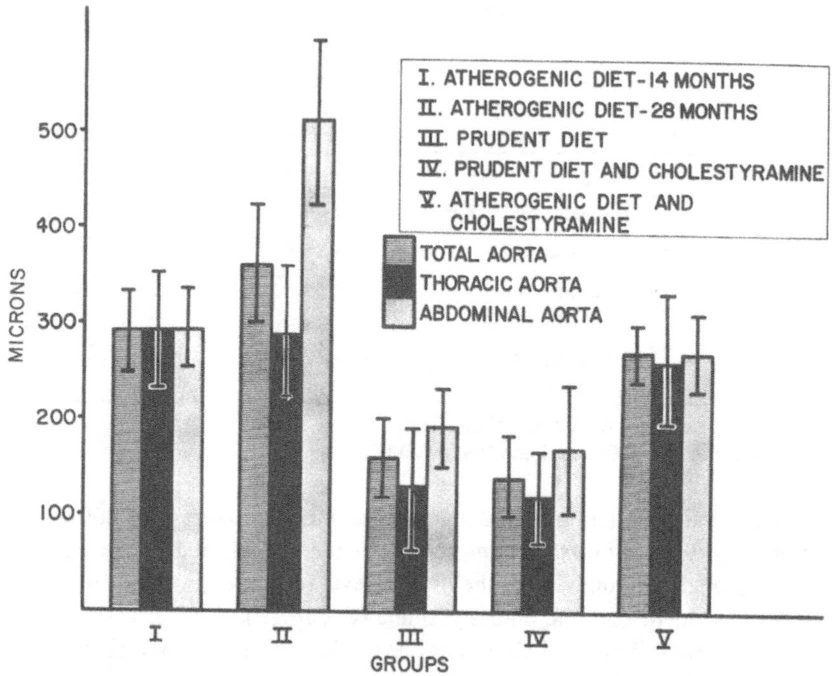

Fig. 3. Bar graph of aortic intimal lesion thickness.

the groups treated with a prudent diet with or without cholestyramine, this percentage was reduced to 10 percent and 40 percent, respectively, of the involvement seen in reference groups. Similarly, the extent of microscopically visible aortic lesions was greatest in monkeys fed the atherogenic diet for 14 or 28 months (Groups I and II). In each of these groups lesions involved 100 percent of the cut intimal surface. In contrast, frequency ratings in the treated groups (III and IV) were substantially lower and averaged only 64 and 52 percent, respectively. Severity ratings paralleled these estimates of surface involvement.

In these, as in previous studies (Wissler et al., 1975; Wissler and Vesselinovitch, 1976; Vesselinovitch et al., 1977b; Wissler and Vesselinovitch, 1977; Vesselinovitch et al., 1978), it was shown that cholestyramine alone has had beneficial effects on the disease process, even when monkeys were continued on the atherogenic diet. Figure 3 is a bar graph showing aortic intimal lesion thickness, as measured by filar micrometer. It is obvious that prudent diet with or without cholestyramine reduced intimal thickness substantially, while the combination of cholestyramine with an atherogenic diet arrested but did not reduce the average thickness of intimal lesions, in comparison to the reference group.

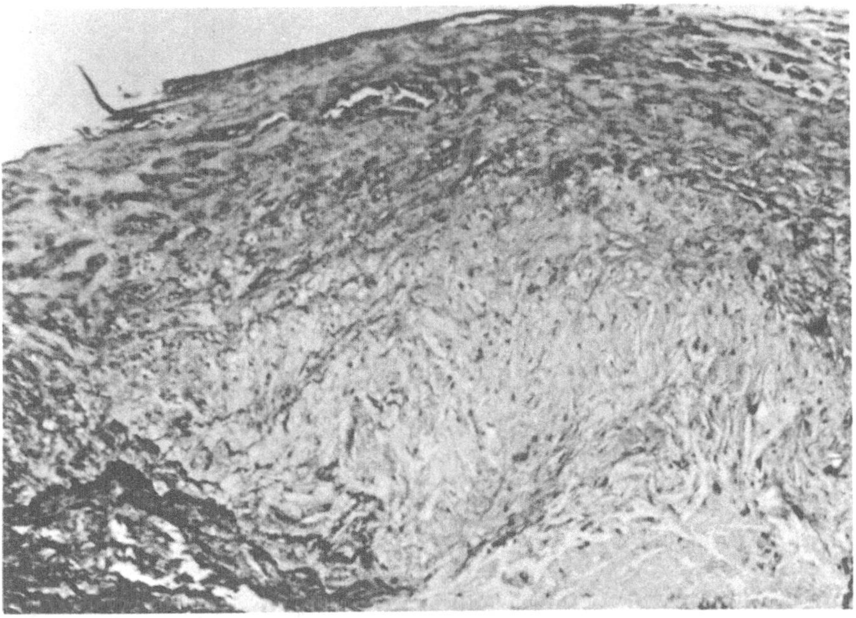

Fig. 4. Average lesions from abdominal aortas of *Macaca mulatta,* fed a 25 percent fat (1:1 coconut oil and butterfat) and 2 percent cholesterol diet for 14 months. Marked intimal proliferation, disruption of internal elastic membrane, lipid-rich cells, and collagen fibers in the upper portions of the lesion are seen. Gomori trichrome aldehyde fuchsin stain. (×40)

Photomicrographs of four representative aortic lesions are shown in Figs. 4 to 7. They represent the type of lesions used for point-counting measurements. Figure 4 is from an average plaque from an animal fed an atherogenic diet during induction time and stained for connective tissue elements using Gomori trichrome aldehyde fuchsin stain. Severe intimal proliferation, abundant lipid accumulation and some necrosis are present. Collagen and elastin fibers mixed with proliferative cells were also easily identified (Fig. 4). Figures 5 and 6 are sections showing lesions from monkeys treated with the prudent diet, either alone or with cholestyramine. These two sections from treated animals show representative lesions with mild to moderate intimal proliferation, with minimal intracellular lipid deposition and no visible necrosis. Figure 7 is a photomicrograph of a typical lesion from a monkey fed the atherogenic diet with cholestyramine during the second part of the study and stained for connective tissue elements (GTAF). Fibrocellular lesions with minimal lipid deposition are seen.

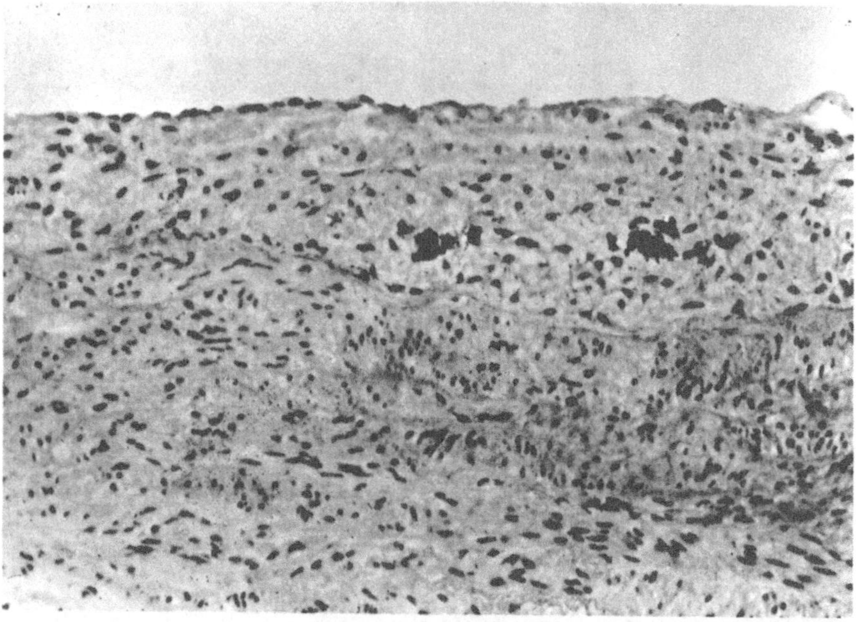

Fig. 5. Abdominal aortic lesion from a *M. mulatta* specimen fed an 18 percent corn oil and 0.05 percent cholesterol (prudent) diet during 14 months of treatment. Mild intimal proliferation is visible. Oil-red-O stain. (×40)

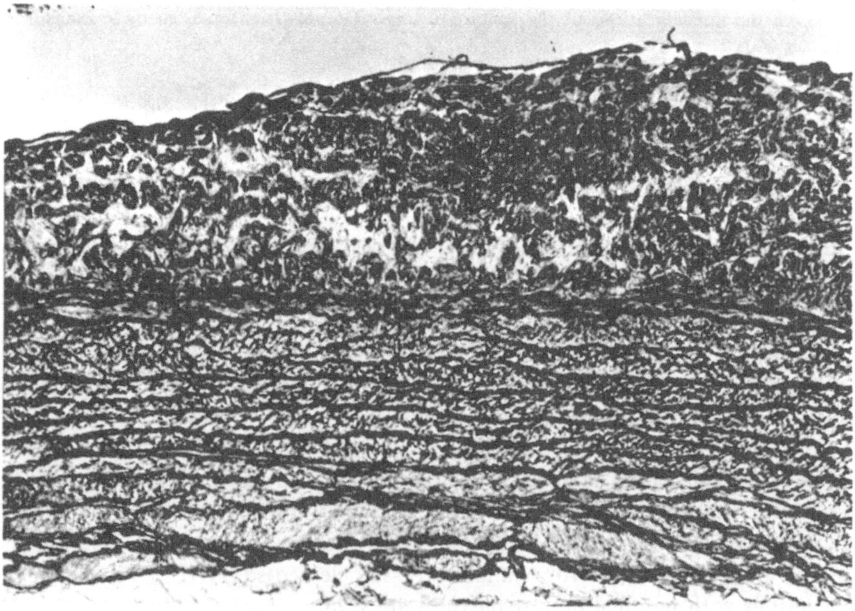

Fig. 6. A representative lesion from the abdominal aorta of a *M. mulatta* specimen fed the 18 percent corn oil, 0.05 percent cholesterol, and 2.5 percent cholestyramine ration for a 14-month treatment period. Again, only a fibrocellular remnant of the lesion with minimal lipid deposition is observed. Oil-red-O. (×40)

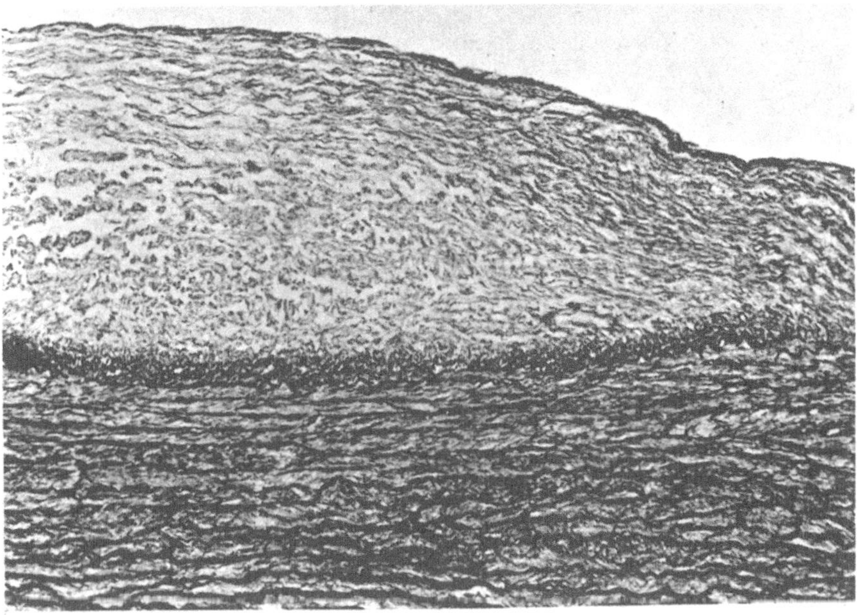

Fig. 7. Lesion from the thoracic aorta of a *M. mulatta* specimen fed an atherogenic diet throughout the experiment but with 2.5 percent cholestyramine added during the last 14 months (treatment period). Moderate intimal proliferation is seen, as well as a mixture of collagen and elastin fibers. Gomori trichrome aldehyde fuchsin stain. (×40)

Coronary Arteries

Table 4 shows some of the results of coronary grading in these animals. Lesions were more frequent in nontreated monkeys (Groups I and II), with an incidence of 98 percent and 100 percent, respectively, whereas in treated animals (Groups III, IV, and V) only 62 percent, 66 percent, and 79 percent, respectively, of the sections included a lesion. The positive results in coronary arteries were obtained in the more objective measurements of luminal

Table 4. Coronary Artery Lesions

Group	*No. of Animals*	*Microscopic*		
		Luminal narrowing	*Frequency (%)*	*Severity*
I	5	45 ± 4.5	98 ± 2.4[a]	1.6 ± 0.2
II	4	59 ± 5.1	100	2.2 ± 0.2
III	5	16 ± 2.9	62 ± 13.8[b]	0.4 ± 0.1[b]
IV	5	18 ± 3.6	66 ± 11.6[b]	0.8 ± 0.1[b]
V	5	29 ± 2.8	79 ± 2.3 [b]	1.0 ± 0.2[b]

[a]Standard error; *p* based on Behrens-Fisher Test.
[b]Different from Groups I and II at $p < 0.05$.

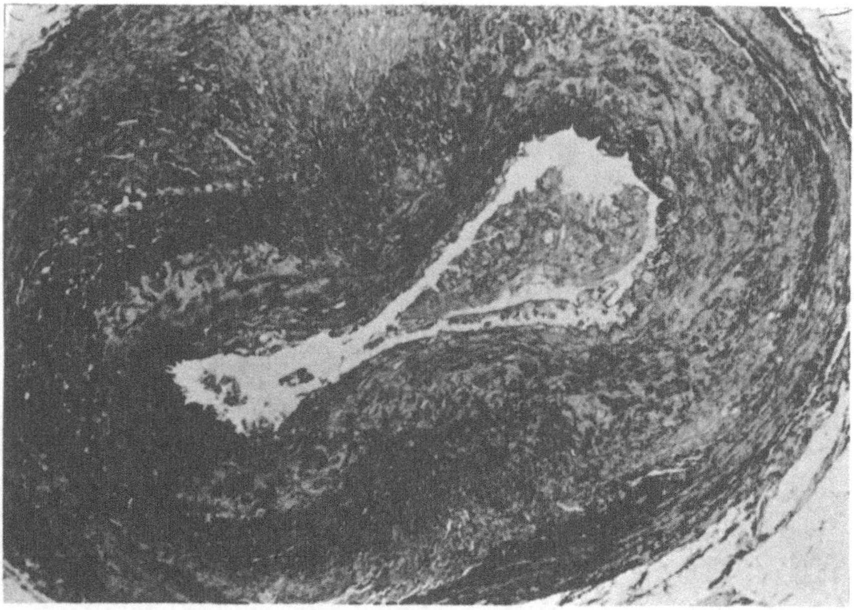

Fig. 8. Severe coronary artery lesion from a monkey fed a 25 percent fat, 2 percent cholesterol diet for 14 months. Marked intimal proliferation, necrosis, mild calcification, and disappearance of internal elastic membrane are observed. Gomori trichrome aldehyde fuchsin stain. (×20)

diameter. These data were made more reliable because the entire coronary artery system was fixed under pressure. As expected, luminal narrowing was greatest in groups fed an atherogenic diet for 14 and 28 months, averaging about 50 percent at this time. Treatment with the prudent diet was most efficient in reducing luminal narrowing. The results of this experiment also indicate that addition of cholestyramine did not significantly enhance the effect of the prudent diet, although it had a beneficial effect when given concurrently with an atherogenic diet.

Figures 8 through 11 are four representative lesions from coronary arteries used for point-counting. Figure 8 is a picture of a lesion stained for lipid from animals fed an atherogenic diet for 14 months. Lesions from untreated animals are characterized by severe intimal proliferation, lipid deposition, disrupted elastic membrane, necrosis, and calcification. In Figures 9, 10, and 11 the photomicrographs of treated animals with prudent diet alone (Group III) (Fig. 9) or with cholestyramine (Group IV) (Fig. 10), as well as monkeys continued on atherogenic diet with cholestyramine (Group V) (Fig. 11) mild to moderate intimal proliferation, minimal lipid deposition and less necrosis were observed.

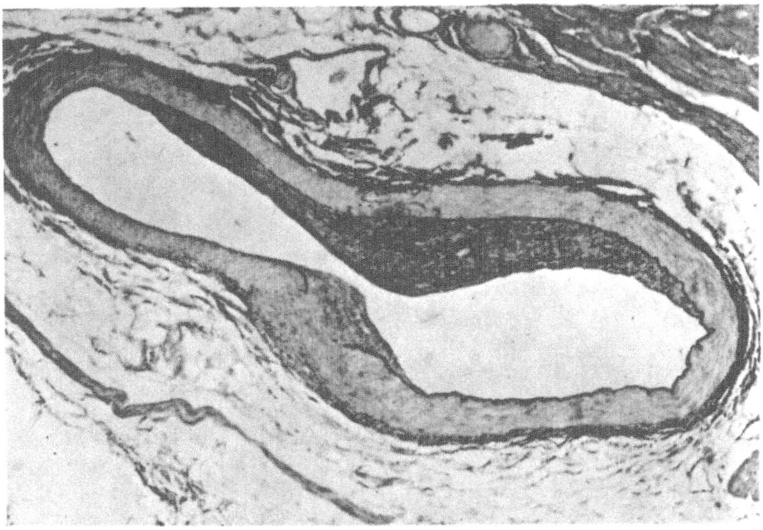

Fig. 9. Coronary artery lesion from a *M. mulatta* fed an 18 percent corn oil and 0.05 percent cholesterol diet during 14-month treatment period. Minimal fibrocellular lesion with focally disrupted internal elastic lamina is seen. Gomori trichrome aldehyde fuchsin stain. (×20)

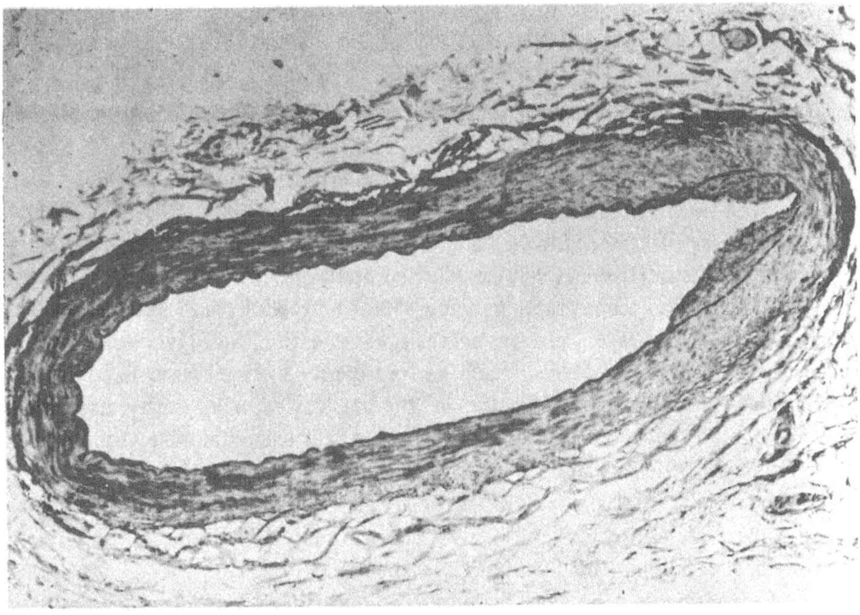

Fig. 10. Coronary artery lesions from a monkey fed the prudent diet with 2.5 percent cholestyramine during the 14-month treatment period. Minimal fibrocellular lesion and continuous internal elastic lamina are observed. Gomori trichrome aldehyde fuchsin stain. (×20)

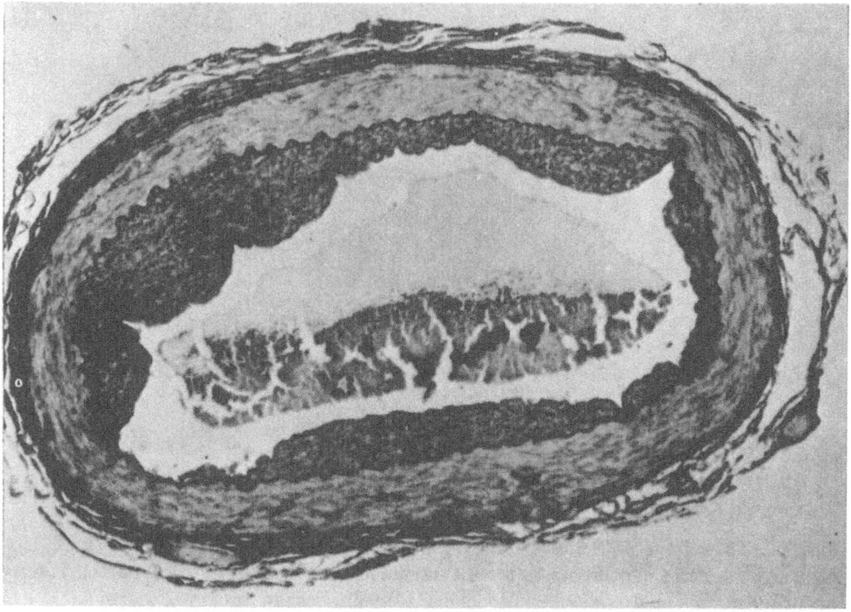

Fig. 11. A typical coronary artery lesion from a *M. mulatta* specimen fed the atherogenic diet throughout the study and receiving 2.5 percent cholestyramine during the 14-month treatment period. Moderate intimal proliferation mixed with connective tissue fibers are seen. Oil-red-O stain. (×20)

Quantitative Measurements of Lesion Components–Point-Counting Method

To extend the microscopic studies, quantitative microscopic measurements were made of lipid, collagen, elastin, necrosis, calcification, and GAGs in the arteries of these animals. Standardized sections of aortas and coronary arteries were stained selectively for desired components.

Figure 12 is a bar graph showing total (intracellular and extracellular) lipid, as well as collagen, elastin, necrosis, calcification, and glycosaminoglycans in aortic intimal lesions. Each bar represents average lesion size for the particular group while each fraction of the bar was adjusted (either expanded or contracted, based on actual point-counting) for each stainable component per unit area of lesion size. It is evident that in all treated groups (Groups III, IV, and V), total stainable lipid, both intracellular and extracellular, as well as necrosis and calcification, were substantially decreased, as was total lesion size, following the 14-month therapeutic period.

Furthermore, it appears that these components were most efficiently reduced in the group receiving a combination therapy of diet and drug (Group IV). However, the differences in results between Groups III and

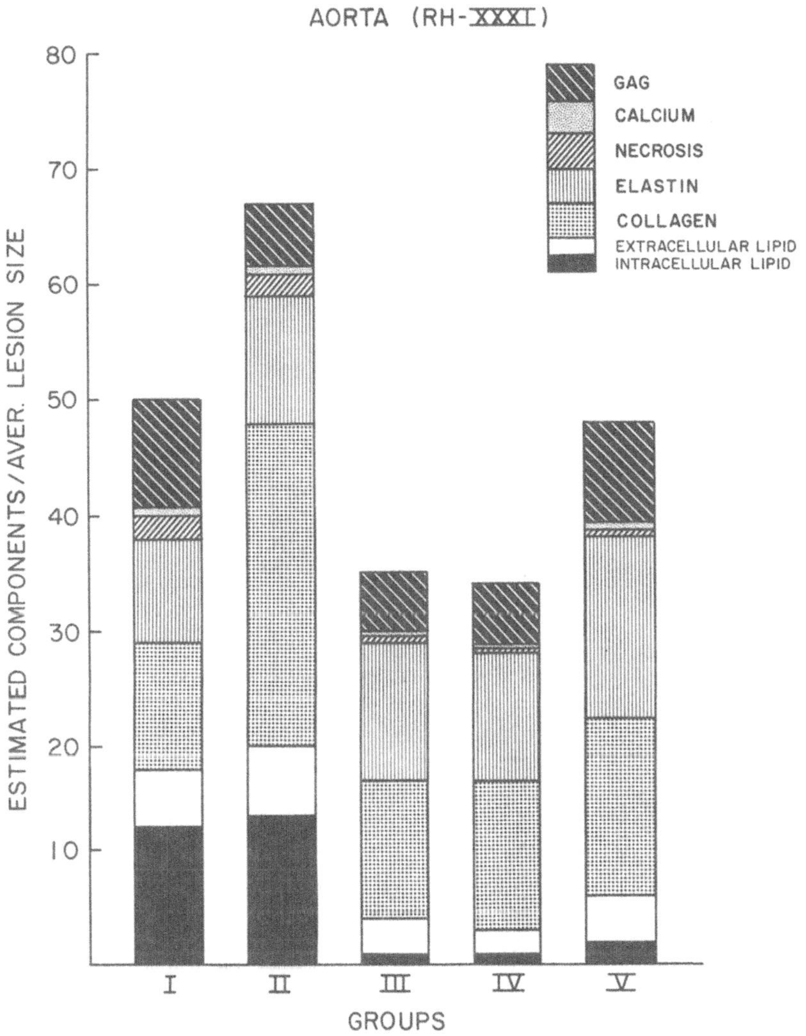

Fig. 12. Bar graph of various components in an aortic intimal lesion, adjusted per unit area of lesion size. Intra- and extracellular lipid, collagen, elastin, necrosis, calcification, and glycosaminoglycans are shown. Each bar represents the average lesion size for each particular group.

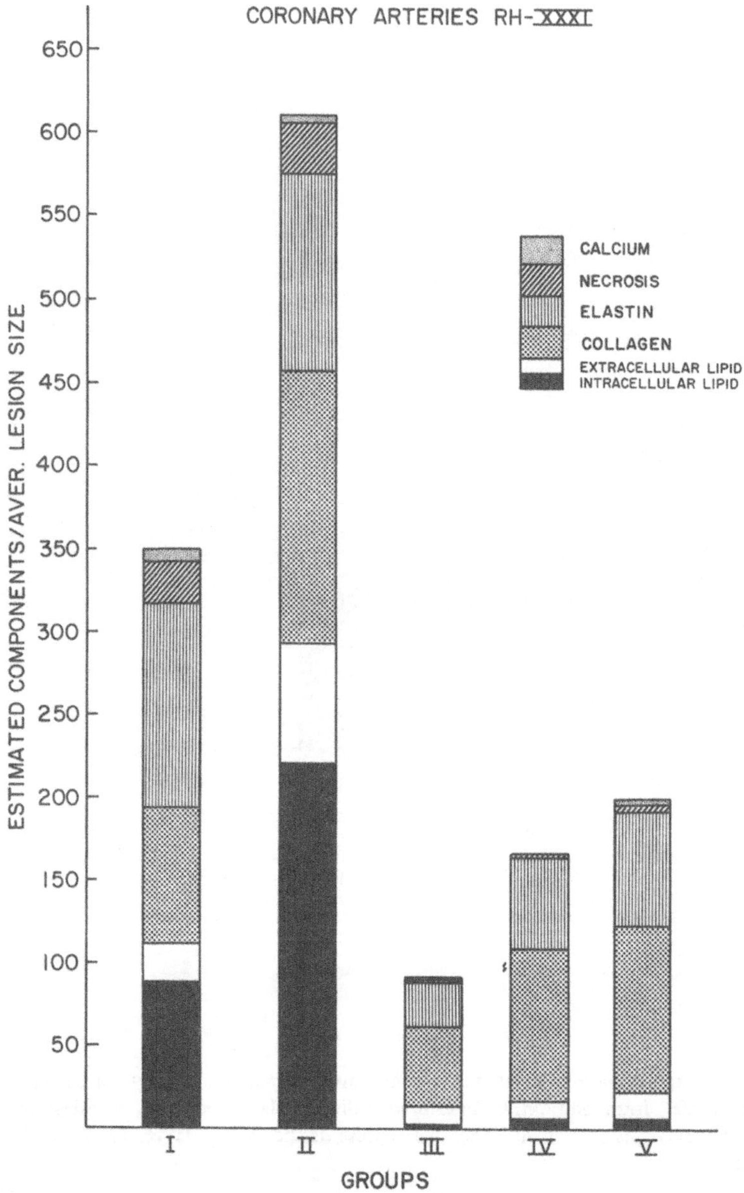

Fig. 13. Similar bar graph representing components in the intimal coronary artery lesions. Calculations of results and grouping is the same as for aortic lesions.

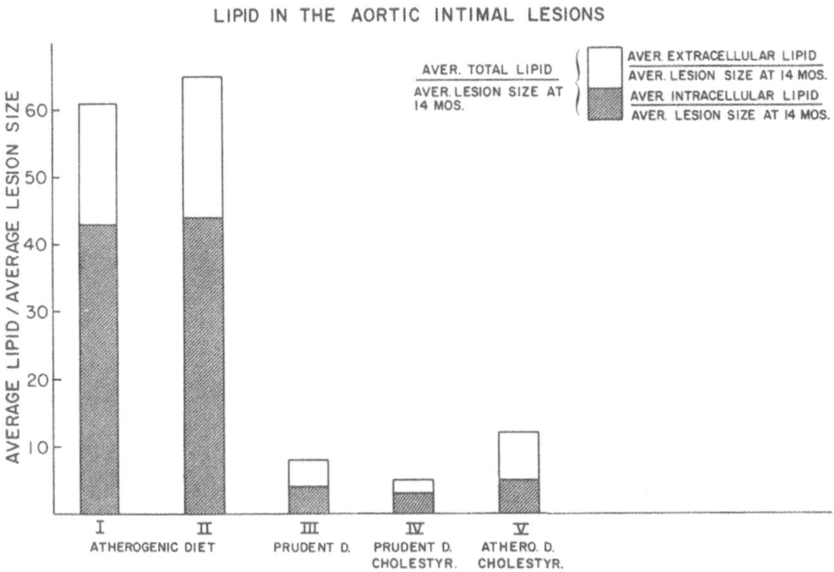

Fig. 14. Bar graph of relative lipid components in intimal aortic lesions. Each cross-hatched part of the bar represents the area occupied by intracellular lipid, while the white part shows area occupied by extracellular lipid. This is shown for each experimental group, divided by the average area of lesion size at the end of induction (14 months).

IV were not great, and most of the slightly greater effect of cholestyramine added to a prudent ration is due to a larger decrease in intracellular lipid. Total GAGs did not seem to be affected, which is in agreement with the biochemical analyses of the same aortas (Radhakrishnamurthy et al., 1977).

Figure 13 shows a similar bar graph of various stainable lesions from coronary artery sections. Portions of the bars represent adjusted amounts of a particular component per average lesion size. Changes are similar to those observed in aortic components but lesions were most reduced in coronary arteries of animals treated only with a prudent diet (Group III).

If one plots individual components shown in the combined bar graphs, the patterns emerge even more clearly. When data for total, intracellular, and extracellular lipid in the aortic intimal lesions are depicted, as shown in Fig. 14, the effect of therapy is quite obvious. The cross-hatched part of the bar represents intracellular lipid, while the white part is extracellular lipid. Lipid components are expressed as the area occupied by fat in any given section, divided by the average area of lesions at 14 months. This calculation was performed to demonstrate the actual decrease of lipids independent of the concomitant decrease in lesion size. It is obvious that in all treated groups

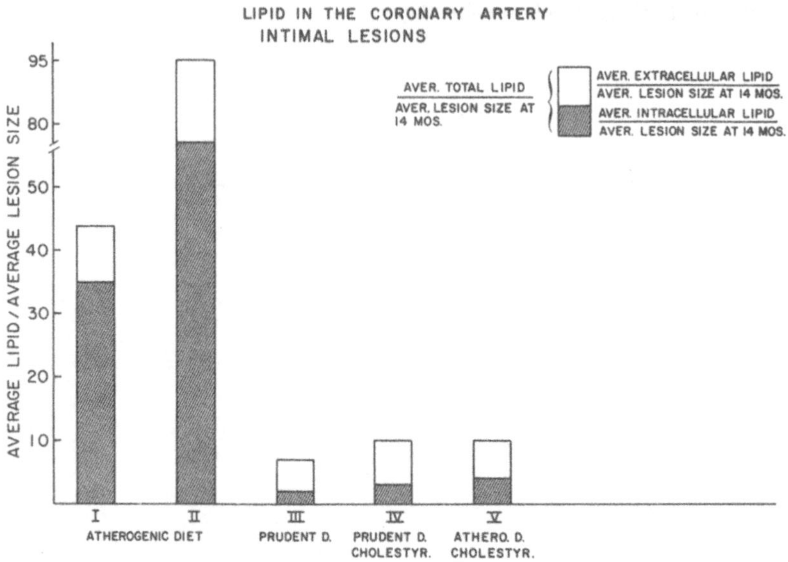

Fig. 15. Bar graph of the intra- and extracellular lipid content in intimal lesions in coronary arteries. Calculations are the same as for aortic lesions. Cross-hatched parts of the bars represent intracellular lipid and white parts indicate extracellular lipid.

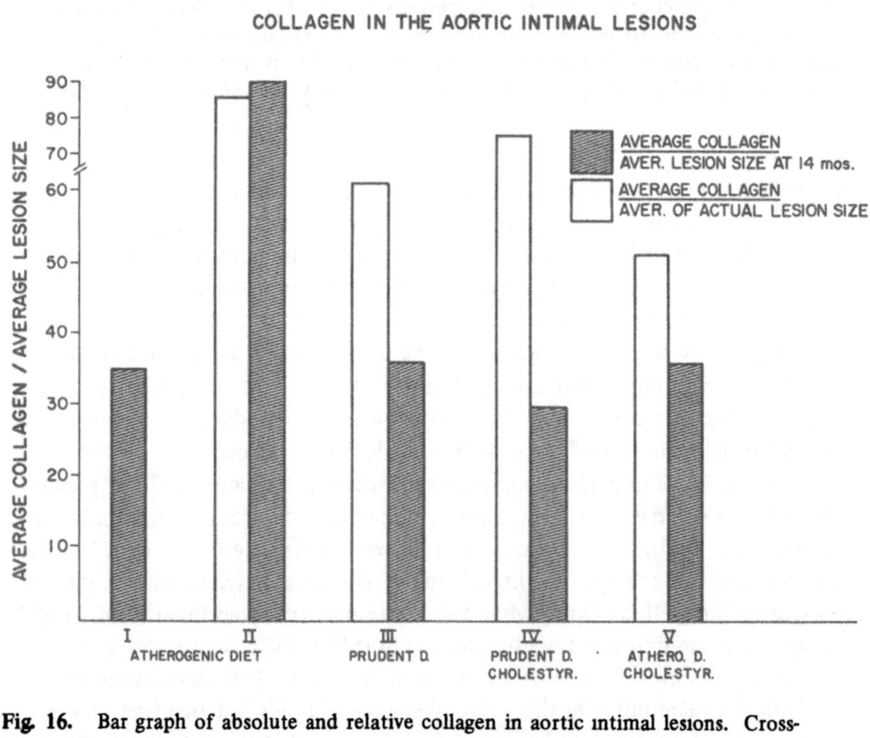

Fig. 16. Bar graph of absolute and relative collagen in aortic intimal lesions. Cross-hatched bars represent average count of stainable collagen per average lesion size at the end of induction (14 months). Light bars show average counts of collagen per average actual lesion size at the end of the experiment (28 months). A slight reduction of collagen is seen in animals fed the prudent diet with 2.5 percent cholestyramine (Group IV) during treatment.

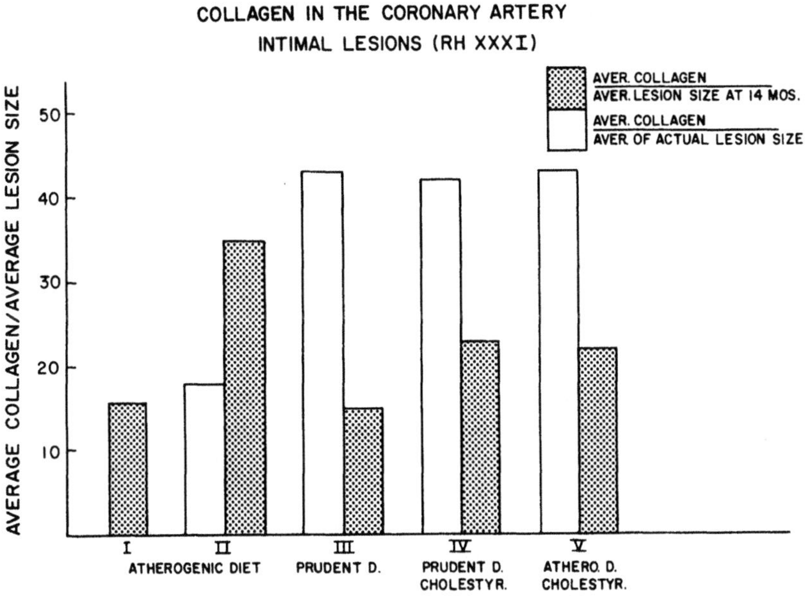

Fig. 17. Bar graph of absolute and relative collagen content in coronary artery intimal lesions. Black bars represent average counts of collagen per average lesion size of 14 months, while light bars are average collagen per average lesion size at 28 months. Relative collagen content (black bars) appears mildly reduced.

(Groups III, IV, and V), total, intracellular and extracellular lipid were substantially decreased. However, it appears that lipid was most effectively reduced in the group receiving combined therapy of diet and drug (Group IV). Figure 15 is a bar graph of lipid content in intimal lesions in coronary arteries. Lipid data from coronary artery and aortic lesions were calculated in the same way. A reduction similar to that seen in aortic lesions was noted, except that prudent diet therapy was apparently most effective. A reversal of the ratio of the prevalence of intra- and extracellular lipid was observed in both the aorta and coronary arteries following regression therapy.

Figure 16 is a bar graph showing areas of stainable collagen in aortic plaques. Crosshatched bars represent average point-counted areas of collagen per average lesion size at 14 months, while light bars represent average collagen calculated as a percentage of the average actual lesion size at 28 months. It is apparent that if we relate the data to the actual lesion size at 28 months (light bars), the collagen appears to have increased in treated groups. If, on the other hand, we assume that lesions are the same size as they were at 14 months when treatment commenced, the collagen content appears unchanged or slightly reduced. Collagenous areas were most prominent in animals fed the atherogenic diet for 28 months (90 percent), and were much smaller in monkeys receiving the combined cholestyramine and prudent diet (30 percent).

Table 5. Percentage of Necrosis in Intimal Lesions in Rhesus Monkeys

Group	*No. of Animals*	*Aorta (%)*	*Coronary Arteries (%)*
I	5	13 ± 2.8[a]	15 ± 5.5
II	4	15 ± 3.4	33 ± 11.5
III	5	3 ± 1.4[b]	0.2 ± 0.2[b]
IV	5	1 ± 0.6[b]	0.7 ± 0.2[b]
V	5	4 ± 1.3[b]	3 ± 1.6[b]

[a]Standard error; p based on Behrens-Fisher Test.
[b]Results different from Groups I and II at $p \geqslant 0.01$.

Another example of this difference between absolute and relative collagen content is presented in Fig. 17. Here the collagen data for coronary artery plaques are similarly presented. Again, if we relate collagen content to the lesions as they appear at 14 months, it appears to remain constant following therapy.

These observations for collagen changes during the regression period are in agreement with chemical analyses of coronary arteries following longer treatment periods as reported by Armstrong and Megan (1975). They indicated that, in general, absolute values of collagen decrease only after prolonged therapy (18 months or more), and that changes are most apparent if expressed in relation to anatomical units, not as milligrams per unit of wet weight.

When stainable collagen in aortic and coronary artery intimal lesions was compared (Figs. 16 and 17), it became apparent that collagen occupied almost double the proportion of space in aortic lesions at the 14-month point.

Table 5 describes in terms of percentages the area of obvious necrosis in aortic and coronary artery intimal lesions. It is obvious that in all treated groups necrosis was substantially reduced. All three treated groups (III, IV, and V) showed significantly decreased areas of necrosis when compared to either of the reference groups (I and II). Similar decreases in stainable calcification were seen in aortic and coronary artery intimal lesions.

Histochemical Evaluation of Acid Lipase in Lesions

Acid lipase activity or acid cholestryl esterase activity (Schaffner et al., 1978) implicated in the pathogenesis as well as the regression of atherosclerotic lesions, was markedly elevated in cholesterol-rich lesions. Histochemical techniques showed this activity to be localized in fat-filled foam cells (Schaffner et al., 1978).

Biochemical determinations of acid lipase activity in total aortic homogenates revealed a striking correlation between enzyme activity and arterial

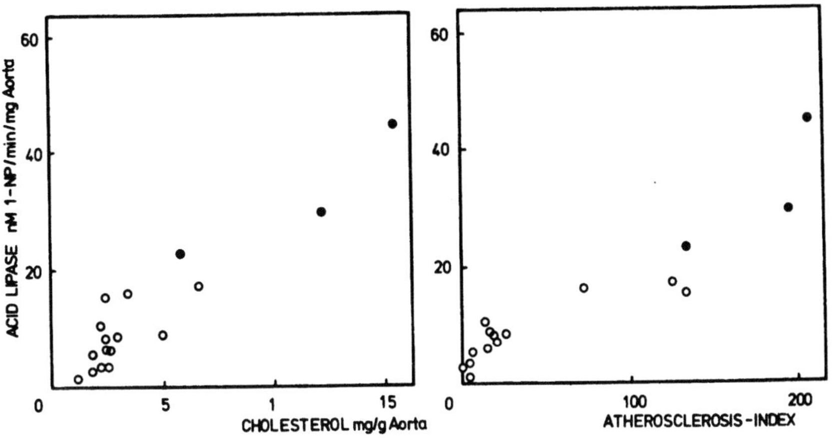

Fig. 18. Acid lipase activity in total aortic homogenates. At left are scatter plots of acid lipase activity and cholesterol content in the aortic arch of a *M. mulatta* specimen treated with three regression regimens (open circles) and an atherogenic diet (black circles) for 28 months. At right are the same enzyme data compared to the atherosclerotic index, obtained by multiplication of lesion severity in the thoracic aorta with the surface area occupied by lesions (Swahn, 1952). Extent of disease and lipid deposition appears closely correlated with the activity of this lysosomal enzyme. Data are expressed per unit of adventitia-free wet weight. Conditions for the enzyme assay were: α-naphtyl palmitate, 5 m*M*, Triton x-100 50 m*M* assayed for 30, 45, and 60 minutes at pH 4.2.

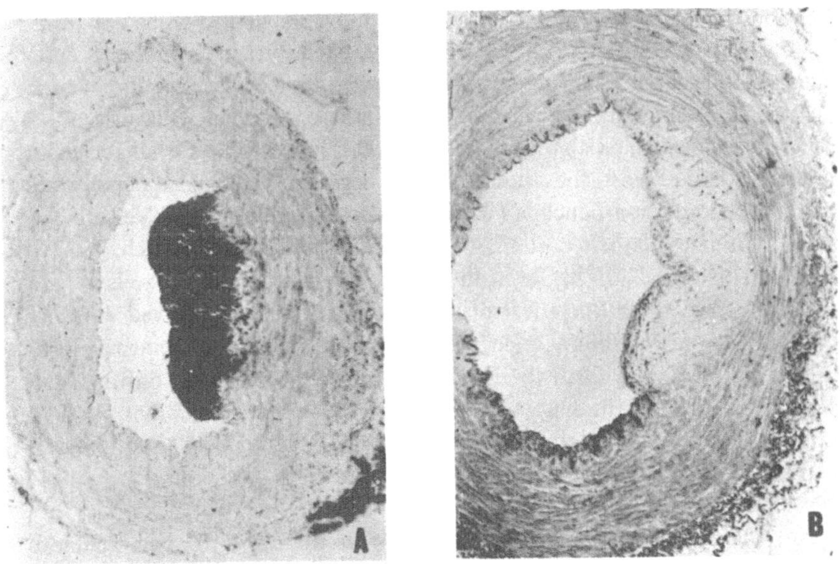

Fig. 19. (a) Acid lipase activity in a carotid artery from a *M. mulatta* specimen fed an atherogenic diet for 14 months. Lipid-laden foam cells are the only cells stained deeply in the intimal lesion. Reacted for 2 hours; methyl green counterstained; (b) acid lipase activity in a carotid artery from a *M. mulatta* specimen fed 18 percent fat, 0.05 percent cholesterol (prudent diet) and 2.5 percent cholestyramine. There were no positively stained cells after 2 hours incubation. (×10)

cholesterol content on the one hand, and the atherosclerosis index on the other (Fig. 18). The range of enzyme activity varied from 3 to 42 nm substrate hydrolyzed per mg wet tissue per minute. After lesion regression this activity was found to have decreased proportionately with the cholesterol content of the lesion. Enzyme activity was found to increase up to 14 times that noted in animals kept on the atherogenic diet when compared to the reactivity of animals whose lesions showed the most marked evidence of regression. Figure 19A is a photomicrograph of a carotid artery from an animal fed an atherogenic diet for 14 months, and Fig. 19B is a section from a similarly sampled carotid artery from a monkey treated with prudent diet and cholestyramine. The difference in extent of the histochemical reaction for acid lipase in the two sections is quite evident.

DISCUSSION

In these studies feeding a prudent diet to rhesus monkeys for 14 months following an equal period of feeding the same animals an atherogenic diet resulted in substantial reversal of arterial atherosclerosis. Evidence of lesion reduction was essentially the same in animals treated with cholestyramine as an adjunct to the prudent diet. The small additional improvement of lesions in this latter group over lesions of animals treated with diet alone was not statistically significant. Surprisingly, cholestyramine produced evidence of substantial lesion regression even when used as the sole therapeutic measure and with continued feeding of the atherogenic diet. Reversal of lesions in animals of this group (Group V) was, however, less dramatic than in animals treated with the prudent dietary regimen. This unexpected finding seems to be quite reproducible (Wissler et al., 1975; Wissler and Vesselinovitch, 1976; Vesselinovitch et al., 1977b; Wissler and Vesselinovitch, 1977; Vesselinovitch et al., 1978), even though the serum cholesterol levels at which this reversal and/or arrest of lesion progression was observed were in a range that we would have expected to promote lesion development. Regression of plaques in this experiment in a rather short period confirms and extends our previous findings with a more rigorous therapeutic diet, used either alone or with cholestyramine (Wissler et al., 1975; Wissler and Vesselinovitch; 1976; Vesselinovitch et al., 1977b; Wissler and Vesselinovitch, 1977; Vesselinovitch et al., 1978).

Although lesion size and extent of disease did not differ when cholestyramine was added to the prudent diet in comparison to diet given alone, there were some definitely ameliorative effects of cholestyramine. However, these emerged only after evaluation of additional lesion parameters, as well as the time course of normalization of the lipoprotein levels. Some of these parameters are a more rapid reappearance of increased high-density lipoprotein (HDL): low-density lipoprotein (LDL) ratios as shown by agarose gel electrophoretic studies (Vesselinovitch et al., 1977a); an accelerated disappearance of cutaneous xanthomas as compared to the effect of either low-fat, low-cholesterol, or prudent diet alone (Vesselinovitch et al., 1977a), and the presence of slightly less necrosis, collagen, and intracellular lipid in the lesions of animals treated with cholestyramine (Vesselinovitch et al., 1977b; Vesselinovitch et al., 1978). It also remains to be seen if there are some additional effects attributable to this bile acid sequestering agent on other components or on metabolic pathways explaining its substantial effects even in the presence of relatively high serum cholesterol levels.

In addition, accompanying quantitative evaluation of lesion components indicates that lesion thickness and composition varied according to treatment. As suspected, different therapies resulted in varying ratios of lesion components: some components, such as total (intracellular and extracellular) lipid, necrosis, and stainable calcium, decreased; some components remained unaffected, such as glycosaminoglycans, and some components, such as collagen and elastin, showed either an increase, were more or less stationary, or decreased slightly, depending on how they were expressed.

A decrease of stainable lipid in general, and intracellular lipid in particular, agrees with previous observations made by us and several other investigators who have studied lesions following regression regimens in nonhuman primates (Armstrong, 1970; Tucker et al., 1971; DePalma et al., 1972; Stary, 1972; Eggen et al., 1974; Stary, 1974; Wissler et al., 1975; Bond et al., 1976; Bullock et al., 1976; Stary et al., 1976; Vesselinovitch et al., 1976; Wissler and Vesselinovitch, 1976; Strong et al., 1977; Vesselinovitch et al., 1977b; Wissler and Vesselinovitch, 1977; Vesselinovitch et al., 1978). Lower lipid content in both intracellular and extracellular sites in treated lesions together with regeneration of endothelial cells (Buonassisi, 1973; Armstrong et al., 1975) and a reduced labeling index of cells in the plaque (Stary, 1974), represent major changes observed in treated lesions. Although stainable lipid in this study was substantially reduced in all treated groups, this reduction was most apparent in aortas of animals receiving combined therapy of diet and drug (Group IV).

It is interesting to note that if elastin and collagen measurements in cross-sectional lesions are expressed in absolute amounts, they do not decrease in treated groups. If, on the other hand, measurements of relative amounts of these fibrous proteins are made in the same groups, a definite decrease is seen when compared with animals fed the atherogenic diet for 28 months (Group V). These observations of collagen changes during regression are in agreement with chemical analyses of coronary arteries with longer treatment periods reported by Armstrong and Megan (1975). They discriminated in their measurements of collagen and elastin between "concentration" and "content." The first represented measurements per unit mass, while the second indicated the absolute amount per unit of vascular anatomy (Armstrong, 1978).

In their measurements of collagen concentration (per unit mass) during three separate regression intervals in *Macaca fascicularis,* it was found to be higher than in lesions from the reference group. Collagen apparently became "a more prominent part of the arterial wall" in regression. If, however, collagen measurements were expressed (for anatomical unit) as content, it was shown to be lower than at the end of the induction period, after a treatment of 18 or more months with a vigorous dietary regimen (Armstrong and Megan, 1975).

Next to decrease in lipid components, the size of necrotic centers of lesions seemed to be the next most responsive part of the advanced lesion and was consistently reduced in all treated groups, even in arteries of animals continued on the atherogenic diet but treated with cholestyramine (Group V). However, this decrease was somewhat less than in the other two treated groups (Groups III and IV). Similar results were observed for stainable calcium, a finding that confirms the observation of Daoud et al. (1976).

Increase of extracellular glycoproteins which correlates with severity of lesions has been observed and described (Stevens et al., 1976; Haust, 1977). However, in experimental regression, proteoglycan matrix does not seem to be affected (Radhakrishnamurthy et al., 1975). Total stained glycosaminoglycans in aortic lesions in this study were also not affected by therapy. This corroborates biochemical analyses of the same aortas (Radhakrishnamurthy et al., 1977). The glycosaminoglycans results are much more revealing when individual GAGs are taken into consideration. By analyzing separate components, Radhakrishnamurthy et al. (1977) reported that concentrations of dermatan sulfate and chondroitin-6-sulfate decreased, while hyaluronic acid and heparin sulfate generally increased in aortas of animals undergoing therapy (Radhakrishnamurthy et al., 1977). It is believed that hyaluronic acid is a product of endothelial cells, thus indirectly indicating their evident healing and regeneration during therapy. This corresponds to the electron microscopic findings made by Weber et al. (1977) and Jones (1978) in our laboratory, where endothelial healing was also observed by scanning and transmission electron microscopy.

Lesion size and components were measured by a simple, inexpensive and reliable quantitative point counting method. Until a computer and digitizer-assisted morphometric instruments are developed, this morphometric approach is still useful in studies of this type. Results obtained compare favorably, we believe, with other methods which are either more costly or more complicated. To our knowledge, quantitative morphometric methods have not been used previously to analyze the response of lesion components to various atherogenic diets or to compare lesion components of established and treated plaques.

Finally, acid lipase activity was determined because of its probable role in neutral lipid removal, especially the removal of cholesterol ester. Enzyme activity was apparently associated with lysosomes of fat-filled cells of the type described by, among others, Gaton and Wolman (1977). These cells are thought to be derived from macrophages and/or blood-borne monocytes (Stary, 1976; Gaton and Wolman, 1977; Schaffner et al., 1980). The number of these elements present could substantially influence the fate and regression potential of lesions (Adams and Bayliss, 1976; Gaton and Wolman, 1977), and a relative scarcity of cells with the associated lack of lipolytic enzyme activities in atheromatous lesions might be an important factor in predicting the regression potential of advanced plaques (Adams and Bayliss, 1976).

Morphometric measurements of atherosclerotic plaque components offer a useful method of quantitating the effects of various methods of producing lesions and of varying methods of reducing the size of plaques. Since space-occupying features and relative, as well as absolute, amounts of various plaque components influence the clinical effects of atherosclerosis, it is important to be able to quantitate these features and to study their interrelationships. Point-counting, intelligently used, together with the results of chemical analyses, constitutes a powerful combination in the study of experimental atherosclerosis.

SUMMARY

The results from this as well as from previous studies in our laboratory (Wissler et al., 1975; Vesselinovitch et al., 1976; Wissler and Vesselinovitch, 1976; Vesselinovitch et al., 1977b; Wissler and Vesselinovitch, 1977; Vesselinovitch et al., 1978) amply demonstrate that dietarily induced atherosclerosis in rhesus monkeys can be arrested and reversed by diet and/or drug therapy. In the study reported here, severe hyperlipemia and moderate to marked atherosclerosis were induced by feeding a diet enriched with coconut oil–butterfat and cholesterol for periods of 14 or 28 months. A subsequent change to a "prudent diet," with or without cholestyramine, after the animals had been fed the atherogenic ration for 14 months, resulted in prompt and sustained lowering of serum cholesterol levels and substantial reversal of arterial atherosclerosis. Induction and regression time periods were equal in this experiment. Furthermore, the bile acid sequestering resin, cholestyramine, had a substantially beneficial effect even when combined with the continued atherogenic ration, although to a lesser extent than when combined with the prudent ration.

Quantitative evaluation of lesion components by point-counting planimetry indicated important effects of atherogenic diet and therapy on individual lesion components. From these studies it became apparent that all the therapeutic regimens resulted in an absolute decrease of some components, such as lipid, necrosis, and calcium in the intima; and only a relative decrease of collagen and elastin, while some components appeared to remain unaffected, such as total glycosaminoglycans. Lysosomal enzyme activities, acid lipase, and acid phosphatase correlated closely with regression as judged by athero-index and biochemical determinations of cholesterol levels.

ACKNOWLEDGEMENTS

Work reported in this chapter was supported in part by United States Public Health Service grant HL 15062 and the Louis A. Block Fund of the University of Chicago.

The authors wish to express their gratitude to three excellent technicians who assisted with much of the laboratory work reported here, Ms. Gabrielle Chassagne, Ms. Dorothy Thomas, and Ms. Manuela Bekermeier. The authors also wish to thank Mr Robert Pisciotta for his assistance with library research and Ms. Judy Johnson for her editorial help.

REFERENCES

Abell, L., Levy, B.B., Bradie, B.B., and Kendall, F.E. A simplified method for the estimation of total cholesterol in serum and demonstration of its specificity. *J. Biol. Chem.* 195, 375–380 (1952).

Adams, C.W.M., and Bayliss, O.B. Detection of macrophages in atherosclerotic lesions with cytochrome oxidase. *Br. J. Exp. Path.* 57, 30–36 (1976).

Armstrong, M.L. Connective tissue in regression, in *Atherosclerosis Reviews,* vol. 3. R. Paoletti and A.M. Gotto, eds. Raven Press, New York (1978), pp. 147–168.

Armstrong, M.L., and Megan, M.D. Arterial fibrous proteins in cynomolgus monkeys after atherogenic and regression diets. *Circ. Res.* 36, 256–261 (1975).

Armstrong, M.L., Warner, E.D., and Connor, W.E. Regression of coronary atheromatosis in rhesus monkeys. *Circ. Res.* 27, 59–67 (1970).

Beadenkopf, W.G., Daoud, A., Marks, R.U., and Kinch, S.H. Epidemiology and pathology of coronary artery disease. I. Method of study. *J. Chron. Dis.* 12, 504–520 (1960).

Bond, M.G., Bullock, B.C., Clarkson, T.B., and Lehner, N.D.M. Effect of plasma cholesterol concentrations on "regression" of primate atherosclerosis. *Am. J. Path.* 82, 69a (1976).

Bullock, B.C., Bond, M.G., Lehner, N.D.M., and Clarkson, T.B. Effect of plasma cholesterol concentration (220 vs. 300 mg/dl) in preexisting coronary atherosclerosis in rhesus monkeys. *Circulation* 54, (suppl. II, 139 (1976).

Buonassisi, V. Sulphate mucopolysaccharide synthesis and secretion in endothelial cell culture. *Exp. Cell Res.* 76, 363–368 (1973).

Classification of Atherosclerosis Lesions. World Health Organization Technical Report Series, No. 143, World Health Organization, Geneva (1958), p. 3.

Cornhill, J.F., and Roach, M.R. Quantitative method for the evaluation of atherosclerotic lesions. *Atherosclerosis* 20, 131–136 (1974).

Cranston, W.I., Mitchell, J.R.A., Russell, R.W.R., and Schwartz, C.J. The assessment of aortic disease. *J. Atheroscler. Res.* 4, 29 (1964).

Crawford, T., Dexter, D., and Teare, R.D. Coronary-artery pathology in sudden death from myocardial ischemia–a comparison by age-groups. *Lancet* I, 181–185 (1961).

Daoud, A., Jarmolych, J., Zumbo, A., Fani, K., and Florentin, R. "Preatheroma" phase of coronary atherosclerosis in man. *Exp. Mol. Path.* 3, 475–484 (1964).

Daoud, A.S., Jarmolych, J., Augustyn, J., Fritz, K.E., Singh, J.K., and Lee, K.T. Regression of advanced atherosclerosis in swine. *Arch. Path. Lab. Med.* 100, 372–379 (1976).

DeHoff, R.T. Quantitative metallography, in *Technique for the Direct Observation of Structure and Imperfections,* vol. 2, part 1. R.F. Bunshqh, ed. Wiley, New York (1968), pp. 221–226.

DePalma, R.G., Insull, W., Bellon, E.M., Roth, T.W., and Robinson, A.V. Animal models for the study of progression and regression of atherosclerosis. *Surgery* 72, 268–278 (1972).

Eggen, D.A., Strong, J.P., and McGill, H.C. An objective method for grading atherosclerotic lesions. *Lab. Invest.* 11, 732–742 (1962).

Eggen, D.A., Strong, J.P., Newman, W.P., Catsulis, C., Malcom, G.T., and Kokatnur, M.G. Regression of diet-induced fatty streaks in rhesus monkeys. *Lab. Invest.* 31, 294–301 (1974).

Gaton, E., and Wolman, M. The role of smooth muscle cells and hematogenous macrophages in atheroma. *J. Path.* 123, 123–128 (1977).

Gore, I., and Tejada, C. The quantitative appraisal of atherosclerosis. *Am. J. Path.* 33, 875–885 (1957).

Hata, Y., Shigematsu, H., Tsushima, M., and Aihara, K. A Xerographic method for the quantitative assessment of atherosclerotic lesions. *Atherosclerosis* 29, 251–258 (1978).

Haust, D. Connective tissue in atherosclerosis, in *Atherosclerosis IV (Proceedings Fourth International Symposium).* G. Schettler, Y. Goto, Y. Hata, and G. Klose, eds. Springer-Verlag, Berlin (1977), pp. 30–35.

Holman, R.L., Brown, B.W., Gore, I., McMillan, G.C., Paterson, J.C., Pollak, O.J., Roberts, J.C., and Wissler, R.W. An index for the evaluation of arteriosclerotic lesions in the abdominal aorta–a report by the Committee on Lesions of the American Society for the Study of Arteriosclerosis. *Circulation* 22, 1137–1143 (1960).

Insull, W. Stain for differentiation and quantitation of gross lesions of atherosclerosis. *Arch. Path.* 83, 474–478 (1967).

Jones, R.M. Ultrastructural studies of regression of advanced atherosclerosis in rhesus monkeys with and without cholestyramine. *Fed. Proc.* 37, 835 (1978).

Lee, J.C., and Downing, S.E. A simplified technique for postmortem evaluation of coronary arteries. *Yale J. Biol. Med.* 49, 273–282 (1975).

McGill, H.C., Brown, B.W., Gore, I., McMillan, G.C., Paterson, J.C., Pollak, O.J., Robert, J.C., and Wissler, R.W. Grading human atherosclerotic lesions using a panel of photographs. *Circulation* 37, 455–459 (1968).

Massmann, J., and Oestreich, S. Angiometric studies of human coronary artery sclerosis. *Atherosclerosis* 20, 287–294 (1974).

Mitchell, J.R.A., and Cranston, W.I. A simple method for the quantitative assessment of aortic disease. *J. Ath. Res.* 5, 135–144 (1965).

Morgan, R.S., and Adams, C.W.M. A graticule for measuring atherosclerosis. *Atherosclerosis* 19, 347–348 (1974).

Noble, R.P. Electrophoretic separation of plasma lipoproteins in agarose gel. *J. Lipid Res.* 9, 693–700 (1968).

Radhakrishnamurthy, B., Eggen, D.A., Kokatnur, M., Jirge, S., Strong, J.P., and Berenson, G.S. Composition of connective tissue in aortas from rhesus monkeys during regression of diet-induced fatty streaks. *Lab. Invest.* 33, 136–140 (1975).

Radhakrishnamurthy, B., Ruiz, H., Dalferes, E.R., Vesselinovitch, D., Wissler, R.W., and Berenson, G.S. The effect of various diets on aorta glycosaminoglycans in rhesus monkeys. *Circulation* 56, suppl. III, 144 (1977).

Roberts, J.C., Moses, C., and Wilkins, R.H. Autopsy studies in atherosclerosis. I. Distribution and severity of atherosclerosis in patients dying without morphological evidence of atherosclerotic catastrophe. *Circulation* 20, 511–519 (1959).

Rodriguez, F.L., and Robbins, S.L. Capacity of human coronary arteries–a postmortem study. *Circulation* 19, 570 (1959).

Schaffner, T., Elner, M.V., Bauer, M., and Wissler, R.W. Acid lipase: a histochemical and biochemical study using triton *x*-100-naphtyl-palmitate micelles. *J. Histochem. Cytochem.* 26, 000–000 (1978).

Schaffner, T., Taylor, K., Bartucci, E.J., Fischer-Dzoga, K., Beeson, J.H., Glagov, S., and Wissler, R.W. Arterial foam cells exhibit distinctive immunomorphologic and histochemical features of macrophages. *Am. J. Path.* 100, 57–80 (1980).

Stary, H.C. Progression and regression of experimental atherosclerosis in rhesus monkeys, in *Medical Primatology, Part III.* E.J. Goldsmith, and J. Morr-Jankowsky, eds. S. Karger, Basel (1972), pp. 356–367.

Stary, H.C. Cell proliferation and ultrastructural changes in regressing atherosclerotic lesions after reduction of serum cholesterol, in *Atherosclerosis III (Proceedings Third International Symposium).* G. Schettler, and A. Weizel, eds. Springer-Verlag, Berlin (1974), pp. 187–190.

Stary, H.C. Coronary artery fine structure in rhesus monkeys: the early atherosclerotic lesion and its progression. *Prim. Med.* 9, 359–395 (1976).

Stary, H.C., Eggen, D.A., and Strong, J.P. The mechanism of atherosclerosis regression, in *Atherosclerosis IV (Proceedings Fourth International Symposium).* G. Schettler, Y. Goto, Y. Hata, and G. Klose, eds. Springer-Verlag, Berlin (1976), pp. 399–404.

Stevens, R.L., Columbo, M., Gonzales, J.J., Hollander, W., and Schmid, K. The glycosaminoglycans of the human artery and their changes in atherosclerosis. *J. Clin. Invest.* 58, 470–481 (1976).

Strong, J.P., Stary, H.C., and Eggen, D.A. Evolution and regression of aortic fatty streaks in rhesus monkeys, in *Atherosclerosis: Metabolic, Morphologic and Clinical Aspects (Adv. Exp. Med. Biol., vol. 82).* G.W. Manning and M.D. Haust, eds. Plenum Press, New York (1977), pp. 603–613.

Swahn, B. A new micromethod for the determination of total lipids in serum. *Scand. J. Clin. Lab. Invest.* 4, 247–251 (1952).

Tucker, C.F., Catsulis, C., Strong, J.P., and Eggen, D.A. Regression of early cholesterol-induced aortic lesions in rhesus monkeys. *Am. J. Path.* 65, 493–514 (1971).

Vesselinovitch, D., Harris, L., and Wissler, R.W. The relationship between lipoprotein levels and xanthomas during progression and regression of atherosclerosis. *Am. J. Path.* 86, 51a (1977a).

Vesselinovitch, D., Wissler, R.W., Borensztajn, J., and Schaffner, T. The effect of diets with or without cholestyramine on the lesion components of atherosclerotic plaques. *Fed. Proc.* 37, 835 (1978).

Vesselinovitch, D., Wissler, R.W., Hughes, R., and Borensztajn, J. Reversal of advanced atherosclerosis in rhesus monkeys, part I. Gross and light microscopic studies. *Atherosclerosis* 23, 155–176 (1976).

Vesselinovitch, D., Wissler, R.W., Schaffner, T., Hughes, R., and Borensztajn, J. Reversal of advanced atherosclerosis in rhesus monkeys by prudent diet with and without cholestyramine. *Circulation* 56, suppl. III, 144 (1977b).

Weber, G., Fabbrini, P., Resi, L., Jones, R., Vesselinovitch, D., and Wissler, R.W. Regression of arteriosclerotic lesions in rhesus monkey aortas after regression diet: scanning and transmission electron microscope observations of the endothelium. *Atherosclerosis* 26, 535–547 (1977).

Wissler, R.W., and Vesselinovitch, D. Studies of regression of advanced atherosclerosis in experimental animals and man. *Ann. N.Y. Acad. Sci.* 275, 363–378 (1976).

Wissler, R.W., and Vesselinovitch, D. Regression of atherosclerosis in experimental animals and man. *Mod. Conc. Cardiovasc. Dis.* 46, 27–32 (1977).

Wissler, R.W., Vesselinovitch, D., Borensztajn, J., and Hughes, R. Regression of severe atherosclerosis in cholestyramine-treated rhesus monkeys with or without a low-fat, low-cholesterol diet. *Circulation* 52, suppl. II, 16 (1975).

Zugibe, F.T., Bourke, D.W., and Brown, K.D. A plastic injection method for grading atherosclerosis of the coronary arteries–a preliminary report. *Am. J. Clin. Path.* 35, 563–571 (1961).

10

Atherosclerosis and Diet

DAVID KRITCHEVSKY

INTRODUCTION

Elevated serum cholesterol levels are one of the principal factors (risk factors) indicating a susceptibility to atherosclerotic heart disease (ASHD). The Framingham, Massachusetts study (Kagan et al., 1962) established three major risk factors: (1) elevated serum cholesterol levels (above 240 mg/dl); (2) elevated systolic blood pressure (above 160 mm Hg); and (3) excessive cigarette smoking (over 20 cigarettes per day). A recent comparison of ASHD death rates in 40-year-old Scottish and Swedish men showed that, while the cholesterol levels of the two groups were similar, the Scots, who had considerably higher coronary mortality, also had significantly higher serum triglyceride levels (Oliver et al., 1975). Strasser (1972) has listed over 30 factors related to the risk of ASHD, ranging from age to water softness, and including items such as blood group, educational level, and personality type. The risk factors represent statistical diagnoses which are accurate for large populations but which may have less predictive value for individuals.

Nichols et al. (1976) analyzed dietary intakes of subjects in the Tecumseh, Michigan study (involving over 4000 individuals) and found no correlations between serum cholesterol and triglyceride levels and intake of fat, sugar, starch, alcohol, coffee, or tea. Furthermore, Slater et al. (1976) and Porter et al. (1977) have been among several groups of investigators who found that the ingestion of one egg per day had no effect on serum cholesterol levels of men. There still seems to be a piece missing from the puzzle.

Table 1. Distribution of Cholesterol between Lipoprotein Fractions[a]

	Total cholesterol (mg/dl)	*α-Lipoprotein (%)*	*β-Lipoprotein (%)*	α/β
Human				
Newborn	65	43	57	0.75
Female				
18–35 yr	187	34	66	0.52
45–65 yr	252	24	76	0.32
Male				
18–35 yr	197	25	75	0.33
45–65 yr	239	22	78	0.28
Nephrotic	577	6	94	0.06
Myocardial infarct	259	14	86	0.16
Rabbit				
Normal	51	53	47	1.13
Atherosclerotic	2000	9	91	0.10
Dog				
Normal	210	83	17	4.88
Atherosclerotic	2000	6	94	0.06

[a]From Barr et al. (1951) and Olson (1958).

Lipids circulate in the serum as a continuum of lipid-protein molecules of varying composition and hydrated density. Gofman et al. (1950) showed that ultracentrifugation of serum in media of varying densities permitted separation of lipoproteins by flotation. These molecules were originally designated by S_f (Svedbergs of flotation) levels, but are now known as very-low-density (VLDL), low-density (LDL), and high-density (HDL) lipoproteins. As density rises, the triglyceride content of the molecules falls and the protein content rises. The size of the molecules and their molecular weight also fall with increasing density. Earlier it had been shown that electrophoretic fractionation of serum yielded rapid- (α-) and slow- (β-) migrating fractions. The α-fraction is related to HDL and the β-fraction to LDL.

A slight variation in the electrophoretic technique (Lees and Hatch, 1963) has permitted separation into α-, β-, and pre-β bands and has led to classification of lipoproteinemias in a manner that has made for more rational diagnosis and treatment (Fredrickson et al., 1967).

Barr et al. (1951) showed that the cholesterol-rich β-lipoprotein fraction was elevated in diseases that lead to ASHD, and that the ratio of β- to α-lipoprotein is also elevated in these disorders. Olson (1958) showed that a high β/α lipoprotein ratio was seen in animals susceptible to atherosclerosis (Table 1).

The relationship between α-lipoprotein levels and protection from coronary disease has recently been rediscovered (Miller and Miller, 1975), and there are now a number of reports in the literature correlating protection from ASHD with serum HDL levels. Treatment of cholesteremia by diet or drugs now aims at affecting HDL levels, rather than simply affecting total cholesterol level. The serum cholesterol/phospholipid ratio, which was widely studied in the 1950s (Morrison, 1952) as a predictive measure and then abandoned, may actually have been a crude measure of the α/β lipoprotein ratio. The cholesterol/phospholipid ratio of LDL is 2.04, and that of HDL is 0.70. Thus, increasing the level of HDL at the expense of LDL would result in a lower cholesterol/phospholipid ratio.

The increasing incidence of ASHD in the United States has been blamed primarily on the American diet, particularly on dietary fat and cholesterol. But many other aspects of the American diet have changed, and all of these changes have played a role in affecting serum cholesterol levels. It should also be pointed out that diet is only one aspect in an individual's lifestyle that may dictate his or her susceptibility to ASHD.

Data compiled by Gortner (1975), Friend (1967), Rizek et al. (1974), and Scala (1975) have indicated the changes that have taken place. Comparison of per capita nutrient availability in 1909 and 1972, respectively, shows that there has been a slight drop in calories (4 percent). The amount of available protein hasn't changed (102 g daily), but the ratio of animal/vegetable protein has. The amount of protein available from animal sources (meat, poultry, fish, eggs, and dairy products) was 53 g in 1909 and 69 g in 1972. The amount of protein available from vegetable sources in 1909 was 49 g and was 32 g in 1972. Thus, the ratio of animal/vegetable protein has risen from 1.08 in 1909 to 2.16 in 1972. Fat consumption increased by 26 percent between 1909 and 1972. The ratio of animal/vegetable fat was 4.9 in 1909 and 1.6 in 1972, the major difference being in the use of oils, which rose by a factor of 10. The dietary ratio of linoleic acid/saturated fatty acids was 0.21 in 1909 and 0.4 in 1972.

The amount of carbohydrate in the American diet fell by 21 percent, and the ratio of starch/sugar fell from 2.15 to 0.89 (Page and Friend, 1974). Thus, the availability of simple sugar has actually risen from 156 g in 1909 to 205 g in 1972. Dietary crude fiber intake fell by about 50 percent. The availability of cholesterol, however, has remained relatively constant, ranging from 509 mg in 1909 to 556 mg in 1972. In the period from 1900 to 1960, the death rate from heart disease rose from 130 to 355 individuals per 100,000. In the decade 1968 to 1978 there has been a remarkable drop (>15 percent) in coronary disease. The data suggest that no single dietary factor can be held solely responsible for the rise in ASHD.

Table 2. Influence of Peanut Oil and Other Fats on Atherosclerosis in Rabbits[a]

Fat	*Number of Animals*	*Serum Cholesterol (mg/dl)*	*Average atheromata*[b]	
			Arch	*Thoracic*
Coconut oil	44/45	1360	2.15 ± 0.16	1.67 ± 0.14
Peanut oil	98/106	1483	1.89 ± 0.10	1.35 ± 0.08
Peanut oil R[c]	31/31	1833	1.31 ± 0.12	1.05 ± 0.10
Corn oil	100/106	1548	1.52 ± 0.10	1.05 ± 0.07

[a]From Kritchevsky et al. (1971, 1973). All diets contained 2 percent cholesterol and 6 percent fat. Fed for two months.
[b]Graded on a scale of 0 to 4.
[c]Randomized (autointeresterified) peanut oil.

LIPIDS

In general, saturated fat is more cholesteremic for humans than is unsaturated fat (Ahrens, 1957). In animals, saturated fat is also more atherogenic than unsaturated fat (Kritchevsky et al., 1954). One oil that doesn't fit this pattern is peanut oil, which has an iodine value of 93 and is still inordinately atherogenic for rats (Gresham and Howard, 1960), monkeys (Vesselinovitch et al., 1974), and rabbits (Kritchevsky et al., 1971). Interesterification of peanut oil affects its structure, but not its fatty acid spectrum, and results in a significant reduction in its atherogenicity (Kritchevsky et al., 1973; see Table 2). Interesteritication of butter or lard has no effect on the atherogenicity of either (Kritchevsky and Tepper, 1977), which suggests that either their levels of saturation are such that alteration of structure has no effect, or that there is something unique about peanut oil. The structures of native and interesterified peanut oil have recently been delineated (Myher et al., 1977) and will perhaps yield a clue to the apparently anomalous behavior of this fat.

In our discussion of lipids, special mention should be made of milk. It has been suggested that milk be deleted from the human diet because of its level of fat (3.7 percent) and its cholesterol content (80 to 90 mg/pint) (Segall, 1977). Sour milk (Mann and Spoerry, 1974), yogurt (Mann, 1977), and whole milk (Howard and Marks, 1977), however, have all been shown to be hypocholesteremic in man. In rats, skim milk (Malinow and McLaughlin, 1975) and whole milk (Kritchevsky et al., 1979) are hypocholesteremic. Milk will inhibit cholesterol synthesis when added to rat liver slices or homogenates (Boguslawski and Wrobel, 1974; Bernstein et al., 1976, 1977). Livers of milk-fed rats exhibit reduced levels of HMG-CoA reductase fatty acid synthetase, and cholesterol 7-α-hydroxylase (Kritchevsky et al., 1979). The hypocholesteremic factor in milk has not been identified, but hydroxymethylglutaric acid (Mann, 1977) and orotic acid (Richardson, 1978) are among the candidate substances.

Table 3. Influence of Protein on Plasma Cholesterol Levels of Rabbits[a]

	Plasma Cholesterol (mg/dl)	
Protein	*14 days*	*28 days*
Casein	140	200
Whole egg	150	235
Skim milk	185	230
Lactalbumin	115	215
Beef protein	150	160
Pork protein	140	110
Egg white	110	105
Wheat gluten	65	80
Peanut protein	90	80
Peanut meal	85	75
Soy concentrate	75	25
Soy isolate	30	15

[a]After Hamilton and Carroll (1976). Diets contained 60 percent dextrose, 30 percent protein, 5 percent cellulose, 4 percent salt mix, 1 percent fat, and a vitamin supplement.

PROTEINS

Ignatowski (1909) postulated that a toxic factor in animal protein was responsible for the development of atherosclerosis. He established atherosclerosis in rabbits by feeding eggs and milk, but the work was questioned because the diets contained cholesterol. Newburgh and Clarkson (1923) showed that a casein diet was hypercholesteremic and atherogenic for rabbits, and Meeker and Kesten (1941) reported that a diet containing casein and cholesterol was significantly more atherogenic for rabbits than one containing soy protein and cholesterol. That the difference did not result from the action of intestinal flora was shown by Kritchevsky et al. (1959), who reported that casein plus cholesterol was considerably more cholesteremic than soy protein plus cholesterol in both conventional and germ-free chickens.

Experiments by Lofland and co-workers (Lofland et al., 1961, 1966), Clarkson et al., (1962), and Strong and McGill (1967) have demonstrated that the quantity of protein may also influence cholesteremia in pigeons or primates. In general, high-protein diets are more cholesteremic and more atherogenic.

Carroll and Hamilton (1975) demonstrated that rabbits exhibited higher cholesterol levels when fed animal protein than when fed vegetable protein. There was a wide range of effects, however, so that beef protein was 20 percent less cholesteremic than casein, but 45 percent more cholesteremic than pork protein. Table 3 summarizes some of their data (Hamilton and Carroll, 1976).

Sirtori et al. (1977) have reported on experiments in which the protein content of the "prudent" diet that is fed to hypercholesteremic subjects was altered. Substitution of vegetable for animal protein rendered the diet much more hypolipidemic. The prudent diet contained 21 percent protein of which 62 percent was of animal origin. On this diet, cholesterol levels fell by 5 percent and triglyceride levels by 11 percent. The vegetable-protein diet also contained 21 percent protein of which only 7 percent was of animal origin. About two-thirds of the other 93 percent of protein was soy protein. When this diet was fed after the prudent diet, cholesterol levels fell by 23 percent and triglyceride levels by 16 percent. When the vegetable-protein diet was fed first, however, cholesterol and triglyceride levels fell by 19 and 17 percent, respectively. Institution of the prudent diet caused triglyceride levels to fall a further 8 percent, but cholesterol levels rose by 9 percent. The ratio of polyunsaturated to saturated fatty acids (P/S) in the diets described above was 2.7, but even when vegetable protein was present in a diet whose P/S ratio was 0.1, the hypolipidemic effect persisted (Sirtori et al., 1979).

CARBOHYDRATES AND FIBER

Dietary carbohydrate affects serum triglyceride levels (Ahrens et al., 1961; Anderson et al., 1963) but does not always seem to have a hypercholesteremic effect. Grande (1974) summarized data showing that isocaloric substitution of starch (from fruit, cereal grains, or legumes) for sucrose lowered cholesterol levels. In the 12 experiments cited, the calories exchanged averaged 23 percent, and an average of 15 subjects were fed for 23 days, with an average cholesterol reduction of 13 mg/dl. Mann and Truswell (1972) conducted a similar exchange and found no hypocholesteremic effect. The observed effect may have been due to the fiber content of the starch-containing diets.

A summary of the literature (Kritchevsky, 1964) showed that saturated fat was atherogenic for rabbits when added to a semipurified diet, but not when added to a stock diet. It was demonstrated that the residue present in the stock diet was responsible for its protective effect (Kritchevsky and Tepper, 1965, 1968; Table 4). Moore (1967) showed that specific types of

Table 4. Influence of Fiber on Atherosclerosis in Rabbits[a]

Diet	*Fat*[b]	*Fiber*	*Serum Cholesterol (mg/dl)*	*Atherosclerosis*
A	14% HCNO	15% Cellulose	207 ± 36	1.7
B	14% HCNO	85% Stock Residue[c]	64 ± 9	0.8
C	2% Stock[d]	98% Stock[d]	40 ± 9	0.3

[a]After Kritchevsky and Tepper (1965, 1968).
[b]HCNO, hydrogenated coconut oil.
[c]Residue from solvent extraction of stock diet.
[d]Stock diet—commercial ration containing 2 percent fat.

Table 5. Influence of Pectin on Serum and Liver Cholesterol Levels in Animals

Species	Pectin (%)	Cholesterol (%)	Cholesterol Changes (%) Serum	Liver	Reference
Rat	2.5	1.0	−15	−36	Wells and Ershoff (1961)
Rat	5.0	1.0	−20	−60	Wells and Ershoff (1961)
Rat	5.0	1.0	−12	−65	Ershoff and Wells (1962)
Rat	5.0	1.0	0	−31	Riccardi and Fahrenbach (1967)
Rat	5.0	1.0	−19	−33	Kiriyama et al. (1969)
Rat	10.0	1.0	− 9	−75	Ershoff and Wells (1962)
Rat	10.0	1.0	−10	−41	Riccardi and Fahrenbach (1967)
Rat	5.0	0.5	+ 3	−75	Story et al. (1977)
Rat	7.0	0.5	−21	−64	Tsai et al. (1976)

nonnutrient fiber when added to a semipurified diet had different effects on cholesteremia and atherosclerosis. Cellophane gave the highest levels of serum and aortic cholesterol, and wheat straw gave the lowest. Aside from the fiber the two diets were identical.

Recent years have seen a great upsurge in interest in dietary fiber and its consequences. The interest stems from the publications of Burkitt et al. (1974) and Trowell (1972), who equate deficiency in dietary fiber with greater susceptibility to colon cancer, heart disease, and other diseases prevalent in the Western world. Earlier, Cleave (1956), Walker and Arvidsson (1954), and Antonis and Bersohn (1962) had suggested that low-fiber diets might have deleterious consequences.

The definition of fiber is still being debated, but the term is generally regarded to mean indigestible plant residues. The principal constituents of fiber are cellulose (an unbranched polymer of 1-4, β-D-galacturonic acid polymer with branches containing rhamnose, arabinose, xylose, and fucose) and lignin (a polymer containing sinapyl, coniferyl, and coumaryl alcohols). Only lignin is not carbohydrate in nature. Experiments with fiber have utilized pure preparations, such as pectin or cellulose, or plant materials, such as alfalfa or bran, which contain several types of fiber along with protein, fat, digestible carbohydrate, and trace minerals.

Cellulose has little effect on lipid metabolism in experimental animals. Wells and Ershoff (1961) added 5 percent cellulose to a semipurified rat diet containing 1 percent cholesterol and found sharp increases in serum and liver cholesterol. A similar effect has been observed by Kiriyama et al. (1969) and Tsai et al. (1976). Story et al. (1977) observed a slight hypercholesteremia in rats fed 1 percent cholesterol and 5 percent cellulose.

Pectin, however, will cause significant reductions in liver cholesterol levels of rats fed semipurified diets containing 1 percent cholesterol (Wells and Ershoff, 1961; Ershoff and Wells, 1962; Riccardi and Fahrenbach, 1967; Kiriyama et al., 1969; Tsai et al., 1976; Chang and Johnson, 1976; Story et al., 1977).

The effects of pectin on serum and liver lipids of rats are summarized in Table 5. Pectin (5 percent) has been shown to increase the excretion of bile acids, but not that of neutral steroids, in rats fed 1 percent cholesterol (Leveille and Sauberlich, 1966). Guar gum has also been found to lower serum and liver cholesterol levels in cholesterol-fed rats (Ershoff and Wells, 1962; Riccardi and Fahrenbach, 1967).

Portman and Murphy (1958) showed that the substitution of a semi-purified diet for laboratory ration in rats resulted in a marked decrease in fecal excretion of bile acids and neutral steroids. Substitution of alfalfa for cellulose in a semipurified diet will increase excretion of bile acids by 49 percent and of neutral steroids by 76 percent (Kritchevsky et al., 1974).

Some effects of fiber on experimental atherosclerosis have been cited earlier in this chapter. Cookson et al. (1967) fed rabbits meal or meal and alfalfa (at a ratio of 1:9) plus a daily dose of 600 mg of cholesterol. After ten weeks, the rabbits which had been fed meal were hypercholesteremic and atherosclerotic; the meal-and-alfalfa-fed animals exhibited normal serum lipids and had no atherosclerosis. Howard et al. (1967) reported that the dilution of an atherogenic diet with an equal weight of stock diet inhibited atherosclerosis in rabbits. Fisher et al. (1966) showed that chickens fed an atherogenic diet containing cellulose exhibited significantly more atherosclerosis than did chickens fed a similar diet containing pectin.

Hardinge and Stare (1954) and Hardinge et al. (1958) reported that vegetarians ingested more fiber and had lower serum cholesterol levels than did subjects eating a mixed diet. Cholesterol levels (mg/dl ± SEM) in purely vegetarian, lacto-ovo vegetarian, and nonvegetarian men were 206 ± 9, 243 ± 5, and 288 ± 13, respectively. In purely vegetarian, lacto-ovo, and nonvegetarian women, cholesterol levels were 206 ± 10, 269 ± 16, and 295 ± 16, respectively.

Walker and Arvidsson (1954) were among the first investigators to suggest that South African blacks had a much lower incidence of heart disease than white South Africans because of their massive daily intake of crude fiber. Keys et al. (1961) found that the addition of 15 percent cellulose to the diet had no effect on cholesterol levels. Truswell and Kay (1976) summarized the literature, and found that bran had virtually no effect on serum lipid levels. They cited ten studies in which an average intake of 37 g per day of bran was fed. Munoz et al. (1978) have reported that bran prepared from red spring wheat is indeed hypocholesteremic.

Pectin has been fed at levels ranging from 6 to 36 g daily and has been shown to be hypocholesteremic. Pectin feeding results in a large increase in bile acid excretion and a small increase in neutral steroid excretion (Kay and Truswell, 1977; Miettinin and Tarpila, 1977).

Table 6. Interaction of Fiber and Protein in Experimental Atherosclerosis in Rabbits[a]

	Serum lipids (mg/dl ± SEM)			α/β Lipoprotein	Average Atheromata	
Fiber	*Protein*	*Cholesterol*	*Triglyceride*	*Cholesterol*	*Arch*	*Thoracic*
Cellulose	Casein	402 ± 40	164 ± 5	0.05	1.81	1.19
Cellulose	Soy	248 ± 44	41 ± 8	0.08	1.50	1.00
Wheat straw	Casein	375 ± 42	94 ± 19	0.05	1.17	0.88
Wheat straw	Soy	254 ± 35	66 ± 9	0.08	1.04	0.77
Alfalfa	Casein	193 ± 34	60 ± 8	0.11	0.70	0.55
Alfalfa	Soy	159 ± 20	62 ± 17	0.14	0.88	0.58

[a]From Kritchevsky et al. (1977). Diets contained 40 percent sucrose, 25 percent protein, 15 percent fiber, 14 percent hydrogenated coconut oil, 5 percent salt mix, and 1 percent vitamin mix, and were fed for ten months.

Guar gum also has a hypocholesteremic effect in humans. At a level of 6 g per day, a 5 percent reduction in cholesterol levels has been observed (Fahrenbach et al., 1965), and at 36 g daily an average serum cholesterol decrease of 16 percent was seen (Jenkins et al., 1975).

Antonis and Bersohn (1962) fed diets that contained either 15 or 40 cal percent fat and 4 or 15 g fiber. When the diet contained 40 cal percent fat, increasing the fiber content had virtually no effect on excretion of acidic steroids, but increased neutral steroid excretion by 50 to 90 percent. On the low-fat regimen, increasing fiber content resulted in increased excretion of both acidic (24 to 43 percent) and neutral (81 to 95 percent) steroids.

Kiehm et al. (1976) changed the 2200-cal diet of 13 diabetic men so that the carbohydrate level was raised by 77 percent. The ratio of complex to simple carbohydrates rose from 1.15 to 2.63 and the fiber content was trebled. Serum cholesterol levels fell by 24 percent, triglyceride levels by 15 percent, and blood glucose levels by 26 percent.

The mechanism(s) of action of fiber is not yet clear. It does reduce intestinal transit time and increase fecal bulk, which may result in reduced availability of nutrients. Many types of grains and fiber bind bile acids and bile salts (Eastwood and Hamilton, 1968; Kritchevsky and Story, 1974; Balmer and Zilversmit, 1974; Birkner and Kern, 1974; Story and Kritchevsky, 1976). Bile salt binding inhibits cholesterol absorption.

The interaction of various nutrients must be considered in assessing the lipidemic or atherogenic potential of diets. Carroll and Hamilton (1975) reported that cholesterol levels of rabbits fed a diet containing casein plus dextrose were triple those of rabbits fed soy protein and dextrose. Substitution of raw potato starch for dextrose resulted in normal cholesterol levels in both groups.

Kritchevsky et al. (1977) fed rabbits a semipurified, cholesterol-free atherogenic diet containing as its protein either casein or soy protein. The type of fiber affected the cholesteremia and atherosclerosis. Thus, when the fiber was cellulose, casein was much more atherogenic than soy protein; when the fiber was alfalfa, the differences were virtually eliminated (see Table 6).

The foregoing discussion has attempted to demonstrate that components of the diet other than fat can affect cholesteremia and atherosclerosis. This fact must be kept in mind in the assessment of dietary effects on cholesteremia. The data on milk serve to show that one cannot indict any foodstuff because of one specific component.

ACKNOWLEDGMENTS

This research was supported in part by grants HL-03299 and HL-05209, and Research Career Award HL-00734, from the National Institutes of Health.

REFERENCES

Ahrens, E.H., Jr. Nutritional factors and serum lipid levels. *Am. J. Med.* 23, 928–952 (1957).

Ahrens, E.H., Jr., Hirsch, J., Oette, K., Farquhar, J.W., and Stein, Y. Carbohydrate induced and fat induced lipemia. *Trans. Assoc. Am. Phys.* 74, 134–146 (1961).

Anderson, J.T., Grande, F., Matsumoto, Y., and Keys, A. Glucose, sucrose, and lactose in the diet and blood lipids in man. *J. Nut.* 79, 349–359 (1963).

Antonis, A., and Bersohn, I. The influence of diet on fecal lipids in South African white and Bantu prisoners. *Am. J. Clin. Nut.* 11, 142–155 (1962).

Balmer, J., and Zilversmit, D.B. Effects of dietary roughage on cholesterol absorption, cholesterol turnover and steroid excretion in the rat. *J. Nut.* 104, 1319–1328 (1974).

Barr, D.P., Russ, E.M., and Eder, H.A. Protein-lipid relationships in human plasma. II. Atherosclerosis and related conditions. *Am. J. Med.* 11, 480–493 (1951).

Bernstein, B.A., Richardson, T., and Amundson, C.H. Inhibition of cholesterol biosynthesis by bovine milk, cultured buttermilk and orotic acid. *J. Dairy Sci.* 59, 539–543 (1976).

Bernstein, B.A., Richardson, T., and Amundson, C.H. Inhibition of cholesterol biosynthesis and acetyl-coenzyme A synthetase by bovine milk and orotic acid. *J. Dairy Sci.* 60, 1846–1853 (1977).

Birkner, H.J., and Kern, F., Jr. *In vitro* adsorption of bile salts to food residues, salicylazosulfapyridine, and hemicellulose. *Gastroenterology* 67, 237–244 (1974).

Boguslawski, W., and Wrobel, J. An inhibitor of sterol biosynthesis present in cow's milk. *Nature* 247, 210–211 (1974).

Burkitt, D.P., Walker, A.R.P., and Painter, N.S. Dietary fiber and disease. *J. Am. Med. Assoc.* 229, 1068–1074 (1974).

Carroll, K.K., and Hamilton, R.M.G. Effects of dietary protein and carbohydrate on plasma cholesterol levels in relation to atherosclerosis. *J. Food Sci.* 40, 18–23 (1975).

Chang, M.L.W., and Johnson, M.A. Influence of fat level and type of carbohydrate on the capacity of pectin in lowering serum and liver lipids of young rats. *J. Nut.* 106, 1562-1568 (1976).

Clarkson, T.B., Prichard, R.W., Lofland, H.B., and Goodman, H.O. Interactions among dietary fat, protein and cholesterol in atherosclerosis-susceptible pigeons: Effects on coronary atherosclerosis. *Circ. Res.* 11, 400-404 (1962).

Cleave, T.L. The neglect of natural principles in current medical practice. *J. R. Nav. Med. Serv.* 42, 55-82 (1956).

Cookson, F.B., Altschul, R., and Fedoroff, S. The effects of alfalfa on serum cholesterol and in modifying or preventing cholesterol-induced atherosclerosis in rabbits. *J. Atheroscler. Res.* 7, 69-81 (1967).

Eastwood, M.A., and Hamilton, D. Studies on the adsorption of bile salts to non-absorbed components of diet. *Biochem. Biophys. Acta* 152, 165-173 (1968).

Ershoff, B.H., and Wells, A.F. Effects of guar gum, locust bean gum and carrageenan on liver cholesterol of cholesterol-fed rats. *Proc. Soc. Exp. Biol. Med.* 110, 580-582 (1962).

Fahrenbach, M.J., Riccardi, B.A., Sanders, J.C., Lourie, I.N., and Heider, J. Comparative effects of guar gum and pectin on human serum cholesterol levels. *Circulation* 32, 11 (abstract) (1965).

Fisher, H., Soller, W.G., and Griminger, P. The retardation by pectin of cholesterol-induced atherosclerosis in the fowl. *J. Atheroscler. Res.* 6, 292-298 (1966).

Fredrickson, D.S., Levy, R.I., and Lees, P.S. Fat transport in lipoproteins–an integrated approach to mechanisms and disorders. *N. Eng. J. Med.* 276, 32-42; 94-103; 148-156; 215-225; 273-281 (1967).

Friend, B. Nutrients in the United States food supply, A review of trends, 1909-1913 to 1965. *Am. J. Clin. Nut.* 20, 907-914 (1967).

Gofman, J.W., Lindgren, F., Elliott, H., Mantz, W., Hewitt, J., Strisower, B., Herring, V., and Lyon, T.P. The role of lipids and lipoproteins in atherosclerosis. *Science* 111, 166-171 (1950).

Gortner, W.A. Nutrition in the United States, 1900-1974. *Cancer Res.* 35, 3246-3253 (1975).

Grande, F. Sugars in cardiovascular disease, in *Sugars in Nutrition.* H.L. Sipple and K.W. McNutt, eds. Academic Press, New York (1974), pp. 401-437.

Gresham, G.A., and Howard, A.N. The independent production of atherosclerosis and thrombosis in the rat. *Br. J. Exp. Path.* 41, 395-402 (1960).

Hamilton, R.M.G., and Carroll, K.K. Plasma cholesterol levels in rabbits fed low fat, low cholesterol diets–Effects of dietary proteins, carbohydrates and fibre from different sources. *Atherosclerosis* 24, 47-62 (1976).

Hardinge, M.G., and Stare, F.J. Nutritional studies of vegetarians. II. Dietary and serum levels of cholesterol. *Am. J. Clin. Nut.* 2, 83-88 (1954).

Hardinge, M.G., Chambers, A.C., Crooks, H., and Stare, F.J. Nutritional studies of vegetarians. III. Dietary levels of fiber. *Am. J. Clin. Nut.* 6, 523-525 (1958).

Howard, A.N., and Marks, J. Hypocholesterolaemic effect of milk. *Lancet* 2, 255-256 (1977).

Howard, A.N., Gresham, G.A., Jennings, I.W., and Jones, D. The effect of drugs on hypercholesterolaemia and atherosclerosis induced by semi-synthetic low cholesterol diets. *Prog. Biochem. Pharm.* 2, 117-127 (1967).

Ignatowski, A. Über die Wirkung des tierischen Eiweisses auf die Aorta und die parenchymatosen Organe der Kaninchen. *Virchows Arch. Path. Anat. Physiol.* 198, 248-270 (1909).

Jenkins, D.J.A., Leeds, A.R., Newton, C., and Cummings, J.H. Effect of pectin, guar gum and wheat fibre on serum cholesterol. *Lancet* 1, 1116-1117 (1975).

Kagan, A., Kannel, W.B., Dawber, T.R., and Revotskie, N. The coronary profile. *Ann. N.Y. Acad. Sci.* 97, 883–894 (1962).

Kay, R.M., and Truswell, A.S. Effect of citrus pectin on blood lipids and fecal steroid excretion in man. *Am. J. Clin. Nut.* 30, 171–175 (1977).

Keys, A., Grande, F., and Anderson, J.T. Fiber and pectin in the diet and serum cholesterol concentration in man. *Proc. Soc. Exp. Biol. Med.* 106, 555–558 (1961).

Kiehm, T.G., Anderson, J.W., and Ward, K. Beneficial effects of a high carbohydrate, high fiber diet on hyperglycemic diabetic men. *Am. J. Clin. Nut.* 29, 895–899 (1976).

Kiriyama, S., Okozaki, Y., and Yoshida, A. Hypocholesterolemic effect of polysaccharides and polysaccharide-rich foodstuffs in cholesterol fed rats. *J. Nut.* 97, 382–388 (1969).

Kritchevsky, D. Experimental atherosclerosis in rabbits fed cholesterol-free diets. *J. Atheroscler. Res.* 4, 103–105 (1964).

Kritchevksy, D., and Story, J.A. Binding of bile salts *in vitro* by non-nutritive fiber. *J. Nut.* 104, 458–462 (1974).

Kritchevsky, D., and Tepper, S.A. Factors affecting atherosclerosis in rabbits fed cholesterol-free diets. *Life Sci.* 4, 1467–1471 (1965).

Kritchevsky, D., and Tepper, S.A. Experimental atherosclerosis in rabbits fed cholesterol-free diets: Influence of chow components. *J. Atheroscler. Res.* 8, 357–369 (1968).

Kritchevsky, D., and Tepper, S.A. Cholesterol vehicle in experimental atherosclerosis. 15. Randomized butter and randomized lard. *Atherosclerosis* 27, 339–345 (1977).

Kritchevsky, D., Tepper, S.A., and Story, J.A. Isocaloric, isogravic diets in rats III. Effect of nonnutritive fiber (alfalfa or cellulose) on cholesterol metabolism. *Nut. Rep. Int.* 9, 301–308 (1974).

Kritchevsky, D., Kolman, R.R., Guttmacher, R.M., and Forbes, M. Influence of dietary carbohydrate and protein on serum and liver cholesterol in germ-free chickens. *Arch. Biochem. Biophys.* 85, 444–451 (1959).

Kritchevsky, D., Tepper, S.A., Vesselinovitch, D., and Wissler, R.W. Cholesterol vehicle in experimental atherosclerosis, II. Peanut oil. *Atherosclerosis* 14, 53–64 (1971).

Kritchevsky, D., Tepper, S.A., Vesselinovitch, D., and Wissler, R.W. Cholesterol vehicle in experimental atherosclerosis, 11. Peanut oil. *Atherosclerosis* 14, 53–64 (1971). 17, 225–243 (1973).

Kritchevsky, D., Tepper, S.A., Williams, D.E., and Story, J.A. Experimental atherosclerosis in rabbits fed cholesterol-free diets. 7. Interaction of animal or vegetable protein with fiber. *Atherosclerosis* 26, 397–403 (1977).

Kritchevsky, D., Tepper, S.A., Morrissey, R.B., Czarnecki, S.K., and Klurfeld, D.M. Influence of whole or skim milk on cholesterol metabolism in rats. *Am. J. Clin. Nut.* 32, 597–600 (1979).

Kritchevsky, D., Moyer, A.W., Tesar, W.C., Logan, J.B., Brown, R.A., Davies, M.C., and Cox, H.R. Effect of cholesterol vehicle in experimental atherosclerosis. *Am. J. Physiol.* 178, 30–32 (1954).

Lees, R.S., and Hatch, F.T. Sharper separation of lipoprotein species by paper electrophoresis in albumin-containing buffer. *J. Lab. Clin. Med.* 61, 518–528 (1963).

Leveille, G.A., and Sauberlich, H.E. Mechanism of the cholesterol-depressing effect of pectin in the cholesterol-fed rat. *J. Nut.* 88, 209–214 (1966).

Lofland, H.B., Jr., Clarkson, T.B., and Goodman, H.O. Interactions among dietary fat, protein and cholesterol in atherosclerosis-susceptible pigeons: Effects on serum cholesterol and aortic atherosclerosis. *Circ. Res.* 9, 919–924 (1961).

Lofland, H.B., Clarkson, T.B., Rhyne, L., and Goodman, H.O. Interrelated effects of dietary fats and proteins on atherosclerosis in the pigeon. *J. Atheroscler. Res.* 6, 395–403 (1966).

Malinow, M.R., and McLaughlin, P. The effect of skim milk on plasma cholesterol in rats. *Experientia* 31, 1012–1013 (1975).

Mann, G.V. A factor in yogurt which lowers cholesteremia in man. *Atherosclerosis* 26, 335–340 (1977).

Mann, G.V., and Spoerry, A. Studies of a surfactant and cholesteremia in the Masai. *Am. J. Clin. Nut.* 27, 464–469 (1974).

Mann, J.I., and Truswell, A.S. Effects of isocaloric exchange of dietary sucrose and starch on fasting serum lipids, postprandial insulin secretion and alimentary lipaemia in human subjects. *Br. J. Nut.* 27, 395–405 (1972).

Meeker, D.R., and Kesten, H.D. Effect of high protein diets on experimental atherosclerosis of rabbits. *Arch. Path.* 31, 147–162 (1941).

Miettinen, T.A., and Tarpila, S. Effect of pectin on serum cholesterol, fecal bile acids and biliary lipids in nonnolipidemic and hyperlipidermic individuals. *Clin. Chim. Acta.* 79, 471–477 (1977).

Miller, G.J., and Miller, N.E. Plasma high density lipoprotein concentration and development of ischaemic heart disease. *Lancet* 1, 16–19 (1975).

Moore, J.H. The effect of the type of roughage in the diet on plasma cholesterol levels and aortic atherosis in rabbits. *Br. J. Nut.* 21, 207–215 (1967).

Morrison, L.M. The serum phospholipid-cholesterol ratio as a test for coronary atherosclerosis. *J. Lab. Clin. Med.* 39, 550–556 (1952).

Munoz, J.M., Sandstead, H.H., Jacob, R.A., Logan, G.M., Jr., and Klevay, L.M. Effects of some cereal brans on glucose tolerance and plasma lipids of normal men. *Fed. Proc.* 37, 755 (1978).

Myher, J.J., Marai, I., Kuksis, A., and Kritchevsky, D. Acylglycerol structure of peanut oils of different atherogenic potential. *Lipids* 12, 775–785 (1977).

Newburgh, L.H., and Clarkson, S. The production of atherosclerosis in rabbits by feeding diets rich in meat. *Arch. Int. Med.* 31, 653–676 (1923).

Nichols, A.B., Ravenscroft, C., Lamphrear, D.E., and Ostrander, L.D., Jr. Independence of serum lipid levels and dietary habits, the Tecumseh study. *J. Am. Med. Assoc.* 236, 1948–1953 (1976).

Oliver, M.F., Nimmo, I.A., Cooke, M., Carlson, L.A., and Olsson, A.G. Ischaemic heart disease and associated risk factors in 40 year old men in Edinburgh and Stockholm. *Eur. J. Clin. Invest.* 5, 507–514 (1975).

Olson, R.E. Atherosclerosis–a primary hepatic or vascular disorder? *Perspect. Biol. Med.* 2, 84–121 (1958).

Page, L., and Friend, B. Level of use of sugars in the United States, in *Sugars in Nutrition.* H.L. Sipple and K.W. McNutt, eds. Academic Press, New York (1974), pp. 94–107.

Porter, M.W., Yamanaka, W., Carlson, S.D., and Flynn, M.A. Effect of dietary egg on serum cholesterol and triglyceride of human males. *Am. J. Clin. Nut.* 30, 490–495 (1977).

Portman, O.W., and Murphy, P. Excretion of bile acids and hydroxysterols by rats. *Arch. Biochem. Biophys.* 76, 367–376 (1958).

Riccardi, B.A., and Fahrenbach, M.J. Effect of guar gum and pectin N. F. on serum and liver lipids of cholesterol-fed rats. *Proc. Soc. Exp. Biol. Med.* 124, 749–752 (1967).

Richardson, T. The hypocholesteremic effect of milk–A review. *J. Food Prot.* 41, 226–235 (1978).

Rizek, R.L., Friend, B., and Page, L. Fat in today's food supply: Level and use of sources. *J. Am. Oil Chem. Soc.* 51, 244–250 (1974).

Scala, J. The physiological effects of dietary fiber, in *Physiological Effects of Food Carbohydrates.* A. Jeanes and J. Hodge, eds. American Chemical Society, Washington, D.C. (1975), pp. 325–335.

Segall, J.J. Is milk a coronary health hazard? *Br. J. Prev. Soc. Med.* 31, 81–85 (1977).

Sirtori, C.R., Agradi, E., Conti, F., Mantero, O., and Gatti, S. Soybean protein diet in the treatment of Type II hyperlipoproteinaemia. *Lancet* 1, 275–277 (1977).

Sirtori, C.R., Conti, F., Sirtori, M. Giantranceschi, G. Zucchi, C. Zoppi, S., Agradi, E., Tavazzi, L., Mantero, O., Gatti, E., and Kritchevsky, D. Clinical experience with a soybean protein diet in the treatment of hypercholesterolemia. *Am. J. Clin. Nut.* 32, 1645–1658 (1979).

Slater, G., Mead, J., Dhopeshwarkar, G., Robinson, S., and Alfin-Slater, R.R. Plasma cholesterol and triglycerides in men with added eggs in the diet. *Nutr. Rep. Int.* 14, 249–260 (1976).

Story, J.A., and Kritchevsky, D. Comparison of the binding of various bile acids and bile salts *in vitro* by several types of fiber. *J. Nut.* 106, 1292–1294 (1976).

Story, J.A., Czarnecki, S.K., Baldino, A.R., and Kritchevsky, D. Effect of components of fiber on dietary cholesterol in the rat. *Fed. Proc.* 36, 1134 (1977).

Strasser, T. Atherosclerosis and coronary heart disease: The contribution of epidemiology. *WHO Chron.* 26, 7–11 (1972).

Strong, J.P., and McGill, H.C., Jr. Diet and experimental atherosclerosis in baboons. *Am. J. Path.* 50, 669–690 (1967).

Trowell, H. Dietary fiber and coronary heart disease. *Eur. J. Clin. Biol. Res.* 17, 345 (1972).

Truswell, A.S., and Kay, R.M. Bran and blood-lipids. *Lancet* I, 367 (1976).

Tsai, A.C., Elias, J., Kelley, J.J., Lin, R.S.C., and Robson, J.R.K. Influence of certain dietary fibers on serum and tissue cholesterol levels in rats. *J. Nut.* 106, 118–123 (1976).

Vesselinovitch, D., Getz, G.S., Hughes, R.H., and Wissler, R.W. Atherosclerosis in the rhesus monkey fed three food fats. *Atherosclerosis* 20, 303–321 (1974).

Walker, A.R.P., and Arvidsson, U.B. Fat intake, serum cholesterol concentration and atherosclerosis in the South African Bantu. I. Low fat intake and age trend of serum cholesterol concentrations in the South African Bantu. *J. Clin. Invest.* 33, 1358–1365 (1954).

Wells, A.F., and Ershoff, B.H. Beneficial effects of pectin in prevention of hypercholesterolemia and increase in liver cholesterol in cholesterol-fed rats. *J. Nut.* 74, 87–92 (1961).

11

Systematic Approach to the Treatment of Hereditary Hyperlipidemia

JEAN DAVIGNON
SUZANNE LUSSIER-CACAN

INTRODUCTION

The central role of plasma cholesterol in atherogenesis has been amply demonstrated. It is also well established that hyperlipidemia is an important risk factor for coronary heart disease. The physician is thus justified in making an all-out effort to reduce elevated plasma lipid levels in the hope of preventing, arresting, or reverting the atherosclerotic process. Indeed, there is considerable evidence in experimental animals (Armstrong, 1976) and in humans (Basta et al., 1976; Gresham, 1976; Barndt et al., 1977) to indicate that lowering of plasma lipid levels will reduce the cardiovascular complications of atherosclerosis and promote the regression of the lesions. While there is much controversy regarding the measures applicable to the general population for the prevention of atherosclerosis (Ahrens, 1976), the importance of treating individuals at risk is not disputed. The following discussion will be concerned mainly with the treatment of patients affected with primary hyperlipidemias, and will describe in general terms the major steps to be taken in a rational and effective therapeutic approach. For further details the reader is referred to a comprehensive review of the subject (Davignon, 1978).

FIRST STEP: MAKE AN ACCURATE DIAGNOSIS

An accurate diagnosis is mandatory if an appropriate treatment is to be instituted. Indeed, the treatment will depend to a large extent on the nature and severity of the plasma lipid disorder. A thorough case history and physical examination, supplemented with a few laboratory tests, should allow the physician to exclude the major secondary causes of hyperlipidemia and detect aggravating factors. Special attention should be given to obesity, diabetes, hypothyroidism, excessive alcohol intake, use of oral contraceptives, pregnancy, nephrotic syndrome, pancreatitis, and biliary obstruction. A good family history and the search for revealing clinical clues will help establish the hereditary nature of the plasma lipid abnormality and help determine its classification into a well defined disease category (Fredrickson et al., 1978). A family history of premature coronary heart disease, or early manifestations of atherosclerosis in a patient in the presence of tendon xanthomas, should orient towards a diagnosis of familial hypercholesterolemia (lipoprotein phenotype II). Attacks of abdominal pain in childhood with eruptive xanthomas and lipemia retinalis are strongly suggestive of familial hyperchylomicronemia (lipoprotein lipase deficiency, Type I). Lipemia retinalis, revealed by ophthalmoscopic examination of the fundi, develops when plasma triglycerides exceed 3000 mg/dl (Vinger and Sachs, 1970), and may also be present in familial mixed hyperlipidemia (Type V). Discrete planar xanthomas along the palmar creases, orange or brownish pigmentation of the palmar creases, brownish tuberoeruptive xanthomas at the elbows, punctate xanthomas at the tip of the fingers, brownish-orange eruptive xanthomas on the buttocks, with or without tendon xanthomas, are features to be found in familial dysbetalipoproteinemia (Type III). A turbid or lactescent plasma (triglycerides above 300 mg/dl), an asymptomatic arterial bruit, xanthelasma of the eyelids or arcus corneae are other less specific clues that may be witness to the presence of an hereditary form of hyperlipidemia. The eye signs may be the only manifestation of familial hyperprebetalipoproteinemia (Type IV) or of familial combined hyperlipidemia (multiple phenotype disease).

It is important to remember that primary hyperlipidemia may be present in the absence of clinical manifestations. It is often revealed by the familial context or, fortuitously, by abnormal plasma cholesterol (>240 mg/dl) or triglyceride (>150 mg/dl) level determinations in the course of a routine or disease-oriented screening. In most cases the knowledge of the clinical setting and measurements of plasma cholesterol (CH) and triglycerides (TG) will suffice to make the diagnosis.

In some instances, more specialized laboratory tests might be needed to refine the diagnosis, to establish it on firmer grounds, or to provide information for a more quantitative assessment of risk. An analysis of the cholesterol content of the major plasma lipoprotein classes, combined with lipoprotein electrophoresis on the separated fractions (Davignon and Langelier, 1971), is most helpful. It is useful especially to assess the concentrations of the *atherogenic* low-density lipoproteins (LDL) or of the *protective* high-density lipoproteins (HDL); to detect the presence of the beta-migrating very-low-density-lipoprotein, or intermediate-density lipoportein (β-VLDL, IDL) of Type III; to measure the VLDL-CH/TG ratio, which is reported to be equal to or greater than 0.3 in familial Type III (when triglycerides are under 1000 mg/dl) (Fredrickson et al., 1975); to get an estimate of risk for coronary heart disease from the CH/HDL or LDL/HDL ratios (Castelli et al., 1977); or to reveal the presence of minor or unusual plasma lipoprotein bands such as the Lp(a) fraction ("sinking" pre-beta-lipoprotein) or the slow-migrating pre-beta band (De Gennes et al., 1975). A deficiency of plasma lipoprotein lipase activity (LPL) measured after an heparin injection will confirm the diagnosis of familial hyperchylomicronemia (Krauss et al., 1974). A polyacrylamide gel electrophoresis of delipidized VLDL may reveal a deficiency of apolipoprotein C-II, an activator of LPL, which leads to an unusual form of familial hyperlipidemia (Breckenridge et al., 1978). Measurement of plasma apolipoprotein E (apo-E) concentrations which are increased in Type III also has its merit (Kushwaha et al., 1977). More importantly, the diagnosis of familial dysbetalipoproteinemia (Type III) will be confirmed by measurement of the isomorphs of apo E by isoelectric focusing of delipidized VLDL and demonstration of a deficiency in apo E-III (Utermann et al., 1977).

Not all primary hyperlipidemias have the same degree of *atherogenicity*, and this should be taken into consideration in a global therapeutic approach. Hypercholesterolemia due to an elevation of the plasma LDL fraction appears to be more deleterious than hypertriglyceridemia secondary to a rise in VLDL (Slack, 1969). Hereditary hyperlipidemias could be ranked in presumed order of increasing atherogenic potential as follows: hyperalphalipoproteinemia, the longevity syndrome, for which no treatment is needed (Glueck et al., 1976); familial hyperchylomicronemia, in which abdominal pain and pancreatitis are more of a problem than atherosclerosis; familial mixed hyperlipoproteinemia (Type V), in which atherosclerotic complications are not abnormally prevalent (Fredrickson et al., 1978), unless it is complicated by diabetes; familial hypertriglyceridemia (Type IV); familial hyperlipidemia with slow-migrating prebetalipoprotein (De Gennes et al., 1975); familial combined hyperlipidemia (Goldstein et al., 1973); Brunzell et al., 1976), and Type III with about the same degree of atherogenicity; the heterozygous form of familial hypercholesterolemia where early atherosclerotic complications are the rule; and, at the top of the list, its homozygous form which is the most lethal, both forms demanding a vigorous treatment.

SECOND STEP: OBTAIN BASELINE PLASMA LIPID VALUES AND CONTROL OTHER RISK FACTORS

In order to assess ably the effectiveness of the lipid-lowering regimen it is important, before initiating treatment, to obtain three to five baseline values of plasma cholesterol and triglycerides over several weeks. This observation period may be useful, not only for later comparison, but also for the valuable detection of unexpected fluctuations in plasma lipids which could be due, for instance, to the spurious use of alcohol or to changes in body weight. It is then time to evaluate the patient's dietary habits, to gain some insight into his or her psychosocial environment, and to determine the patient's level of understanding of the disease and his or her ability to comply. Body weight should be monitored throughout the follow-up period.

The decision to treat, as well as the modality and extent of the therapeutic regimen, must not rest solely on the degree of elevation of plasma lipid concentrations. The nature of the hyperlipidemia, the familial incidence of coronary heart disease, the age and sex of the patient, and whether clinical manifestations of atherosclerosis and associated risk factors are present must be taken into account. The treatment must not be applied without regard to the psychosocial, economic, and nutritional status of the patient, and without securing his or her understanding of both the condition and its treatment.

It is well known that major risk factors for coronary heart disease potentiate one another (Stamler, 1978). It would be futile to spend a considerable amount of time and energy at lowering plasma lipid levels while neglecting other risk factors which could also be corrected. Particular attention should be given to hypertension, cigarette smoking, diabetes, and obesity in the course of treatment of hyperlipidemia. It must be remembered that hypertension developing in a previously normotensive hyperlipidemic subject might be the first indication of the atheromatous involvement of a renal artery.

Following plasma lipid changes is not the only way of assessing the effectiveness of the treatment; xanthelasmas and other skin and tendon xanthomas must be carefully examined for signs of regression. On occasion, skin lesions may regress before any lowering of plasma lipid is achieved (Palmer and Blacket, 1972). Radiologic techniques used to obtain a more objective evaluation of the changes in size of tendon xanthomas have been described (Gattereau et al., 1973).

THIRD STEP: INSTITUTE A LIPID-LOWERING DIET TAILORED TO THE PLASMA LIPOPROTEIN ABNORMALITY

The first attempt at lowering plasma lipids in primary hyperlipidemias should be dietary. If the patient is both obese and hypertriglyceridemic, a low-calorie diet is likely to be successful. Plasma triglyceride levels are very sensitive to weight changes, (Fig. 1) whereas LDL cholesterol is the least affected.

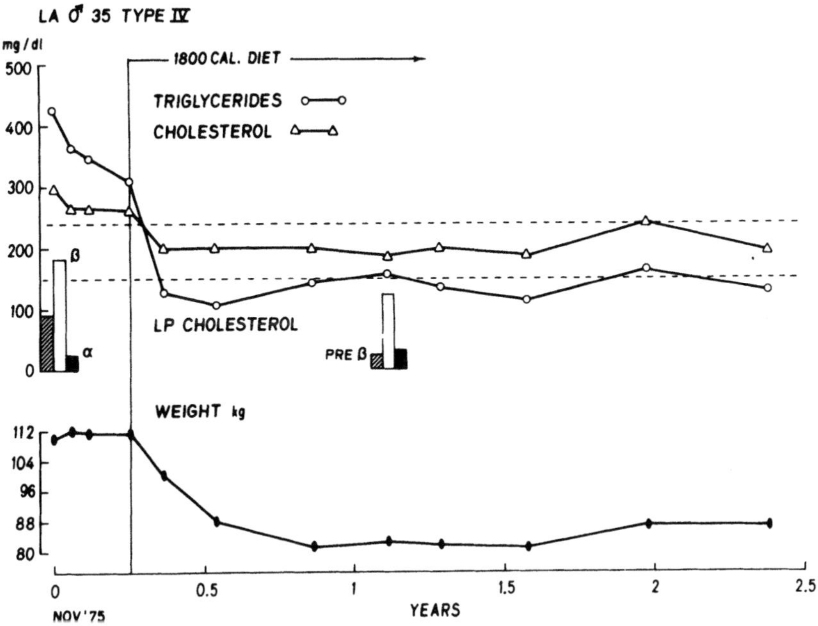

Fig. 1. Sustained effect of body weight reduction on plasma lipid levels in familial hypertriglyceridemia (Type IV). A 35 percent fall in body weight was accompanied by a 48 percent reduction in plasma triglycerides, but only a 7 percent fall in plasma cholesterol in this 35-year-old man when his daily caloric intake was reduced from 2700 to 1800 calories. The bar graphs depict the changes in the cholesterol content of plasma lipoproteins. In this instance, there was a concomitant decrease in the level of beta-lipoprotein- (or LDL-) cholesterol as the pre-beta-lipoprotein (or VLDL-) cholesterol level was lowered.

In the nonobese hyperlipidemic subject the choice of the dietary regimen should be guided by the plasma lipoprotein abnormality. Exogenous fats, whether saturated or not, contribute to the formation of chylomicrons and should be limited in the diet of patients who have an excess of these particles in their fasting plasma (phenotypes I and V). This is the basis for the treatment of familial lipoprotein lipase deficiency (Type I). Medium-chain triglycerides which are absorbed and transported to the liver through the portal system do not contribute to chylomicron formation, and may be used as a substitute for vegetable oil in this disease (Furman et al., 1965). The total daily fat intake should be kept between 25 and 35 g per day and no alcohol should be permitted, since it may promote or enhance pancreatitis.

Saturated fats ingested in large amounts increase the cholesterol fraction which is transported by LDL. Their intake should thus be reduced whenever hyperbetalipoproteinemia is present (phenotypes IIa and IIb), as in familial hypercholesterolemia and in familial combined hyperlipidemia. Fats and oils containing polyunsaturated fatty acids are recommended as substitutes. Indeed, their high linoleic acid content contributes its own cholesterol-lowering effect in addition to a potential antithrombogenic activity (Hornstra and Vles, 1978). The cholesterol content of the diet should also be reduced in these high-risk individuals (<300 g per day). Although the effect of dietary cholesterol on plasma cholesterol concentrations is controversial (Glueck and Connor, 1978), it remains that some individuals might be highly susceptible to its hypercholesterolemic effect. Rhomberg and Braunsteiner (1976) have reported the development of marked hypercholesterolemia and skin xanthomas in an individual who had ingested large amounts of cholesterol in the form of egg yolks (one egg yolk contains 250 mg of cholesterol) for an extended period of time. This effect was reversible. In addition, the feeding of an excess of dietary cholesterol has been shown recently to induce the formation of an apo-E-rich, cholesterol-ester-rich lipoprotein fraction (HDL_c) in humans, the significance and consequences of which remain to be determined (Mahley et al., 1978).

An excess of simple carbohydrates in the diet usually enhances the endogenous hypertriglyceridemia which is found in phenotypes IIb, III, IV, and V (Lussier-Cacan et al., 1977). Affected patients should be encouraged to limit their intake of simple sugars. In some cases, a dietary intake reduced in simple sugar, without a reduction in total caloric intake, may completely correct an endogenous hypertriglyceridemia (Fig. 2).

The dietary management of primary hyperlipidemias constitutes a major challenge for the patience and the perseverance of the physician. It is a task which is to be shared with a dietitian to revise the dietary habits, give detailed instructions to the patients, monitor adherence to the regimen, make the diet more appealing, adapt it to the cultural and socioeconomic context, and provide support and counseling. The person responsible for the preparation of the meals should be present when dietary instructions are given to the patient. It is important to make both of them realize that many of the dietary changes imposed may often be adopted for the benefit of the entire family. In order to maintain a high degree of motivation and insure compliance, it is mandatory that the follow-up visits not be too far apart, especially in the first few years of treatment.

FOURTH STEP: ADD LIPID-LOWERING DRUGS (IF NEED BE) WITHOUT DISCONTINUING THE DIET

When the physician is convinced that the prescribed dietary regimen has been well understood and rigorously followed, the results obtained are

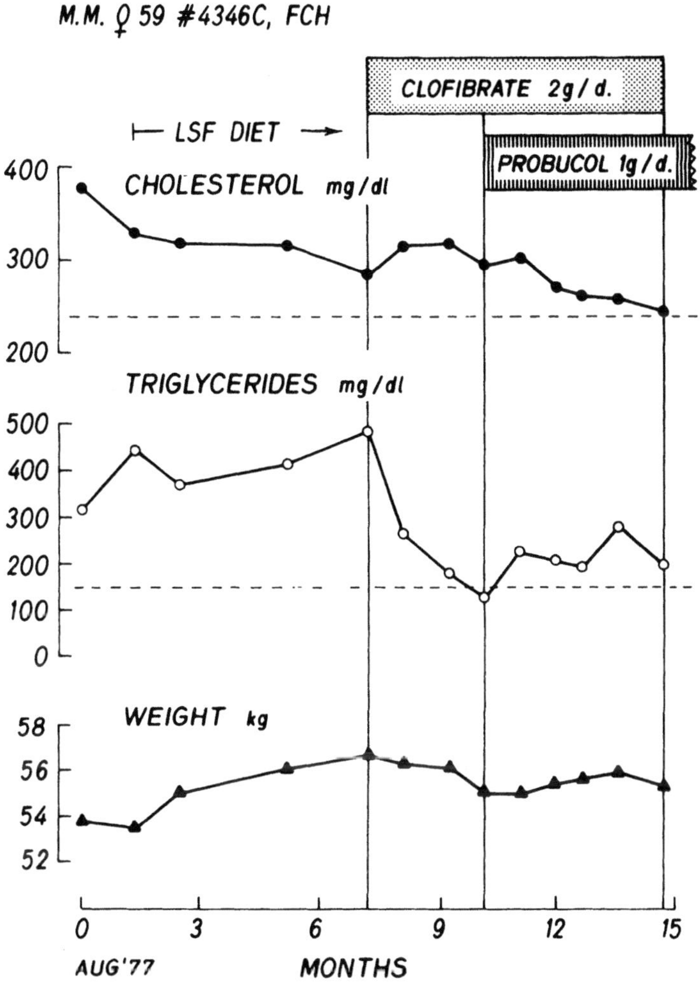

Fig. 2. Effect of an isocaloric restriction of simple carbohydrates in the nonobese hypertriglyceridemic patient. An isocaloric dietary regimen limited in refined and concentrated simple sugars (R-CHO) with a moderate restriction in saturated fats and cholesterol normalizes plasma triglycerides (familial Type IV), while body weight is maintained constant in this 21-year-old man. The bar graphs demonstrate that the reduction of the cholesterol content of the pre-beta-lipoproteins (LP) is compensated by an increase in the cholesterol of both beta- and alpha-lipoproteins in this case. Levels attained, however, remain within the normal range.

Table 1. Response of Plasma Cholesterol to Clofibrate in 37 Patients[a] with Familial Hypercholesterolemia (Type II)[b]

Type of Response	*Number of Subjects (%)*	*Number of Females*
Sensitive ↓ ⩾20%	12 (32.4%)	9
Intermediate ↓ ⩾10% <20%	15 (40.6%)	9
Resistant ↑ or ↓ <10%	10 (27.0%)	4

[a]15 males, 22 females.
[b]From Davignon et al., 1971.

evaluated after five or six months. The decision to add a drug is made after taking into account the degree of plasma-lipid lowering achieved with the diet, as well as the age of the individual, the nature of the hyperlipidemia, its effect in the family and in the patient in terms of atherosclerotic cardiovascular disease, the presence of associated risk factors and aggravating factors, and the ability to comply. As a rule drugs are not a substitute for the diet, but an addition.

Drugs are of no value in *familial hyperchylomicronemia* and there is currently no alternative to the dietary regimen. In *familial hypercholesterolemia* (FH) it is often necessary to add drugs, since the dietary approach is not usually very effective. In our diet-probucol study on 30 heterozygous FH patients (LeLorier et al., 1977), a mean reduction of only 6.5 percent for plasma cholesterol and 3.0 percent for plasma triglycerides was obtained when a low-cholesterol- (⩽300 mg per day) low-saturated-fat (P/S [polyunsaturated to saturated fatty acid ratio] ⩾ 1.8) regimen given for 12 weeks replaced a standard North American diet (cholesterol ⩾600 mg per day; P/S ⩽ 0.3; duration of diet was eight weeks). This is especially true in the homozygous form of FH, which is the most difficult to treat. The drugs of choice are: cholestyramine (24 g per day in two to four doses) or one of its analogues; clofibrate (1 g twice a day), when it can be shown that LDL-cholesterol is responsive to its effect (Davignon et al., 1971) (about one-third of the cases, especially women; see Table 1) or one of its more potent derivatives available in some countries; and probucol (0.5 g twice a day), singly or in combination. A cholestyramine-clofibrate combination may be quite effective in some cases. Nicotinic acid has many side effects and must be given in high doses (2 to 4 g per day in four doses), but it has its usefulness when other drugs fail. Dextrothyroxin, neomycin, beta-sitosterol, and para-aminosalicylic acids are second-line drugs which may be added to enhance the effect of some first-line drugs. Much caution should be exerted, however, with the use of dextrothyroxin (6 to 8 mg per day, starting with 2 mg per day with increments of 2 mg every four to five weeks), since it may exacerbate symptoms of angina pectoris and favor the induction of cardiac arrhythmias. If no combination of drugs is satisfactory, one must consider performing a partial ileal bypass operation (Buchwald et al., 1974) as a last resort in high-risk individuals. The effectiveness of portacaval shunt (Starzl et al., 1978) in homozygous FH is unpredictable; and this approach is still experimental.

Familial dysbetalipoproteinemia (Type III) is usually quite responsive to clofibrate, which is the drug of choice. In some instances, estrogens might be beneficial (Kushwaha et al., 1977). In treating *familial hypertriglyceridemia* (Type IV), clofibrate is also a first-line drug if the response to the diet has been inadequate. In case of resistance to this medication one is left with the use of nicotinic acid as a major hypotriglyceridemic agent. In treating *familial combined hyperlipidemia* (FCH), the approach should be guided by the phenotype. An occasional patient may be remarkably responsive to probucol (LeLorier et al., 1977; Enjalbert et al., 1980). If plasma cholesterol or LDL-cholesterol levels tend to increase during clofibrate reduction of the hypertriglyceridemia (see below) in the presence of hypercholesterolemia, a combination of another cholesterol-lowering agent might help correct this effect. This is illustrated in Fig. 3, where we see the result of combining probucol with clofibrate. In treating *familial mixed hyperlipidemia,* nicotinic acid, norethindrone acetate (Glueck et al., 1969), and oxandrolone (Glueck, 1971) have been used with some success.

The list of lipid-lowering agents developed over the past 20 years is overwhelmingly large (Bencze, 1975; Kritchevsky, 1975), and bears witness to the fact that the ideal drug has not yet been discovered. Only a few drugs have met with some popularity because of their effectiveness, but they all have some drawbacks. Since their effect is not curative and they must be given for extended periods of time, it is imperative to select the most potent agent with the least side effects or which is the least likely to be a potential health hazzard. Some comments should be made on the use of clofibrate, which has been a matter of controversy in recent years.

Clofibrate is a potent lipid-lowering and antiatherogenic agent in animals (Bencze, 1975). When it was introduced for the treatment of hyperlipidemia in humans it was found to be well tolerated and was quite effective at reducing plasma triglycerides; thus, it became widely employed. It is only with usage that some of its side effects, and some other of its pharmacologic properties (De Gennes et al., 1969) became known. Early it was found that it potentiated the effects of anticoagulants of the coumarin type (Solomon et al., 1968), and that its cholesterol-lowering effect was opposed by some oral contraceptive drugs (Smith and Prior, 1968). Later on, the myalgic syndrome—a rare occurrence which necessitates discontinuation of the drug—was described by Langer and Levy (1968). At the conclusion of the large-scale Coronary Drug Project (CDP) Study (Coronary Drug Project Research Group, 1975), other side effects emerged in a small proportion of cases (e.g.,

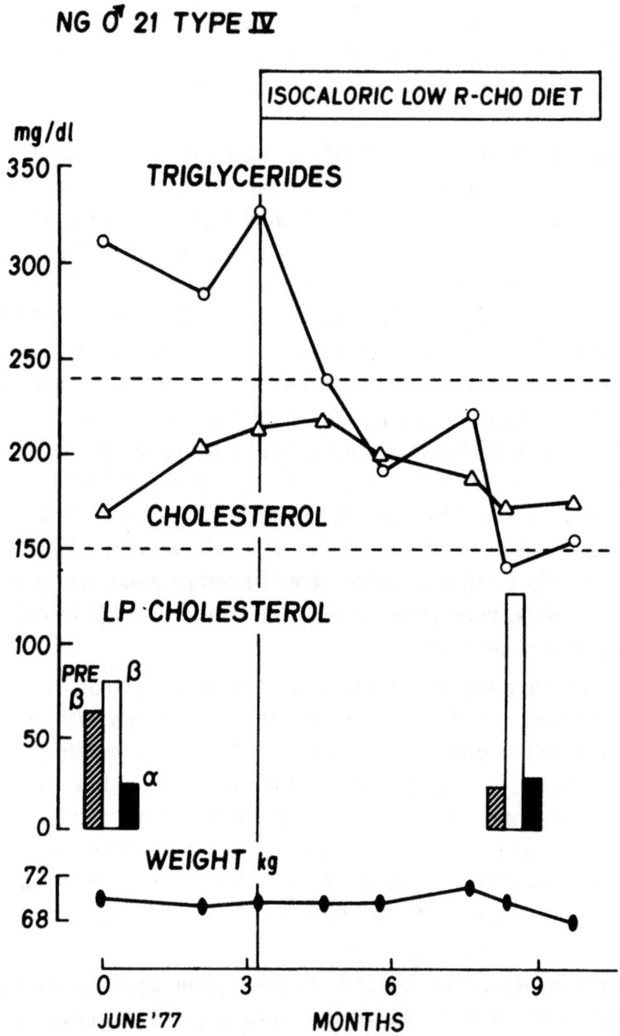

Fig. 3. Control with probucol of persistant hypercholesterolemia after reduction of plasma triglycerides with clofibrate. Clofibrate induced a 53 percent fall in plasma triglycerides in this 54-year-old woman with familial combined hyperlipidemia. In spite of a slight reduction in weight, plasma cholesterol remained elevated. When probucol was added this residual hypercholesterolemia was normalized within five months. A low-cholesterol–low-saturated-fat (LSF) diet was instituted from the sixth week onward and followed adequately throughout the two drug periods.

loss of libido, increase of appetite, palpable spleen, cholelithiasis, etc.), and clofibrate was considered ineffective at reducing the cardiovascular mortality in patients who had already suffered a myocardial infarction. A more recent multicenter primary prevention trial of the World Health Organization (Oliver et al., 1978) confirmed that cholelithiasis was indeed an important side effect, and the opinion was expressed that clofibrate should not be used for the primary prevention of coronary heart disease in the population at large. Nevertheless, this study found a reduction in the incidence of nonfatal myocardial infarction in proportion with the extent of cholesterol-lowering achieved, which demonstrated the merit of reducing plasma cholesterol as a preventive measure and strengthened the lipid hypothesis. The investigators were hasty, however, at drawing their conclusions (Oliver, 1978) and at condemning a drug which still had major indications. Their study design introduced the same mistake we had already pointed out (Pichardo et al., 1977) for the CDP: the indiscriminate use of clofibrate without regard to the degree of resistance or sensitivity to its cholesterol-lowering effect (regardless of its effect on triglycerides). We have clearly established in well-characterized cases of familial hypercholesterolemia (but this is also true of other categories of hyperlipidemia) that a good proportion of patients treated with clofibrate respond by an increase in LDL-cholesterol while their triglycerides are lowered or unchanged (see Table 1) (Davignon et al., 1971; Pichardo et al., 1977). Since such an effect is likely to be deleterious, it constitutes an absolute indication for the discontinuation of clofibrate use (at least when plasma LDL-CH levels are reaching values over 190 mg/dl). As a rule of thumb we have recommended that clofibrate be discontinued if total cholesterol (or LDL-CH when it is measured) is increased or shows only a slight decrease (<8 percent) in familial hypercholesterolemia, or reaches the upper limits of normal in familial hypertriglyceridemia (Davignon, 1978). In contrast, in responsive subjects, the fall in plasma LDL-CH may reach 30 percent, a highly desirable effect. Thus, it is not unexpected that the cholesterol-lowering achieved in both studies should have been so low (6.5 percent in the CDP, and 9 percent in the WHO multicenter trial) and that little benefit had been obtained from the cardiovascular standpoint, the investigators not having taken care to identify and exclude subjects who were resistant to the cholesterol-lowering effect of the drug. Indeed if we look in three different trials at the degree of cholesterol-lowering achieved and at the changes in mortality rate of nonfatal myocardial infarction, as compared to a control group, we can readily see that they are closely related: in the CDP a 6.5 percent fall in cholesterol corresponded to an insignificant 5 percent lower incidence of mortality, in the WHO multicenter trial an 8.8 percent fall corresponded to a 25.8 percent lowering, and in the United Airlines Study (Krasno and Kidera, 1972) the fall in cholesterol and the lowering of mortality were 19.8 percent and 71.4 percent, respectively (after 3.2 years, in this case). Thus, with time the effects of clofibrate and its drawbacks are becoming better known. The indications are becoming better delineated and the task of the attending physician is being facilitated. Clofibrate remains the prototype of the modern lipid-lowering agent. Work devoted at modifying its formula to improve its effectiveness and reduce its untoward side effects should be pursued and encouraged.

SUMMARY AND CONCLUSIONS

A systematic approach to the treatment of primary hyperlipidemias must begin with an accurate diagnosis. When the nature and severity of the plasma lipid disorder are well established, the decision to treat must rest on a careful assessment of the clinical context. Since in most instances the ultimate goal is to prevent complications from atherosclerosis, the other risk factors for coronary heart disease must be taken care of simultaneously. The dietary approach precedes the use of drugs and must take into account the current knowledge relating dietary factors to the pathogenesis of atherosclerosis. The use of drugs must be individualized, and one is often compelled to proceed by trial and error until the most effective combination of drugs is found, or the physician must resort to a surgical approach (if the need arises) in severely resistant cases. At all times treatment must be adapted to the type of plasma lipoprotein abnormality. With experience, as one goes over and over again this type of approach, some golden rules seem to emerge which it might be worthwhile remembering:

1. Treatment may be assessed accurately only if enough plasma lipid values are obtained in each treatment period (baseline, diet alone, diet plus drug A, etc.).
2. Weight loss comes first in overweight hypertriglyceridemic patients.
3. Incidence of coronary heart disease in the family and/or the presence of atherosclerosis in the patient are most important in assessing the risk and deciding on the extent of the treatment.
4. Visits with the physician should not be too far apart to insure motivation and compliance (the "out-of-sight, out-of-mind" rule).
5. Drugs are added to the dietary regimen; they do not substitute for it.
6. Effectiveness of treatment should be assessed not only from changes in plasma lipids, but also from regression of the skin lesions.
7. Potential benefits to the patient should always be weighed against drawbacks and potential hazards of the treatment.

REFERENCES

Ahrens, E.H., Jr. The management of hyperlipidemia; whether, rather than how. *Ann. Int. Med.* 85, 87–93 (1976).

Armstrong, M.L. Evidence of regression of atherosclerosis in primates and man. *Postgrad. Med. J.* 52, 456–461 (1976).

Barndt, R., Jr., Blankenhorn, D.H., Crawford, D.W., and Brooks, S.H. Regression and progression of early femoral atherosclerosis in treated hyperlipoproteinemic patients. *Ann. Int. Med.* 86, 139–146 (1977).

Basta, L.L., Williams, C., Kioschos, J.M., and Spector, A.A. Regression of atherosclerotic stenosing lesions of the renal arteries and spontaneous cure of systemic hypertension through control of hyperlipidemia. *Am. J. Med.* 61, 420–423 (1976).

Bencze, W.L. Hypolipidemic agents, in *Hypolipidemic Agents.* D. Kritchevsky, ed. Springer-Verlag, Berlin (1975), pp. 349–408.

Breckenridge, W.C., Little, A.J., Steiner, G, Chow, A., and Poapst, M. Hypertriglyceridemia associated with deficiency of apolipoprotein C-II. *New Eng. J. Med.* 298, 1265–1272 (1978).

Brunzell, J.D., Schrott, H.G., Motulsky, A.G., and Bierman, E.L. Myocardial infarction in the familial forms of hypertriglyceridemia. *Metabolism* 25, 313–319 (1976).

Buchwald, H., Moore, R., and Varco, R.L. Surgical treatment of hyperlipidemia. *Circulation* 49 (suppl. 1), 1–37 (1974).

Castelli, W.P., Doyle, J.T., Gordon, T., Hames, C.G., Hjortland, M.C., Hulley, S.B., Kagen, A., and Zukel, W.J. HDL cholesterol and other lipids in coronary heart disease. *Circulation* 55, 767–772 (1977).

Coronary Drug Project Research Group. Clofibrate and niacin in coronary heart disease. *J. Am. Med. Assoc.* 231, 360–381 (1975).

Davignon, J. The hyperlipoproteinemias, in *Current Therapy.* H.F. Conn, ed. W.B. Saunders, Philadelphia (1978), pp. 430–440.

Davignon, J., and Langelier, M. Electrophorèse et ultracentrifugation combinées dans le diagnostic des hyperlipidémies primaires. *Union Méd. Canad.* 100, 2120–2128 (1971).

Davignon, J., Aubry, F., Noël, C., Lapierre, Y., and Lafortune, M. Heterogeneity of familial hyperlipoproteinemia type II on the basis of fasting plasma triglyceride/cholesterol ratio and plasma cholesterol response to chlorophenoxyisobutyrate. *Revue Canad. Biol.* 30, 307–318 (1971).

De Gennes, J.L., Truffert, J., and Colas-Belcourt, J.F. Détection et distribution de la prébêtalipoprotéine lente en électrophorèse sur gel d'agarose du sérum total dans 204 cas. *Ann. Méd. Interne* 126, 19–26 (1975).

De Gennes, J.L., Bertrand, C., Bigorie, B., and Truffert, J. Première démonstration de l'activité antidiurétique, pharmacologique et thérapeutique du clofibrate (Atromide-S) dans le diabète insipide pitresso-sensible. *C.R. Acad. Sci. (Paris)* 269, 2607–2610 (1969).

Enjalbert, M., Lussier-Cacan, S., Quidoz, S., LeLorier, J., and Davignon, J. Usefulness of probucol in treating primary hypercholesterolemia. *Canad. Med. Assoc. J.* 123, 754–757 (1980).

Fredrickson, D.S., Goldstein, J.L., and Brown, M.S. The familial hyperlipoproteinemias, in *Metabolic Basis of Inherited Disease.* J.B. Stanbury, J.B. Wyngaarden, and D.S. Fredrickson, eds. McGraw-Hill, New York (1978), pp. 604–655.

Fredrickson, D.S., Morganroth, J., and Levy, R.I. Type III hyperlipoproteinemia: An analysis of two contemporary definitions. *Ann. Int. Med.* 82, 150–157 (1975).

Furman, R.H., Howard, R.P., Brusco, O.J., and Alaupovic, P. Effect of medium-chain-length triglycerides (MCT) on serum lipids and lipoproteins in familial hyperchylomicronemia (dietary-fat-induced lipemia) and dietary-carbohydrate-accentuated lipemia. *J. Lab. Clin. Med.* 66, 912–926 (1965).

Gattereau, A., Davignon, J., Langelier, M., and Levesque, H.P. An improved radiological method for the evaluation of Achilles tendon xanthomatosis. *Canad. Med. Assoc. J.* 108, 39–43 (1973).

Glueck, C.J. Effects of oxandrolone on plasma triglycerides and postheparin lipolytic activity in patients with types III, IV, and V familial hyperlipoproteinemia. *Metabolism* 20, 691–701 (1971).

Glueck, C.J., and Connor, W.E. Diet-coronary heart disease relationship reconnoitered. *Am. J. Clin. Nut.* 31, 727–737 (1978).

Glueck, C.J., Brown, V.W., Levy, R.I., Greten, H., and Fredrickson, D.S. Amelioration of hypertriglyceridemia by progestational drugs in familial type V hyperlipoproteinemia. *Lancet* 1, 1290–1291 (1969).

Glueck, C.J., Gartside, P., Fallat, R.W., Sielski, J., and Steiner, P.M. Longevity syndromes: familial hypobeta and familial hyperalphalipoproteinemia. *J. Lab. Clin. Med.* 88, 941–957 (1976).

Goldstein, J.L., Hazzard, W.R., Schrott, H.G., Bierman, E.L., and Motulsky, A.G. Hyperlipidemia in coronary heart disease. II. Genetic analysis of lipid levels in 176 families and delineation of a new inherited disorder, combined hyperlipidemia. *J. Clin. Invest.* 52, 1544–1568 (1973).

Gresham, G.A. Is atheroma a reversible lesion? *Atherosclerosis* 23, 379–391 (1976).

Hornstra, G., and Vles, R. Effects of dietary fats on atherosclerosis and thrombosis, in *International Conference on Atherosclerosis.* L.A. Carlson, R. Paoletti, C.R. Sirtori, and G. Weber, eds. Raven Press, New York (1978), pp. 471–476.

Krasno, L.R., and Kidera, G.J. Clofibrate in coronary heart disease. *J. Am. Med. Assoc.* 219, 845–851 (1972).

Krauss, R.M., Levy, R.I., and Fredrickson, D.S. Selective measurement of two lipase activities in post heparin plasma from normal subjects and patients with hyperlipoproteinemia. *J. Clin. Invest.* 54, 1107–1124 (1974).

Kritchevsky, D. Newer hypolipidemic compounds. *Adv. Exp. Med. Biol.* 63, 135–150 (1975).

Kushwaha, R.S., Hazzard, W.R., Wahl, P.W., and Hoover, J.J. Type III hyperlipoproteinemia: diagnosis in whole plasma by apolipoprotein-E immunoassay. *Ann. Int. Med.* 86, 509–516 (1977).

Langer, R., and Levy, R.I. Acute muscular syndrome associated with administration of clofibrate. *New Eng. J. Med.* 279, 856–858 (1968).

LeLorier, J., Dubreuil-Quidoz, S., Lussier-Cacan, S., Huang, Y.S., and Davignon, J. Diet and probucol in lowering cholesterol concentrations. *Arch. Int. Med.* 137, 1429–1434 (1977).

Lussier-Cacan, S., Beaudoin, R., Gattereau, A., and Davignon, J. Hypertriglycéridémie induite par les glucides dans les hyperlipoprotéinémies primaires. *Union Méd. Canad.* 106, 474–484 (1977).

Mahley, R.W., Innerarity, T.L., Bersot, T.P., Lipson, A., and Margolis, S. Alterations in human high-density lipoproteins with or without increased plasma cholesterol, induced by diets high in cholesterol. *Lancet* 2, 807–809 (1978).

Oliver, M.F. Cholesterol, coronaries, clofibrate and death. *New Eng. J. Med.* 299, 1360–1362 (1978).

Oliver, M.F., Heady, J.A., Morris, J.N., and Cooper, J. A cooperative trial in the primary prevention of ischaemic heart disease using clofibrate–Report from the committee of principal investigators. *Br. Heart J.* 40, 1069–1118 (1978).

Palmer, A.J., and Blacket, R. Regression of xanthomata of the eyelids with modified fat diet. *Lancet* 1, 66–68 (1972).
Pichardo, R., Boulet, L., and Davignon, J. Pharmacokinetics of clofibrate in familial hypercholesterolemia. *Atherosclerosis* 26, 573–582 (1977).
Rhomberg, H.P., and Braunsteiner, H. Excessive egg consumption, xanthomatosis and hypercholesterolemia. *Br. Med. J.* 1, 1188–1189 (1976).
Slack, J. Risks of ischaemic heart disease in familial hyperlipoproteinaemic states. *Lancet* 2, 1380–1382 (1969).
Smith, R.B.W., and Prior, I.A.M. Oral contraceptive opposition to hypocholesterolaemic action of clofibrate. *Lancet* 1, 750–751 (1968).
Solomon, H.M., Schrogie, J.J., and Williams, D. The displacement of phenylbutazone-^{14}C and warfarin-^{14}C from human albumin by various drugs and fatty acids. *Biochem. Pharm.* 17, 143–151 (1968).
Stamler, J. Lifestyles, major risk factors, proof and public policy. *Circulation* 58, 3–19 (1978).
Starzl, T.E., Putman, C.W., and Koep, L.J. Portacaval shunt and hyperlipidemia. *Arch. Surg.* 113, 71–74 (1978).
Utermann, G., Hees, M., Steinmetz, A. Polymorphism of apolipoprotein E and occurrence of dysbetalipoproteinemia in man. *Nature* 269, 604–607 (1977).
Vinger, P.E., and Sachs, B.A. Ocular manifestations of hyperlipoproteinemia. *Am. J. Ophth.* 70, 563–573 (1970).

12

Nutritional Modification for Prevention and Treatment of Hyperlipidemia and Hyperlipoproteinemia

HERBERT K. NAITO

INTRODUCTION

Although intensive research efforts have begun to elucidate various facets of the etiology, development, and prognosis of the pathogenesis of atherosclerosis, we are still not sure how the initiating and accelerating factors associated with this degenerative disease process interact and manifest themselves. One reason is that the disease process itself is complex, probably developing through a multitude of processes. Early in 1954, Dr. Page introduced the "filtration concept," which is based on the view that atherogenesis is a result of tissue reaction to substances filtered from plasma by lateral arterial pressure, and deposited in the intima as "foreign" lipid. He was careful to list the multitude of factors predisposing to experimental atherogenesis (Page, 1954). Since that time, other predisposing factors have been added to the list (Fig. 1). These factors may not be *causes,* yet because of their close association, demonstrated by statistical means with cardiovascular disease, they were called "risk factors." Since the filtration concept, many hypotheses on the etiology of atherogenesis have been advanced. However, it appears that no single concept is correct, emphasizing the complexity of the disease; the etiology is probably a multifactorial one, adding to the difficulty in understanding the specific role each predisposing factor has in the initiation, development, and regression of the disease process.

Another difficulty is that statistically valid data obtained on large populations and in prospective epidemiological studies are not necessarily directly applicable to an individual. As discussed by Blackburn (1974), there is a large variation among individuals in these predisposing factors and within a

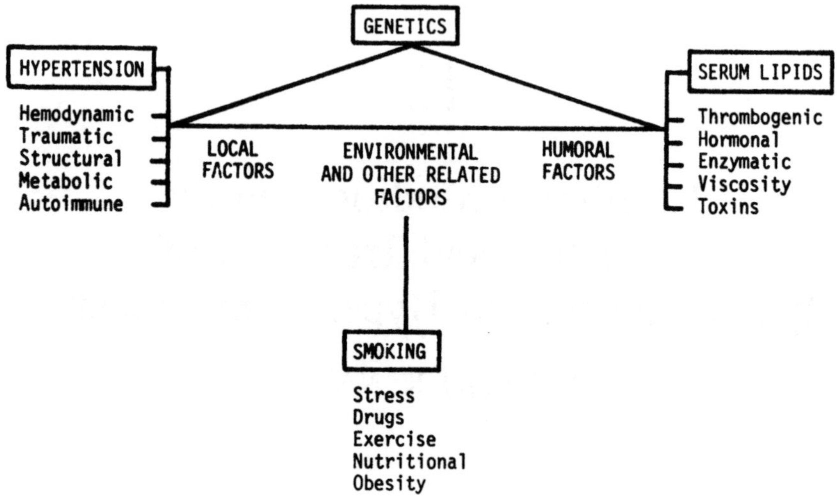

Fig. 1 Primary and secondary factors associated with the etiology, development, and regression of atherosclerosis.

single individual during his or her life span. Factors acting throughout the entire period of the developing degenerative disease are difficult, if not impossible, to evaluate. At any one time, primary risk factors (hypertension, smoking, elevated blood cholesterol level, family history for coronary artery disease) and secondary risk factors (obesity, lack of physical activity, chronic stress, and patients afflicted with gout, diabetes mellitus, hypothyroidism, renal failure and on hemodialyses), (see Fig. 1) are simultaneously involved in the pathogenesis.

Still another difficulty is that differences in food habits have not been adequately demonstrated within the United States between people with and without coronary disease, although habitual diet is related to serum cholesterol concentrations in different populations. The Framingham (Massachusetts) Study seems to suggest that individual genetic, personal, and environmental differences may override the small differences in dietary intake within any one culture (Kannel et al., 1971).

In spite of these possible overriding factors, there can be little doubt that the initiation, development, progression, and regression of atherosclerosis are closely associated with nutritional factors. The evidence accumulated over the last 40 years in animal, clinical, and epidemiologic studies is impressive and persuasive. Nutrition has an important influence on several of the risk factors, particularly serum lipids, lipoproteins, overweight, hypertension, endocrine imbalance, and other metabolic conditions closely associated with atherosclerosis. With appropriate nutritional adjustments, these conditions associated with degenerative vascular disease can be altered and controlled.

Whether the modification of these risk factors by diet will ultimately lead to lower mortality and morbidity from coronary heart disease (CHD) is yet to be proven. Four primary prevention studies (Los Angeles Veterans Administration Study, Finnish Diet Study, Oslo Diet–Heart Study, U.S. Diet–Heart Study) using dietary measures have shown a trend toward favorable results (Laren, 1966; National Diet Heart Study Final Report, 1968; Dayton et al., 1969; Miettinen et al., 1972). Frantz et al. (1975), from the Minnesota Coronary Survey, reported that in the dietary trial of a cholesterol-lowering diet, men <50 years of age showed less mortality and morbidity from CHD events than the control group.

I would like to devote this chapter to nutrition and the nutritional modification of atherosclerosis by diet.

Before discussing the role of various dietary factors on serum lipids and atherosclerosis, it must be emphasized that under practical conditions one cannot examine each dietary factor as a separate entity; the effect of each factor on serum lipids is the result of the total composition and amount of each dietary component in a meal. Proteins, carbohydrates, fats, minerals, and vitamins all have effects of their own and can have additional effects on other dietary components, especially on the efficiency of intestinal absorption, transport, and metabolism of lipids. Thus, it is important to understand the interdependence of nutrients that are manipulated in fat-controlled diets. In this chapter, the simplistic approach will be taken in discussing each nutritional factor as a separate entity. On occasion, attention will be drawn to the need for viewing the various nutritional components in relationship to each other.

Rationale for Control of Blood Lipids and Lipoproteins

There is abundant evidence that elevated serum cholesterol concentration is associated with increased risk of atherogenesis and CHD. Recent articles by Nichols et al. (1977), Davis and Havlik (1977), Glueck and Conner (1977), and Grundy (1977) can be referred to for reviews on the relationship between diet and CHD. Persons with disorders characterized by elevated levels of low-density lipoprotein (LDL), that is, β-lipoprotein, have a strikingly high incidence of CHD, which often is evident at a young age (Stone and Levy, 1972). If the familial β-hyperlipoproteinemic condition is of a homozygote origin, fatal complications of premature atherogenesis occur before age 30 (Fredrickson et al., 1967; Fredrickson and Levy, 1972). From epidemiologic studies and basic and clinical research, there appears to be little doubt that hypercholesterolemia exists as an independent risk factor for coronary artery disease (CAD) (Johnson et al., 1968; Medalie et al., 1973;

Wilhemsen et al., 1973; Gordon et al., 1974). Data from mainland China show that the mean serum cholesterol level in normal people is 136 mg/dl, while in CHD patients it is 190 mg/dl (Van Die Redaskie, 1973). Thus, in a country with a low rate of CHD, there also appears to be a positive relationship between CHD and cholesterol levels.

Evidence on the role of hypertriglyceridemia as an independent risk factor is not yet conclusive. In the Framingham Study, the serum triglyceride level was a risk factor for CHD, but only because of the associated hypercholesterolemia (Kannel et al., 1971). It is not uncommon to find that a markedly increased very-low-density lipoprotein (VLDL) level can also be associated with slightly elevated cholesterol concentration. In the Stockholm Prospective Study, the serum triglycerides and cholesterol levels were found to be independent risk factors for CHD, the highest risk being associated with the elevation of both lipids (Carlson and Bottiger, 1972).

Recently, reappraisal of the importance of high-density lipoproteins (HDL) and/or HDL-cholesterol levels as predictors of CHD has created much interest. According to the Framingham data, there is a clear gradient of CHD incidence rates on serum HDL-cholesterol concentrations (Gordon et al., 1977). Persons with levels below 35 mg/dl have eight times the CHD rate of persons with HDL-cholesterol levels of 65 mg/dl or greater. It was Barr et al. (1951) who first pointed out that a high proportion of serum total cholesterol carried in HDL in babies was similar to that found in animals that appear to have a high resistance to atherosclerotic disease. Many animal studies also support this hypothesis. Nicolosi et al. (1977) reported on squirrel and cebus monkeys fed a semipurified coconut oil diet for a period of three to four years from birth, and found that both species of monkeys developed comparable hypercholesterolemia. However, the squirrel monkey primarily expanded its LDL-cholesterol pool, whereas the cebus monkey primarily increased its HDL-cholesterol pool. There was a greater accumulation of aortic lipids, particularly cholesteryl ester, in the atherosclerotic-susceptible squirrel monkeys. It has recently been shown that, like the rat and dog, the ground squirrel has predominantly HDL (Naito and Gerrity, 1979). All three animal models are resistant to atherosclerotic lesions. Furthermore, when hypercholesterolemia is induced by dietary means, most of the cholesterol in these species is carried in the HDL, thus causing an even greater elevation of the serum HDL levels, which may explain, in part, why the prolonged hyperlipidemia (one year) did not induce any fatty streaking or unusual structural changes in the arterial wall related to coronary or thoracic atherosclerosis. These findings tend to support the hypotheses on the atherogenicity of LDL and the seemingly protective effect of HDL. It has been demonstrated that LDL from hypercholesterolemic serum stimulates growth of smooth muscle cells in tissue culture and leads to intracellular lipid accumulation, while HDL has little effect (Ross and Glomser, 1973; Fischer-Dzoga and Wissler, 1976). One possible mechanism for the protective role of HDL is that HDL competes with LDL for cell-surface receptors and may not be internalized as extensively as the latter lipoprotein, in effect reducing the cholesterol uptake and accumulation in the smooth muscle cell (Carew et al., 1976). It is also possible that HDL, in concert with phospholipids, may remove cholesterol from cholesterol-laden tissues, such as the arterial intima (Bondjer and Bjökerud, 1974; Stein et al., 1975; Stein et al., 1976). Although the mechanism of cholesterol removal from cells is still not known, Glomset suggested that lecithin cholesterol acyl transferase (LCAT) enzyme may play a role in the transport of cholesterol from peripheral tissues to the liver (Glomset, 1968; Glomset and Norum, 1973). While some studies (Rhoads et al., 1976; Castelli et al., 1977; Miller et al., 1977; Stanhope et al., 1977) agree with the Framingham Study (Gordon et al., 1977), others do not support the HDL concept (Mjøs et al., 1977). At the time of writing, there are no clinical studies that correlate myocardial infarction (MI) with HDL-cholesterol levels or coronary lesion formation (determined by cineangiography) with the HDL-cholesterol concentration. In the evaluation of the risk factors associated with lipid or lipoproteins and CHD, there is no single parameter that is the best predictive serum constituent. One should always consider the risks of both cholesterol and triglycerides, as well as all of the major lipoprotein fractions. It has been noted, for example, that Trappist monks have relatively lower serum cholesterol levels than civilian people in the Cleveland, Ohio area, but have not been protected from atherosclerosis (McCullagh and Lewis, 1960). However, because the investigators quantitated the α-lipoprotein concentration by the analytical ultracentrifugal method, it was noted that the α-lipoprotein level was lower than that of the control subjects. This may help to explain why the monks were not protected against CHD.

Before addressing the question of what is adequate dietary or drug therapy for the control of serum lipid and lipoprotein levels, one needs to first consider the degree to which blood lipids should be lowered. In other words, at what level should the clinician consider a sample hyperlipidemic? Many clinical laboratories and practicing physicians still use normal ranges in evaluating whether or not a sample can be considered normal or abnormal. These normograms are based on sampling of "apparently normal" individuals and on arbitrarily defining hyperlipidemia as being present when the plasma cholesterol and/or triglycerides are above the ninety-fifth percentile value for the population to which the person belongs. Unfortunately, because of the way we have defined *normal* in the past, many abnormal test results do not predict disease states or health-risk conditions. Thus, the normal range may not be a healthy level. While a cholesterol value of 250 to 280 mg/dl may be within the ninety-fifth percentile value of the distribution of an apparently normal male population between the ages of 51 to 59 in the United States, about 40 to 50 percent of these individuals develop CHD. One of the most frequent (and perhaps most frustrating) questions confronting the clinician regarding laboratory tests is, "What is normal?" In recent years the term *normal range* has been replaced by the term *reference range*. *Upper limit of normal* is being replaced by *referent value, critical value*, or *cut-off point*. There are at least five major considerations that the reference values depend upon: (1) the reference population and the way that it was chosen; (2) the environmental and physiologic conditions under which the specimens were obtained; (3) the techniques and timing of specimen collection, transportation, preparation, and storage; (4) the analytic method that was used, with data regarding its accuracy, precision, and quality control; and (5) the data set that was observed and the reference intervals that were derived (Galen, 1977). There also is the consideration for subselection based on ethnic background, geographical location, occupation, body weight, sex, age, and other factors such as smoking, alcohol intake, and dietary habits. The reference intervals, 2.5 to 97.5th percentiles, can be compared to the Gaussian estimation of 95 percent of the population, which is included within ± 2 S.D. from the mean. The 2.5 and 97.5th and 0.5 and 99.5th percentiles are frequently used to define the laboratory reference intervals for a chemistry test. The clinician dealing with a single patient, however, does not really care about standard deviations or percentiles. He or she is most interested in knowing whether the test result predicts a particular disease state or implies risk of morbidity or mortality. It is here that the predictive value approach may prove to be of utmost significance. Referent values for serum lipids and lipoproteins should be established that are highly predictive of disease or disease risk, irrespective of the normal distribution.

There are four components that are important in determining the accuracy of a laboratory diagnostic test: (1) sensitivity; (2) specificity; (3) predictive value, and (4) efficiency. Sensitivity indicates the frequency of positive test results in patients with a particular disease, whereas specificity indicates the frequency of negative test results in patients without that specific disease. The predictive value of a positive test result indicates the frequency of diseased patients in all patients with positive test results. The predictive value of a negative test result indicates the frequency of non-diseased patients in all patients with negative test results. The efficiency of a test indicates the percent of patients correctly classified by the test. In screening for disease, we are most interested in the predictive value of the positive result. In CHD, this means establishing predictive values for total cholesterol, triglycerides, LDL, LDL-cholesterol, HDL, HDL-cholesterol, etc. Epidemiologic studies (Kannel et al., 1971; Glueck et al., 1976) show that CHD risk is linear down to a cholesterol concentration of 180 mg/dl. It is now believed that dietary treatment in this country should be initiated when the serum cholesterol level is >220 mg/dl in adults and above 200 mg/dl in children (Food and Nutrition Board, 1972; Connor et al., 1973; Laner et al., 1975). The upper limit of serum triglyceride levels is less clear. Perhaps levels in excess of 150 to 200 mg/dl can be considered unhealthy (Rhoads et al., 1976). The rationale for initiating dietary therapy when the above limits are exceeded is to prevent or minimize the development of CHD, since atherosclerosis seldom occurs with total cholesterol concentration <200 mg/dl over the life span of an individual (Connor and Connor, 1972), unless other risk factors such as genetics, high blood pressure, smoking, and obesity are playing a dominant role.

While serum lipids are not to be neglected, the influence of other risk factors associated with CHD should be simultaneously considered. They include smoking, hypertension, obesity, stress, lack of physical activity, hormonal imbalances, and other primary disease states directly or indirectly associated with abnormal lipid and lipoprotein metabolism.

From a physiologic viewpoint, it is difficult to talk about lipids as a separate entity from lipoproteins, since all lipids are associated with protein components to form soluble complexes in aqueous milieus (see Table 1). While it is easy and convenient to consider only the serum lipid levels when monitoring the effects of a prescribed diet, attention should be focused on the serum lipoproteins for at least two reasons: (1) Lipids are transported as lipoproteins and should be considered as a lipid abnormality that is classifiable as different types of dyslipoproteinemic conditions; and (2) LDL-cholesterol concentration is positively related to the risk of CHD, while HDL-cholesterol concentration is negatively related to the risk of CHD. Thus, the progress of an individual on the diet should be assessed by not only the serum total cholesterol levels, but by the LDL or LDL-cholesterol, and HDL or HDL-cholesterol levels.

Generally speaking, when lowering one serum lipid level (i.e., either cholesterol or triglyceride), the level of the other decreases also. Concomitantly, the concentration of lipoprotein fractions rich in these materials (chylomicron, pre-β- or β-lipoprotein) drop also. Serum total phospholipid levels usually parallel the changes in serum total cholesterol concentration; the cholesterol/phospholipid ratios under normal conditions remain about unity. However, the α-lipoprotein level may not be as predictable. For years the importance of α-lipoproteins in the evaluation of dyslipoproteinemias has usually been neglected, mainly because more emphasis was given to the lipoproteins that carried the greatest proportion of triglycerides and cholesterol, namely chylomicron, pre-β-lipoprotein, and β-lipoprotein. Nikkila (1953) and other investigators (Brunner et al., 1962) recognized many years ago that MI subjects had lower α-lipoprotein and higher β-lipoprotein values

Table 1. Physical, Chemical, and Physiologic Description of Serum Lipoproteins[a]

	Chylomicron	*Very-low-density Lipoproteins*	*Intermediate-density Lipoproteins*	*Low-density Lipoproteins*	*High-density Lipoproteins*
Electrophoretic nomenclature	Chylomicron	Pre-β-lipoprotein	Midband-lipoprotein or remnant-lipoprotein	β-Lipoprotein	α-Lipoprotein
Density (g/ml)	0.95	0.95–1.006	1.006–1.019	1.019–1.063	HDL_2 = 1.063–1.10 HDL_3 = 1.10–1.2
S_f rate[b]	>400	20–400	12–20	0–10	–
Electrophoretic mobility (paper)	Origin	β-Globulin	β-Globulin	β-Globulin	α_1-Globulin
Molecular diameter (Å)	300–5000	~400	~245	200	70–100
Major lipid transported	Exogenous triglycerides	Endogenous triglycerides	Cholesterol	Cholesterol	Phospholipids
Major apoproteins	Apo-B Apo-C-I Apo-C-II Apo-C-III	Apo-B Apo-C-I Apo-C-II Apo-C-III Arginine-rich peptide	Apo-B	Apo-B	Apo-A-I Apo-A-II
Minor apoproteins	Apo-A-I Apo-A-II	Thin-line protein Apo-A-I Apo-A-II	–	–	Apo-C-I Apo-C-II Apo-C-III Thin-line protein Arginine-rich protein

[a]From Jackson et al. (1976), Osborne and Brewer (1977), and Minamisono et al. (1978).
[b]S_f = Svedberg floatation.

than did the normal controls. The point is that it is important to examine the entire lipoprotein spectrum in evaluating a person's risk of CHD (Corday and Corday, 1975). A person may have a normal total cholesterol or β-lipoprotein concentration, but his or her HDL-cholesterol level may be inordinately low, thus placing the individual in a high-risk category for CHD. Whether having a moderately elevated serum cholesterol level (i.e., 275 to 325 mg/dl) with a high HDL-cholesterol level (i.e., >65 mg/dl) places the individual in a non-risk category cannot be answered at this time.

There are other reasons for lowering serum lipids besides the association of high lipid levels with increased incidence in CHD. Hypertriglyceridemia increases the chances for development of pancreatitis, which is a very serious complication of hyperchylomicronemia. Individuals with marked hyperchylomicronemia (Type I hyperlipoproteinemia) may develop eruptive xanthomatosis and lipemia retinalis. With hypercholesterolemia, xanthomas may develop, the most common type being tendon xanthomas. Other forms that can develop are xanthoma tuberosum, planar xanthoma, tuberoeruptive xanthoma, and xanthelasma. Corneal arcus due to lipid deposits in the corneal stroma may occur.

Effects of Specific Nutritional Substances on Serum Lipid Levels

There is little question that nutritional factors can affect serum lipid and lipoprotein levels and patterns. However, it is difficult to predict accurately the size of these changes, since the results are influenced by individual genetic differences in metabolism. Even in animals, such genetic differences occur. In a study (Malinow et al., 1976a), monkeys on a basal chow diet supplemented with 0.5 percent cholesterol for 30 days showed a wide range of serum cholesterol values (110 to 1180 mg/dl). The monkeys were then arbitrarily separated into hypo-, normo- and hyper-responders, depending upon their cholesterol level; the dividing concentrations were <290 and >990 mg/dl, respectively. It is clear that hypo- and hyper-responders differ greatly in their response to dietary cholesterol and that, when they ingest a diet almost free of cholesterol, their basal cholesterol level is also lower in hypo- than in the hyper-responders (Fig. 2). Similar findings have been reported in dogs (Mahley et al., 1974), rabbits (Fillins and Mann, 1956), rats (Imai and Matsumara, 1973), rhesus monkeys (Cox et al., 1958), and squirrel monkeys (Lofland et al., 1972), and humans are no exception.

Second, the effect of each individual nutritional component is influenced by other nutritional components in the diet. It is important to understand the interdependence of nutrients that are manipulated in fat-controlled diets. None of these factors (i.e., total calories, total fat, cholesterol, saturated fat, polyunsaturated fat, protein, carbohydrate, fiber) can be con-

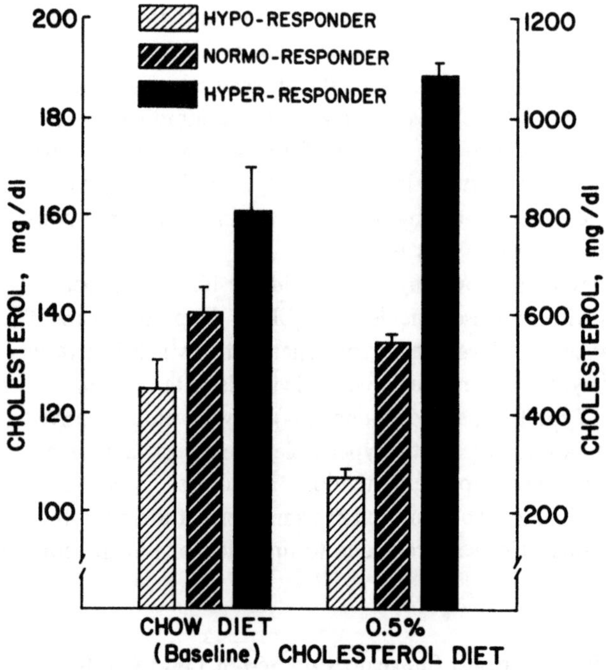

Fig. 2 Serum total cholesterol levels of monkeys on chow diet or cholesterol diet. The response of the animals seems to be dependent on whether they are normo-, hyper- or hyporesponders.

sidered alone. For example, feeding a high-cholesterol diet with low total fat will produce different degrees of hypercholesterolemia as compared to a diet high in cholesterol and high in total fat. Furthermore, the proportion of saturated fat versus mono- and polyunsaturated fats in the total fat component of the diet will have differing degrees of influence. Hegsted et al. (1965) have shown that serum cholesterol levels change at various levels of dietary cholesterol with three different dietary fats (coconut, olive, and safflower oils). All diets had 38 percent of the total calories as fat. In each series, three levels of cholesterol (100, 300, and 700 mg) were given to the subjects, who were fed a diet containing 38 percent, 17 percent and 48 percent of total calories as fat, protein, and carbohydrates, respectively. Aside from the fat in lean meat, fish, and poultry, all fat came from one of the three oils. The changes in serum cholesterol levels were compared to levels established when control subjects were fed a typical American diet. Regardless of the kind of oil in the diet, serum cholesterol concentration was reduced about 5 mg/dl for every 100 mg decrease in dietary cholesterol intake. With the olive oil (26 percent of calories as monounsaturated fat, with a P/S [polyunsaturated to saturated fat] ratio of 0.72), the cholesterol level was similar to that of the control subjects. With the coconut oil (32 percent of calories as saturated fats, with a P/S ratio of 0.03), serum cholesterol increased by 40 mg/dl above control levels, while the safflower oil (25 percent of calories as polyunsaturated fats with a P/S ratio of 5.00) was 40 mg/dl below the control group at each of the respective levels of cholesterol intake.

Studies with various animal models also have shown similar findings. For example, adult, male ground squirrels were fed a rat chow diet (4 percent total fat) supplemented with 2 percent cholesterol (by weight) for half a year and no elevation in serum cholesterol or triglycerides was observed (Naito and Gerrity, 1969). Like other previous studies, the following experiment emphasized the role of fats in influencing the coefficient of absorption of dietary cholesterol and/or decreased cholesterol catabolism and excretion to cause an elevation in the serum cholesterol level. Feeding a diet high in fat and cholesterol, resembling a typical American diet, produced hypercholesterolemia in this animal model (the ground squirrel). The diet, in fact, was 50 percent lower in cholesterol content (1.0 percent by weight), but much higher in fat—particularly in saturated fat—than that used in the previous study. The diet was composed of 30.4 percent fat, 38 percent carbohydrate, 25 percent protein, and 1.5 percent fiber; the remainder was ash.

While the effects of dietary cholesterol in inducing hypercholesterolemia in laboratory animals are convincing, the dietary cholesterol effects in humans are less clear. Certain animals, such as the rat and dog, are resistant to hypercholesterolemia by cholesterol feeding alone. The coefficient of absorption of these two animal models is high (i.e., about 80 to 90 percent), but their ability to completely suppress cholesterol synthesis and increase cholesterol catabolism and excretion is remarkably high, thus enabling them to maintain serum cholesterol homeostasis (Dietschy and Wilson, 1970). The rabbit, on the other hand, readily absorbs cholesterol, but seems to have difficulty in catabolizing and excreting exogenous cholesterol. The prairie dog may fit into this category since it, too, is extremely responsive to cholesterol feeding (Holzbach et al., 1976). In humans, the coefficient of absorption is around 40 percent, depending upon the composition of the diet and the amount of dietary cholesterol. There is still some controversy as to how well the suppression of cholesterol synthesis works by the negative feedback system in humans. It is believed that 3-hydroxy-3-methyl-glutaryl CoA reductase, the rate-limiting enzyme for cholesterol synthesis, can be suppressed by the end-product negative feedback system, but only partially in humans (Grundy et al., 1969). Mattson et al. (1972) have shown that by increasing the cholesterol content of a diet originally low in cholesterol, the serum cholesterol level increases by 5 to 12 mg dl^{-1} 100 mg dietary $cholesterol^{-1}$ 1000 $kcal^{-1}$, providing all other dietary constituents remain unchanged. When the original diet contains substantial amounts of cholesterol, additional dietary cholesterol does not seem to greatly effect the serum levels (Kummerow et al., 1977). However, not all authors agree (Connor and Connor, 1977).

Plant sterols (i.e., campesterol, stigmasterol, and β-stitosterol) are observed in the blood only to a slight extent, since most of them pass out in the stool. Of these phytosterols, β-stitosterol usually predominates in the blood, constituting 60 to 90 percent of the total plant steroids. In a typical American diet, which may contain between 200 to 400 mg of β-stitosterol/day, its coefficient of absorption is about 20 to 30 percent. In pharmacologic amounts, β-stitosterol has been known to have a hypocholesterolemic effect because of interference with the absorption of cholesterol. Mattson et al. (1977) suggested that the extensive solubility of the phytosterol esters in fat, in contrast to the limited solubility of their unesterified form, provides a means for administering effective amounts of these hypocholesterolemic agents in dietary therapy.

First described by Feigle (1918), alcoholic hyperlipemia has been subject to extensive investigations during the 1960s and 1970s (Leiber et al., 1962; Schapiro et al., 1965; Mistius and Ockner, 1972; Lifton and Scheig, 1978). Studies by Losowsky et al. (1963), Schapiro et al. (1965), and Lifton and Scheig (1978) demonstrated that alcohol ingestion in chronic alcoholics can cause hypertriglyceridemia. This lipid abnormality is resolved rapidly with abstention from alcohol and is apparently not provoked by a high-carbohydrate diet. The sera of chronic alcoholics frequently show a Type IV hyperlipoproteinemic pattern with high levels of very-low-density β-lipoprotein, along with elevated triglycerides and cholesterol. The alcohol-related Type IV hyperlipoproteinemia appears different from the carbohydrate-induced Type IV and is independent of acute pancreatitis, liver dysfunction, and obesity. Often, some normolipidemic individuals who have imbibed heavily on the weekend will show marked hypertriglyceridemia lasting for several days. It is not uncommon to observe levels in excess of 1000 mg/dl in these individuals, particularly if they are hypertriglyceridemic subjects who are sensitive to caloric excess, causing hyper-pre-β-lipoproteinemia (unpublished report). Leiber (1974) and Bouchier and Dawson (1964) suggested that alcohol might effect serum lipid levels by impairment of plasma triglyceride removal and increased synthesis of triglyceride-rich lipoproteins.

According to Connor and Connor (1977), the type of protein consumed in mixed human diets has been shown to have no significant effect upon plasma lipid levels in humans. However, casein appears to be more cholesterolemic and/or atherogenic than soya protein for chickens (Kritchevsky et al., 1959) and rabbits (Newburgh and Squire, 1920; Meeker and Kesten, 1940). Dietary protein influences blood lipids, particularly cholesterol levels, in growing animals (Leveille and Fisher, 1958; Nishida et al., 1958; Yeh and Leveille, 1969). In individuals with kwashiorkor, there appears to be decreased serum β-lipoprotein, total cholesterol, triglycerides, and albumin, but α-lipoprotein and lecithin levels are not reduced (Onitiri and Boyo, 1975). It has been suggested that the decreased synthesis of the apoprotein moiety of LDL is the limiting factor for the low lipid level (Flores et al., 1970) in protein deficiency. The impaired rate of synthesis of the lipoprotein would cause triglycerides to accumulate in the liver.

Purified cholesterol is quite unstable when stored in air at room temperature. Recent data on the cytotoxic effects of products of cholesterol autooxidation (namely 25-hydroxycholesterol and cholestane-3β,5α,6β-triol) on aortic smooth muscle cells warrant mention (Imai et al., 1976; Peng et al., 1978), since it is conceivable that the effects might lead to initial lesion of atherosclerosis. Imai et al. (1976) showed that impurities in old USP-grade cholesterol stored at room temperature caused aortic lesions when a total of 1 g of concentrated autooxidative products of cholesterol/kg body weight was administered to rabbits over a seven-week period. The possible implication of these findings is that foods containing cholesterol, particularly those that receive heat and oxygen treatment during processing (e.g., spray-dried eggs and whole milk) could prove to be hazardous to one's health. Their work further suggests that pure cholesterol (either endogenously synthesized by the animal or chemically isolated, purified cholesterol) is not atherogenic. Only when cholesterol becomes a mixture of cholesterol plus spontaneously produced toxic derivatives does it become highly atherogenic. It appears that future studies should include an evaluation of commercially available foods that probably contain toxic derivatives of cholesterol.

Related to the cytotoxic effects of cholesterol autooxidation products is hypervitaminosis D. Vitamin D_3 feeding (intermittent or continuous) does not appear to influence serum cholesterol levels, but does result in development of atherosclerosis and calcified coronary arteries in animals with normal lipid levels (Taura et al., 1978). Kummerow (1977) has reported the presence of cellular debris in the abdonimal aortas of swine when given higher levels of vitamin D_3 than the National Research Council recommends for swine. Additional findings by Kummerow et al. (1976) suggest that high intake of vitamin D_3 will cause degeneration of smooth muscle cells in the aorta.

Nutritional Modification for the Prevention and Treatment of Hyperlipidemia and Dyslipoproteinemia

With the development of the original concepts of the five recognized types of dyslipoproteinemic conditions by Fredrickson et al. (1967), five types of diets were formulated and prescribed (Fredrickson et al., 1974). The different diets have about the same fat composition when available food products are used, except for the Type I diet. All have less than 300 mg of cholesterol and are similar in their P/S ratio. Thus, a single-diet concept for

Table 2. Nutrient Composition of the Master Food Plan

Food Patterns	*Fat (% Calories)*	*Carbohydrate (% Calories)*	*Protein (% Calories)*	*P/S Ratio*	*Cholesterol (mg/day)*
Typical American diet	40	45	15	0.4	750
Moderate-fat diet	40	40	20	1.3	<300
Semi-low-fat diet	35	50	15	2.0	100–300
Low-fat diet	15	65	20	1.3	<300

the treatment of hyperlipidemia is emerging that should be simpler and more practical. Connor and Connor (1977) suggested an "alternative diet," in which cholesterol intake is 100 mg/day, and protein, carbohydrate, and fat intake are 15, 65, and 20 percent, respectively. The P/S ratio is 1.3 and crude fiber intake of 12 to 15 g/day is recommended. The Inter-Society Commission for Heart Disease Resources recommends the use of a moderate-fat diet, suggesting the use of 30 to 35 percent of the total calories as fat (<10 percent saturated fat and ⩾10 percent as polyunsaturated fat). Cholesterol intake is maintained below 300 mg/day. Originally, the Cleveland Clinic used two different diets (Brown, 1971). One was low in fat, with 15 percent of the total calories as fat, and the other was a vegetable oil diet, with 38 percent of the total calories as fat. Serum lipids were equally reduced with either diet in hypercholesterolemic subjects (Brown et al., 1973). In hypertriglyceridemic patients (Types IIb and IV) serum lipids were reduced with greater effectiveness with the 38 percent fat diet than with the 15 percent fat diet. Recently, the Cleveland Clinic has increased the fat content of the Basic Master Food Plan (semi-low-fat diet) from 33 percent to 35 percent, with an elevation of the P/S ratio to 2.0 (Table 2). The Basic Master Food Plan may be used as a guide with which to commence treatment of most patients with the various forms of primary hyperlipoproteinemias (Table 3). The fat content may be varied as best suits a person's needs. The Master Food Patterns include a range of fat-containing diets, from one with a very low fat content (15 percent), but which is high in carbohydrate (65 percent), to one with a fat content near that of the American diet (40 percent), but which is low in carbohydrate (40 percent).

Patients with hypercholesterolemia will respond to a diet with a fat concent of 35 percent of the total calories and with a P/S ratio of 2:1. The quality of the dietary fat is exceedingly important. The intake of animal fat, which is generally high in saturated fat should be minimized; about 7 ounces of low-fat meats (Table 4) per day is the suggested maximum. The polyunsaturated fats (liquid vegetable oils, with the exception of coconut and plam oils) should be substituted for animal fats in the diet. Not all vegetable oils have the same quality of fat. Safflower oil has the highest content of polyunsaturated fats (Table 5), while coconut and palm oils have the lowest.

Table 3. Classification of Types of Primary Hyperlipoproteinemia[a,b]

Clinical manifestations	*Type I*	*Type IIa*	*Type IIb*	*Type III*	*Type IV*	*Type V*
Incidence	Rare	Common	Common	Uncommon	Common	Uncommon
Lipoprotein abnormalities by ultracentrifuge[c]	Severe chylomicronemia	↑LDL	↑LDL, ↑VLDL	VLDL + LDL of abnormal composition	↑VLDL	↑VLDL ↑chylomicrons
Lipoprotein abnormalities by electrophoresis[d]	Chylomicron band at origin	↑B-band	↑B ↑Pre-B band	Broad B (or floating B)	↑Pre-B-band	↑Chylomicrons ↑Pre-B band
Plasma appearance	Creamy layer over clear plasma	Clear or slightly turbid	Clear or slightly turbid	Turbid	Turbid	Creamy layer over turbid plasma
Cholesterol	↑↔	↑	↑	↑	↔	↔
Triglyceride	↑↑	↔	↑	↑	↑	↑
Age of onset	Infancy and childhood	At birth, if genetic; early childhood	At birth, if genetic; early childhood	Third decade, often after menopause in women	Third decade or later; can occur in children with obesity or diabetes	Early adulthood; rare in children
Familial forms	Deficiency of lipoprotein lipase	Familial hyperlipoproteinemia also called familial hypercholesterolemia, most common hyperlipoproteinemia, expressed in two forms; heterozygote (more common disorder, cholesterol concentration elevated but LDL not grossly abnormal), homozygote (less common but cholesterol and LDL levels markedly exaggerated)		Genetic mode uncertain; often called Broad B disease or remnant disease. B-Lipoprotein electrophoretic mobility, but has Pre-B density characteristics. This fraction has	Second most common form; often half of adult close relatives will also have Type IV	When familial, more than half of close relatives have either Type IV or Type V

Table 3. (Continued)

Clinical manifestations	*Type I*	*Type IIa*	*Type IIb*	*Type III*	*Type IV*	*Type V*
				a high amount of triglycerides and low amounts of cholesterol		
Clinical presentation	Episodes of abdominal pain associated with ingestion of dietary fat, pancreatitis, eruptive xanthomas, hepatosplenomegaly, lipemia retinalis, serum lupus erythematosus, lymphoma	Premature vascular disease; tendon and tuberous xanthomas, arcus cornea in 50% of patients	Severe forms are like Type IIa; milder Type IIb patterns tend to be accompanied by glucose intolerance, overweight	Glucose intolerance, tuberoeruptive or planar xanthomas, premature vascular disease, worsened by alcohol excess	Abnormal insulin levels, glucose intolerance in about 50%; excess caloric intake common; occasionally eruptive xanthomas, hyperuricemia, hepatosplenomegaly; worsened by alcohol excess	Bouts of abdominal pain and pancreatitis, eruptive xanthomas, premature atherosclerotic heart disease, hepatosplenomegaly; excess caloric intake common; hyperuricemia, most patients have glucose intolerance, worsened by alcohol excess

Table 3. (Continued)

Clinical manifestations	*Type I*	*Type IIa*	*Type IIb*	*Type III*	*Type IV*	*Type V*
Rule out[b]	Dysgammaglobulinemia, diabetes mellitus, pancreatitis	Thyroid dysfunction, nephrotic syndrome, obstructive liver disease		Dysgammaglobulinemia, thyroid dysfunction	Diabetes mellitus, glycogen storage disease, nephrotic syndrome, pregnancy, Werner's syndrome	Multiple myeloma macroglobulinemia, nephrotic syndrome, alcoholism, pancreatitis, gout
Drug therapy	No effective drug therapy at present	May require combination of diet and drug therapy		–	–	–

[a]From Cleveland Clinic Foundation Diet Manual (1978).

[b]Primary (familial) forms of hyperlipoproteinemia are genetically defined as those which result from the genetic defect and are not the result of separate endocrine disorders, metabolic disorders, improper nutrition, drug interference, and the like, which are secondary (or acquired) hyperlipoproteinemias. All secondary forms of hyperlipoproteinemia must be ruled out before considering treatment of primary hyperlipoproteinemia.

[c]LDL = low-density (beta) lipoproteins; VLDL = very-low-density (pre-beta) lipoproteins; B = beta.

[d] $\uparrow$ = increased concentration; $\downarrow$ = decreased concentration; $\leftrightarrow$ = no change.

Table 4. Fat Content of Meat, Fish, and Poultry

Low-fat meats	Poultry, veal, fish
Medium-fat meats	Roasts, steaks, hamburger, lamb, pork, ham
High-fat meats	Bacon, salt pork, sausages, duck, goose, luncheon meats, frankfurters, beef marbled with fat, chicken and turkey fat

Table 5. Fatty Acid Content of Some Food Products[a,b]

Food Item	*Saturated Fatty Acids*	*Monounsaturated Fatty Acids*	*Polyunsaturated Fatty Acids*
Oils, salad or cooking			
Safflower	8	15	72
Corn	10	28	53
Soybean	15	20	52
Cottonseed	25	21	50
Sesame	14	38	42
Peanut	18	47	29
Olive	11	76	7
Coconut	86	7	–
Beef products[c]			
Porterhouse	36	17	16
Sirloin	29	14	13
Round	12	6	5
Hamburger, lean	10.0	5	4
Hamburger, regular	21.2	10	9
Pork[c]			
Ham	10	11	2
Loin	25	9	10
Fish[c]			
Trout	3	2	–
Salmon	5	5	–
Chicken[c]			
Dark meat, with skin	6	2	2
Dark meat, without skin	4	1	1
Cheeses			
Cheddar	18	11	1
Cottage	2	1	–
Cream	21	12	1
Swiss	15	9	1
Butter	46	27	2
Margarine	18	47	14
Milk, whole	2	1	–
Egg, whole	4	5	1

[a]In percentages.
[b]From Watt and Merrill (1963).
[c]Uncooked.

Olive and peanut oil may be used occasionally. Only special margarines containing large amounts of unhydrogenated liquid vegetable oils are suitable for the diet. Brown et al. (1971) have suggested that knowing the P/S ratio is not sufficient for planning an effective diet because it alone does not indicate the level of fatty acids. When 36 to 42 percent of the calories come from fat, the critical limit of saturated fat in the diet must be <14 percent and the polyunsaturated fat must be >15 percent. In the semi-low-fat diet, in which 35 percent of the calories is derived from fat, the maximum allowable amount of saturated fat is 12 percent and the minimum allowable amount of polyunsaturated fat is 13 percent. As can be seen, the critical limits account for the proportion of fatty acids in relation to the total fat, which will vary from one prescribed diet to another to suit each individual need. Eggs should be limited to 2 to 3 per week. Careful attention should be given to shellfish, sardines, and liver for the high-cholesterol content (Table 6). Notice that crab and shrimp are also high in cholesterol content. Liver contains five times as much cholesterol as beef (steaks). Therefore, when adding liver to the diet, careful attention should be given to the cholesterol and fat composition. Type IIa hyperlipoproteinemic subjects, particularly homozygous hyper-β-lipoproteinemic, may be very resistant to this diet and require further reduction in cholesterol intake from 300 to 200 or even 100 mg/day, followed by drug therapy if necessary.

Hypertriglyceridemia and hyper-pre-β-lipoproteinemia (Type IV) are reduced by a diet low in carbohydrates and require a carbohydrate intake of less than 50 percent, of which the simple refined sugars should be substituted with complex carbohydrates (starches, dietary fiber). The Cleveland Clinic's basic moderate-fat diet calls for 40 percent of the total calories as fat and carbohydrates. If hypertriglyceridemia and hypercholesterolemia (Type V) exist, the semi-low-fat diet should be utilized to reduce the exogenous fat intake to 30 percent of the total calories and the carbohydrate intake to 50 percent. The other two mixed hyperlipidemias (Types IIb and III) respond to the moderate-fat diet. Table 6 gives suggestions on how the Master Food Plan may be applied to the various dyslipoproteinemic conditions. It is imperative that the proper diagnosis be made and that all acquired disorders be corrected before instituting the prescribed diets. It must be remembered that the caloric intake of the diets is calculated on the basis of obtaining and maintaining ideal body weight. Since the serum lipids and lipoproteins usually respond to the prescribed dietary therapy within three weeks, a follow-up program is necessary. Continuing encouragement and reassurance are needed, along with reliable information, if the program is to be successful.

When formulating a particular diet, it is important that a conscious effort be made to decrease the simple sugar consumption and replace it with complex carbohydrates. Consumption of fruits and vegetables should be

Table 6. Meats, Fish, and Poultry[a,b]

Food Item	*Cholesterol/100 g*	*Fat/100 g*
Beef	91	5.3
Chicken		
Light meat	79	3.4
Dark meat	91	6.3
Clams	63	1.6
Crab	101	1.9
Haddock	60	0.5
Halibut	50	7.0
Lamb	100	7.5
Lobster	85	1.5
Oysters	50	1.8 (raw)
Pork	88	8.6
Rabbit	91	5.0 (raw)
Salmon	47	5.9
Scallops	53	1.4
Tuna	63	0.8
Turkey		
Light meat	77	3.9
Dark meat	101	8.3
Veal	99	6.0
Sardines	140	8.6 (raw)
Shrimp	150	0.8 (raw)
Liver	438	3.8 (raw)
Average of beef	91	6
Average of beef and liver	125.5	5.8
Average of fish	64	2.5
Average of poultry	87	5.5
Average of fish and poultry	71	3.5

[a]From Feeley et al. (1972), and Watt and Merrill (1963).
[b]Lean (where possible) and cooked.

Table 7. Summary: Use of the Master Food Plan for Primary Dyslipoproteinemias

Type of Hyperlipidemia	*Elevation of Lipoproteins*	*Type of Hyperlipoproteinemia*	*Diet (P/S Ratio)*
Exogenous triglycerides	Chylomicron	I	Low-fat, 15% (P/S = 1.3%)
Endogenous triglycerides	Pre-β-Lipoprotein	IV	Moderate fat, 40% (P/S = 1.3%)
Cholesterol	β-Lipoprotein	IIa	Semi-low-fat, 35% (P/S = 2.0%)
Mixed hyperlipidemia	β-Lipoprotein Pre-β-Lipoprotein	IIb	Moderate fat, 40% (P/S = 2.0%)
Mixed hyperlipidemia	– Intermediate-Density Lipoprotein	III	Moderate fat, 40% (P/S = 1.3%)
Mixed hyperlipidemia	– Pre-β-Lipoprotein Chylomicron	V	Semi-low-fat, 30% (P/S = 1.3%)

highly encouraged. At present, the average American consumes about 2 to 4 g of dietary fiber daily, while vegetarians consume about 24 g/day. Perhaps the dietary fiber intake should be increased to about 10 to 15 g/day for adequate nutrition. During the past century, composition of the average American diet has changed; complex carbohydrates (fruits, vegetables, and grain products), which once were the mainstay of the diet, now play a minor role. At the same time, fat and sugar consumption have risen markedly; these two dietary elements alone now comprise more than 50 percent of our total caloric intake, up 50 percent from the early 1900s (Dietary Goals for the United States, 1977).

Since plant proteins have a plasma-cholesterol-lowering effect, as compared with animal proteins, the diet should be comprised of at least 50 percent plant protein, as compared to 30 percent in the standard American diet.

It is important that alcohol intake be restricted, especially by the Type I and V patient, when following the prescribed diets. Patients with the other dyslipoproteinemic forms may tolerate alcohol if taken only occasionally, and providing it does not interfere with the weight reduction program or with maintaining ideal body weight.

Table 7 summarizes the use of the Master Food Plan for the various hyperlipidemic and hyperlipoproteinemic conditions.

Since elevated blood pressure may accompany hyperlipidemia in 15 to 20 percent of the patients, salt intake should also be monitored. Salt (sodium chloride) consumption in the United States is estimated to be between 6 and 18 g/day. The Select Committee on Nutrition and Human Needs suggests reducing salt consumption by about 50 to 85 percent, to approximately 3 g/day (Dietary Goals for the United States, 1977).

In the last analysis, it is preventive measures through public education that will best enable us to achieve our ultimate goal of minimizing the risk to atherosclerosis. It is particularly important that parents be educated so that proper behavior patterns and preferences are taught to children by the age of six, an age when acquired traits are probably well implanted.

Role of Physician and Dietitian in Dietary Management

The ideal approach in attempting to lower a patient's risk to CHD is a team approach, particularly when considering dietary management for treating hyperlipidemia. An intimate working relationship should exist between the physician(s), dietitian, and patient. It is imperative that the physician recognizes the importance of nutrition in the overall health care of the patient, has a full understanding and working knowledge of nutritional factors that have been associated with high risk for CHD, and has current knowledge on the most effective way(s) to control the lipid abnormalities via proper dietary management. In the development of this intimate relationship, the first step is close communication of all these people with one another. The physician must adopt the attitude that he or she can depend upon the professional knowledge and experiences of the dietitian in helping the goal of effective patient care to be achieved. The dietitian should be as familiar with the patient as is the physician. Information on the patient's lifestyle, eating habits, likes and dislikes, food practices, and CHD risks should be apparent to both the physician and dietitian in order that they can plan the most effective means of reducing the patient's risk to CHD. With this approach, the responsibility of the dietitian should not only encompass the control of elevated serum lipids through dietary management, but should also include the consideration of diet in the control of elevated blood pressure and body weight, and advice concerning excessive smoking and lack of physical activity as a comprehensive health care therapy for the patient.

For this system of therapy to succeed, it is important that the patient be informed of the seriousness of his or her physical condition and the logic behind instituting the various approaches to minimize the associated risk factors for premature coronary events. Patient education is sadly lacking in most institutions. Unless the physician and dietitian are confident, knowledgeable, and enthusiastic about the effectiveness of minimizing the risk of CHD through dietary management, the patient will not develop the attitude necessary to comply with the prescribed diets and possible altered lifestyle. During instruction, it is most important that the patient help in planning his or her diet; the person buying the food and preparing the meals should also be present. While hyperlipidemia can be genetically determined, in many instances it is also due to environmental conditions, especially improper food habits. If the latter condition applies to the patient, the acquired hyperlipidemic condition of the patient can also be potentially manifested in the other members of the family, particularly the children. Therefore, nutritional education directed toward all members of the family, particularly those who purchase and prepare the meals, is beneficial to all. The prepared meals should, ideally, include the rest of the family members, unless the prescribed diet is drastic and applies only to a person with severe risk factors. It is our experience that group instruction is more effective than individual instruction because of the beneficial effects of interaction among members of the group.

One of the reasons for the poor compliance with diets is the poor design, or even lack of design, of a follow-up period. This is important for both the physician and patient. The physician needs to monitor the blood lipids and lipoproteins to determine the effectiveness of the prescribed diet, while the patient needs further instructions, information on the progress made, and positive reinforcement. In the follow-up period, visits at two, four, and six weeks after the initial two- to three-hour instruction should be adequate. After the initial follow-up period, less frequent visits (perhaps once a year) are required to insure adherence to the diet pattern. The continued objective is to follow through with the measurements that test adherence to the diet, including: body weight, blood lipids and lipoproteins, and blood pressure. The examination should also include discussion of alcohol consumption and smoking patterns. Finally, the patient must always receive encouragement to stay on the diet and physical exercise program.

SPECIAL CONSIDERATIONS

Vitamin C and Lipid Metabolism

Since the late 1970s, there has been considerable interest in vitamins and their role in lipid metabolism; vitamin C, in particular, has received much attention. Biochemical progress on the investigation of vitamin C has advanced rapidly since the isolation and identification of the vitamin by King and Waugh (1932). Vitamin C seems to be involved in at least two systems: (1) the maintenance of vascular wall integrity; and (2) the metabolism of cholesterol to bile acids. Knowledge concerning the basic physiology of its effects on the vascular system, however, has failed to keep pace with the progress of chemical information. It is known that the requirement for ascorbate in collagen biosynthesis is due to its involvement in the hydroxylation of proline and lysine to collagen hydroxyproline and hydroxylysine, respectively (Gould, 1961; Robertson and Van, 1961; Barnes et al., 1970). There is evidence to suggest not only that collagen biosynthesis in inhibited, but that there is an increasing degree of degradation of partially hydroxylated collagen to diffusible peptides in scorbutogenic guinea pigs. It is also known that there is an increase in vascular permeability in animals maintained on atherogenic diets (Gould, 1961; Friedman and Byers, 1963; Veress et al., 1970), drugs (Harman, 1962; Shimamoto, 1966; Robertson and Khairallah, 1973), hormones (Eades, 1966; Koletsky et al., 1966; Robertson and Khairallah, 1971), elevated blood pressure (Esterly and Glagov, 1963; Giese, 1964; Wiener et al., 1969), and possible vitamin C deficiency (Lee, 1961). Since the rat has the ability to synthesize ascorbate, the study (Lee, 1961) on permeability changes due to low vitamin C intake is questionable.

The etiology of atherogenesis is not fully understood. There appear to be several possible mechanisms for the initial development of the arterial vascular disease, but one possible common denominator is a change in vascular permeability (Gore and Stefanovic, 1967). Since collagen is a major component in the arterial blood vessel, it is not unreasonable to suspect that a dysmetabolism of collagen may later alter the arterial wall structure and ultimately affect vascular wall permeability, predisposing the blood vessel to the development of atherosclerotic lesion formation.

The guinea pig, like humans, nonhuman primates, certain birds, and the Indian fruit-eating bat, but unlike most other species, cannot synthesize vitamin C, and is therefore dependent upon exogenous sources for meeting its daily requirements. It has been reported that there is an inverse relationship between liver ascorbic acid concentration and hepatic cholesterol concentration in guinea pigs (Ginter et al., 1967; Ginter and Ondreicka, 1971). Cholesterol accumulation in the liver during low ascorbate intake did not appear to originate from increase synthesis or absorption during times when liver ascorbate was low. However, decreased liver ascorbate appeared to decrease the conversion of cholesterol to bile acids for excretion via the bile (Ginter et al., 1971). Vitamin C may be a necessary cofactor for the hydroxylation of the cholesterol nucleus to form bile acids. It was concluded that this decreased rate of cholesterol catabolism and excretion leads to hypercholesterolemia.

There is a wide divergence of opinion concerning the significance of vitamin C levels in relation to atherosclerosis in human beings. Willis (1953) noted that there frequently was a deficiency of ascorbic acid in the arterial wall of hospitalized patients, and that old age seemed to accentuate the deficiency. He also noted that the lowest levels were in areas most prone to development of atherosclerosis (Willis and Fishman, 1955). Sokoloff et al. (1967) reported that of 20 atherosclerotic, hypercholesterolemic patients, the serum cholesterol decreased 30 percent and the β-lipoprotein decreased 25 percent after a 30-day course of 0.5 g of ascorbic acid three times a day. Normal subjects showed a significant decrease in serum cholesterol levels when 1.0 g ascorbic acid was added to their diet, while those with atherosclerosis receiving clofibrate for treatment of hyperlipidemia or anticoagulant therapy tended to show increased cholesterol levels with high vitamin C intake (Spittle, 1972). Young, normal subjects, when given 1.0 g ascorbic acid per day for 6 weeks in addition to their usual dietary intake, failed to show any significant change in serum cholesterol level (Anderson et al., 1972). Ginter et al. (1970) found decreased plasma cholesterol levels after ascorbic acid therapy in hypercholesterolemic subjects (>200 mg/dl) with initial low blood ascorbic acid levels. In another study, Ginter (1975) reported that 1 g of ascorbic acid daily for a period of three months given to subjects 50 to 75 years of age with a mean cholesterol level of <200 mg/dl had no effect on plasma cholesterol levels. Peterson et al. (1975) administered 4 g of ascorbic acid daily for two months to hypercholesterolemic patients and found no effect on serum lipids.

Since there are conflicting reports on the effects of ascorbate on serum cholesterol levels, we examined the relation of varying intake of ascorbate on serum lipid levels, first in the guinea pig, and second in human beings.

Some of the confusion in the literature appears to be related to the fact that several studies focused upon acute avitaminosis C rather than chronic hypovitaminosis C. Furthermore, the studies used different means of ascorbate administration (via drinking water, gastric intubation, or intraperitoneal injection). Another factor that may have influenced the results is the vehicle that was used in the vitamin C solution. Some investigators used ascorbate in water, while others used sucrose to increase the palatability of the ascorbate. In the present study, a commercial source was used (Ce-Vi Sol from Mead Johnson and Co., Evansville, Indiana), in which ascorbic acid was diluted in a glycerine solution to minimize the oxidation of L-ascorbate to dehydroascorbate, a reaction that occurs extremely rapidly. It is possible that those who provided ascorbate in the drinking water did not obtain the result of ascorbate, but rather the dehydroascorbate effect. Furthermore, when vitamin C is provided in drinking-water bottles, it is not possible to predict the exact amount of ascorbate intake, because there is much spillage when the animals drink. There is also the problem of varying water intake by different animals.

In the first experiment, an acute vitamin C deficiency study was made by feeding ten adult male guinea pigs (English short-hair strain) a chow diet (Reid-Briggs guinea pig diet, ICN Pharmaceutical Co.; Inc., Cleveland, Ohio) completely devoid of vitamin C (Table 8). Ten age-matched control male guinea pigs fed a guinea pig chow containing vitamin C were used to obtain baseline values. Ascorbate content in tissues and sera was measured by the

Table 8. Composition of the Reid-Briggs Scorbutogenic Diet[a,b]

Nutrients	*Percentage by Weight*
Alphacel	15.0
Corn oil	7.3
Glucose	7.8
Salt mixture	6.0
Starch, corn	20.0
Sucrose	10.3
Vitamin-free casein	30.0
Magnesium oxide	0.5
Potassium acetate	2.5
Vitamin fortification mixture[c]	0.6

[a]From Reid and Briggs (1953).
[b]Semisynthetic diet was made by Nutritional Biochemicals Co., Cleveland, Ohio.
[c]Vitamin C fortification, normally consisting of 0.2 percent, was omitted when the diet was made.

method described by Roe and Kuethner (1943). All lipid analyses were done on fasting samples. A detailed description of the methods is described elsewhere (Naito et al., 1977). The results are presented in Table 9. After two weeks on the experimental diet, signs of acute scurvy were demonstrated by microhemorrhages of the small blood vessels of the tibia-femur joint. After two weeks on the scorbutogenic diet, there was a significant reduction in body weight. The level of vitamin C in most organs reached scorbutogenic levels. However, the acute avitaminosis C condition did not appear to be associated with changes in serum lipid levels. Because the animals demonstrated signs of metabolic distress (e.g., cessation of eating, loss of body weight, and lethargy), it appears that these types of acute studies may yield misleading results. This was confirmed after examination of data that was collected by repeating the experiment; it was found that the avitaminosis C

Table 9. Acute Study: Effects of Acute Avitaminosis C for 14 Days ($\bar{X} \pm$ S.D.)[a]

Analytes	*Initial Day 0*[b] *(Baseline Values)*	*Final Day 14*[b]	*Significance*
Total weight change (grams)	800 – 1000	– 47.3 ± 33	$p < .05$
Serum ascorbate (mg/dl)	0.64 ± 0.41	0.052 ± .04	$p < .01$
Urine ascorbate (mg/dl)	1.37 ± 0.79	0.86 ± 0.55	N.S.
Liver ascorbate (mg/100 g)	12.37 ± 6.11	1.15 ± 0.38	$p < .01$
Adrenal ascorbate (mg/100 g)	86.77 ± 29.22	8.05 ± 2.45	$p < .01$
Spleen ascorbate (mg/100 g)	36.11 ± 11.8	4.17 ± 0.6	$p < .01$
Serum cholesterol (mg/dl)	44.7 ± 13.3	58.0 ± 4.4	N.S.
Liver cholesterol (mg/100 g)	302.6 ± 62.8	328.8 ± 26.5	N.S.
Serum triglycerides (mg/dl)	61.8 ± 26.7	146.6 ± 50.3	$p < .1$

[a]Animals were fed the Reid-Briggs guinea pig scorbutogenic diet.
[b]N = 10 animals per group.

Table 10. Experimental Design–Guinea Pig Study

Ascorbate Intake (mg animal^{-1} day^{-1})	*No. Animals (N)*	*Group*	*Diet*
0.5	6	Hypovitaminosis C	Scorbutogenic[a]
5.0	6	Experimental control	Scorbutogenic
50.0	6	Hypervitaminosis C	Scorbutogenic
Normal	6	Control	Chow[b]

[a]Animals were fed the Reid-Briggs guinea pig scorbutogenic diet (with and without cholesterol supplementation) and given vitamin C via tubal intubation.
[b]Animals were fed the Reid-Briggs guinea pig chow diet with 0.2 g percent (w/w) vitamin C fortification.

condition resulted in a 21 percent elevation of the serum cholesterol concentration (unpublished report).

A follow-up study was designed to examine the chronic effects of varying levels of vitamin C (Ce-Vi Sol from Mead-Johnson Laboratories, Evansville, Indiana) intake on serum and liver cholesterol concentration in adult male guinea pigs fed either a chow diet or a 2.0 percent cholesterol- (by weight) supplemented chow diet. The experimental design of this study is presented in Table 10. Since it has been reported that 5 to 10 mg animal^{-1} day^{-1} is the recommended requirement for vitamin C for adult guinea pigs (Banerjec and Singh, 1958; Ginter and Ondreicka, 1971), that daily dose was arbitrarily adopted for the present studies. They are referred to here as "experimental" controls. The 0.5 mg animal^{-1} day^{-1} group, then, was considered the hypovitaminosis C group, and the 50 mg animal^{-1} day^{-1} group was considered the hypervitaminosis C group. A fourth group (control) was fed the standard guinea pig diet (Reid-Briggs), which contained about 0.2 g percent of vitamin C (by weight). The first three groups were fed the Reid-Briggs scorbutogenic diet (Table 8) and were given daily vitamin C via gastric intubation for six weeks, after which time the study was terminated. After

Table 11. Effect of Different Levels of Ascorbate Intake on Serum Lipid Concentration of Guinea Pigs Fed Chow Diet ($\bar{X} \pm$ S.E.M.)

		Ascorbate	
Ascorbate Intake (mg animal^{-1} day^{-1})[a]	*Body Weight (g)*	*Serum (mg/dl)*	*Liver (mg/100 g tissue)*
0.5	498 ± 36	0.028 ± 0.006	1.001 ± 0.187
5.0	590 ± 44	1.068 ± 0.01	5.467 ± 0.176
50.0	535 ± 27	0.1475 ± 0.04	8.649 ± 1.720
Normal[b]	661 ± 33.2	0.35 ± 0.02	9.18 ± 1.0

[a]Animals were fed Reid-Briggs scorbutogenic diet and given Vitamin C via tubal intubation.
[b]Animals were fed Reid-Briggs guinea pig chow diet with 0.2 g percent (by weight) Vitamin C fortification.

Table 12. Effect of Different Levels of Ascorbate Intake on Serum Lipid Concentration of Guinea Pigs Fed Chow Diet ($\bar{X} \pm$ S.E.M.)

Ascorbate Intake	*Serum Lipids (mg/dl)*			*Liver Lipids (mg/100 g tissue)*		
(mg animal^{-1} day^{-1})	*Chol*[a]	*TG*[b]	*PL*[c]	*Chol*	*TG*	*PL*
0.5	110.7 ± 13.2	168 ± 58.1	88.0 ± 14.3	570.1 ± 95.3	1887.3 ± 444.4	3710.2 ± 130.5
5.0	73.8 ± 15.7	87.3 ± 14.9	22.8 ± 10.4	366.7 ± 39.6	3133.2 ± 1175.4	3063.2 ± 54.6
50.0	61.0 ± 3.5	102.0 ± 35.0	47.6 ± 1.7	372.7 ± 31.7	1426.5 ± 334.6	3738.4 ± 153.4
Normal[d]	44.8 ± 5.0	77.2 ± 19.1	68.8 ± 6.6	275.3 ± 4.0	4227.9 ± 591.4	3824.3 ± 101.6

[a]Chol = Total cholesterol.
[b]TG = Triglycerides.
[c]PL = Total phospholipids.
[d]Fed Reid-Briggs guinea pig chow diet with 0.2 g percent (by weight) Vitamin C fortification.

removing 2.5 ml of blood (for lipid studies) via the jugular vein, an equal amount of Evans blue dye was infused and allowed to circulate for two hours while the animals were under amytol anesthesia. The animals were then sacrificed and the tissues removed, frozen with liquid nitrogen, and stored until analyzed. The aorta of each animal was removed quickly, rinsed in buffered 1.3 percent formaldehyde solution, and cut longitudinally, and the intima was examined for Evans blue uptake.

The effects of different levels of vitamin C intake on body weight, serum and liver ascorbate, and cholesterol concentrations of guinea pigs fed a low-cholesterol diet are shown in Tables 11 and 12. All animals gained body weight except the hypovitaminosis C group, which lost weight. The liver ascorbate concentration correlated positively with the increasing dietary intake of vitamin C, while the serum ascorbate levels did not. It is interesting that the 50-mg vitamin C group had a hepatic ascorbate concentration similar to that of the control group. Through feed-intake studies, it was estimated that 40 to 50 mg of vitamin C was consumed per day by the control animals on the Reid-Briggs chow diet containing 0.2 percent vitamin C (by weight). The presumed euvitaminosis C group, 5 mg/day, had a significantly lower liver vitamin C content than the control group. The serum cholesterol level was lowest in the 50 mg/day group and highest in the 0.5 mg/day group, suggesting an inverse relationship between vitamin C intake and serum cholesterol level. The hepatic cholesterol was higher in all three experimental groups when compared to the control group, but the 0.5 mg/day group had the most accumulation of hepatic cholesterol.

In another experiment, the Reid-Briggs chow diet supplemented with 2 percent cholesterol (by weight) was fed to three groups of guinea pigs provided with different levels of vitamin C intake for six weeks. The control group from the previous study was used since this study was conducted during the same time period. The 50 mg/dl group maintained body weight, whereas the 5.0 and 0.5 mg/day groups lost weight (Tables 13 and 14). It appears that with the consumption of a high-cholesterol diet, the consumption of larger amounts of vitamin C may be necessary to prevent the loss of body weight. Like the group fed the low-cholesterol diet, those groups of guinea pigs fed the high-cholesterol diet and given daily vitamin C of varying amounts via stomach intubation showed a positive correlation with the intake and hepatic ascorbate level, and not with the serum ascorbate concentration (see Tables 13 and 14). Thus, it appears that while the serum ascorbate level is not a good index for vitamin C intake, hepatic ascorbate levels are. Again, the 50 mg/day group had a hepatic vitamin C content comparable to that of the controls. Feeding the 2 percent cholesterol diet resulted in an increase in serum cholesterol levels in all three experimental groups as compared to

Table 13. Effect of Different Levels of Ascorbate Intake on Body Weight and Serum and Liver Vitamin C Concentration of Guinea Pigs Fed a Scorbutogenic Diet with 2.0 Percent Cholesterol Supplementation ($\bar{X}$ ± S.E.M.)

Ascorbate Intake (mg animal^{-1} day^{-1})[a]	*Final Body Weight (g)*	*Change in Body Weight (g)*	*Ascorbate*	
			Serum (mg/dl)	*Liver (mg/100 g tissue)*
0.5	381 ± 24	− 96	0.052 ± 0.016	1.232 ± 0.419
5.0	414 ± 5	− 48	0.045 ± 0.369	4.389 ± 1.041
50.0	544 ± 28	− 7	1.392 ± 0.078	8.774 ± 1.391
Control[b]	661 ± 33	+183	0.350 ± 0.020	9.180 ± 1.000

[a]Animals were fed Reid-Briggs scorbutogenic diet with 2.0 percent cholesterol supplementation and given vitamin C via tubal intubation.
[b]Animals were fed Reid-Briggs diet with 0.2 g percent (by weight) vitamin C fortification and no cholesterol supplementation. Calculated intake = 40–50 mg animal^{-1} day^{-1}.

Table 14. Effect of Different Levels of Ascorbate Intake on Serum Cholesterol Concentration of Guinea Pigs Fed a Scorbutogenic Diet with 2.0 Percent Cholesterol-Supplementation ($\bar{X}$ ± S.E.M.)

Ascorbate Intake (mg/animal/day)[a]	*Serum Cholesterol (mg/dl)*	*Liver Cholesterol (mg/100 g tissue)*
0.5	463.8 ± 57.1	4803.5 ± 326.2
5.0	322.7 ± 40.8	4539.9 ± 450.5
50.0	229.3 ± 29.7	3371.7 ± 736.9
Control[b]	44.8 ± 5.0	275.3 ± 4.0

[a]Fed Reid-Briggs scorbutogenic diet with 2.0 percent cholesterol supplementation. Vitamin C given via tubal intubation.
[b]Fed Reid-Briggs diet with 0.2 g percent (by weight) vitamin C fortification and no cholesterol supplementation. Calculated intake = 40 to 50 mg/animal/day.

animals on a chow diet alone (Tables 13 and 14). The data suggested that an inverse relationship existed between vitamin C intake and serum cholesterol level. However, even the intake of 50 mg/day was not sufficient to normalize the serum cholesterol levels. Similarly, the high vitamin C intake had little effect on the accumulation of hepatic cholesterol. The Evans blue dye study indicated that the guinea pigs fed the no-cholesterol diet showed no evidence of dye uptake. However, about 30 percent of the animals in the 0.5 and 5.0 mg ascorbate per day groups fed 2 percent cholesterol showed evidence of Evans blue dye uptake, as exhibited by areas of streaking in the thoracic aorta. The 50 mg/day group and the control animals did not demonstrate any Evans blue dye uptake by the intima. It can be concluded from this study that:

1. Liver ascorbate level correlated with the amount of oral intake of vitamin C, while the serum ascorbate level did not.
2. 5 mg vitamin C per animal per day was not an adequate amount for maintaining normal health and body weight in this strain of guinea pigs; 50 mg per animal per day may have represented a more adequate intake.
3. Cholesterol feeding caused a loss of body weight, particularly in the animals with insufficient vitamin C intake.
4. Vitamin C insufficiency caused an increase in serum and heaptic cholesterol concentrations over a six-week period in both cholesterol-fed guinea pigs and those fed no cholesterol.
5. About one-third of the animals in the 0.5 and 5.0 mg ascorbate per day groups fed the cholesterol diet showed Evans blue dye uptake in the thoracic aorta. The guinea pigs receiving no cholesterol showed no indication of such changes. The 50 mg ascorbate per day group fed cholesterol also showed no uptake of Evans blue dye.
6. This study suggested that vitamin C, in some way, does influence cholesterol metabolism in guinea pigs. Further studies are necessary to define precisely the role of vitamin C in cholesterol metabolism and arterial wall integrity.

It appears that a bolus dose of 50 mg vitamin C via stomach intubation provided a sufficient amount of ascorbate to maintain hepatic vitamin C levels comparable to those of control animals who had vitamin C fortified in their diet. By bolus dose, it is difficult to determine how much vitamin C was actually absorbed by the gastrointestinal tract. The level of 8 to 9 mg ascorbate/1000 g liver probably represents the saturated level. The question arises whether two 25-mg doses or five 10-mg doses per day lead to greater coefficient of absorption of vitamin C, thus leading to more effective action of ascorbate on cholesterol metabolism.

Since the 50 mg/day dose was effective neither in inhibiting nor lowering the serum cholesterol levels in the cholesterol-fed pigs, it would be interesting to determine whether pharmacologic or mega dosages, that is, 250 or 500 mg/day vitamin C, can be effective (see Fig. 3). However, because our attempts to administer 250 mg/day to the animals resulted in animals showing signs of diarrhea, it appears to be physiologically unpractical to experiment with higher dosages.

Results of our study with guinea pigs suggest that insufficient vitamin C intake causes a rise in serum cholesterol levels. Since scurvy or hypovitaminosis C in humans is rare today, it is difficult to extrapolate the usefulness of these animal studies to man. It is probably more important to know whether large dosages can act as hypocholesterolemic agents in humans, especially when previous studies are in conflict (Willis and Fishman, 1955;

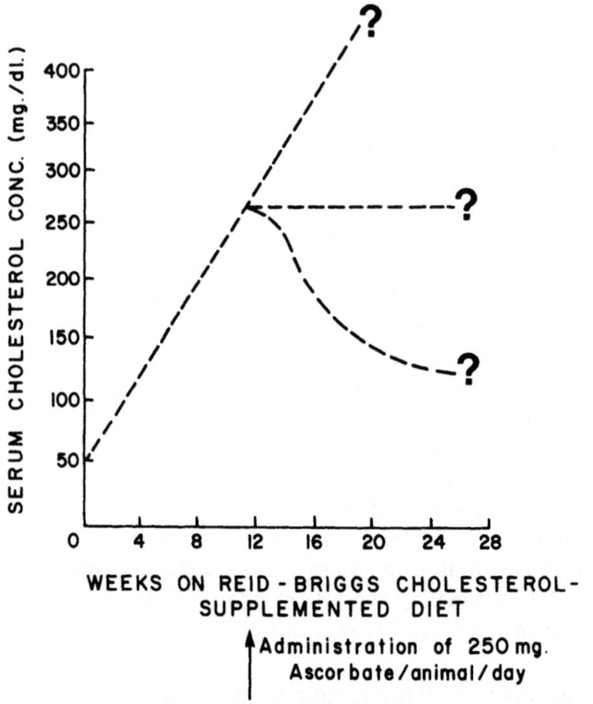

Fig. 3 Schematic diagram illustrating whether large consumption of vitamin C (i.e., 250 mg animal^{-1} day^{-1}) can inhibit the rise of serum total cholesterol level in guinea pigs fed a cholesterol-supplemented diet.

Sokoloff et al., 1967; Ginter et al., 1970; Anderson et al., 1972; Spittle, 1972; Ginter, 1975; Peterson et al., 1975), as discussed earlier.

Since there are conflicting reports on the effect of vitamin C on serum lipids in human beings, a study was designed to determine whether 1 g (500 mg in the morning and 500 mg in the evening) of vitamin C intake per day would lower serum lipids in persons with hyper-β-lipoproteinemia. The double-blind, double-crossover experimental design is shown in Tables 15 and 16. The ten male participants (mean age = 45 years; all had cholesterol concentration >300 mg/dl) were divided into two groups, one of which (Group A) started with the vitamin C period first (two 250-mg tablets in the morning and two 250-mg tablets in the evening), followed by the placebo period (calcium lactate), and ending with the vitamin C period. The second group (Group B) started with the placebo period first, followed by the vitamin C period and ending with the placebo period. Each period but the baseline period (four weeks) lasted six weeks. A baseline period consisting of two bleedings about two weeks apart was set up at the initiation of the experimental period. During each of the three experimental periods, fasting blood samples were collected at two-week intervals. The means of the three bleedings for each period were used to express the effect or lack of effect of

Table 15. Effect of Vitamin C on Serum Lipid and Lipoprotein Concentrations in Hyper-β-Lipoproteinemic Patients[a]
Group A

	Period 0			Period 1			Period 2			Period 3		
Time Period	*1st week*	*2–3 weeks later*	*4th week (time zero)*	*End of 10th week*			*End of 16th week*			*End of 22nd week*		
Treatment	*No vitamin C or placebo (maintain regular diet)*			*On vitamin C*			*Off vitamin C (placebo)*			*On vitamin C*		
				2nd	*4th*	*6th*	*2nd*	*4th*	*6th*	*2nd*	*4th*	*6th*
Physical exam	–	–	X	–	–	–	–	–	–	–	–	–
Dietary history	Briefing	–	X	–	–	X	–	–	X	–	–	X
Laboratory Tests												
(need blood and urine)	–	–	–	–	–	–	–	–	–	–	–	–
Cholesterol	From chart	X	X	X	X	X	X	X	X	X	X	X
Triglyceride	From chart	X	X	X	X	X	X	X	X	X	X	X
Phospholipid	–	X	X	X	X	X	X	X	X	X	X	X
Lipoprotein electrophoresis	From chart	X	X	X	X	X	X	X	X	X	X	X
Total protein	From chart	X	X	–	–	X	–	–	X	–	–	X
Protein electrophoresis	From chart	X	X	–	–	X	–	–	X	–	–	X
SMA-12/60	From chart	X	X	–	–	X	–	–	X	–	–	X
SMA-6/60 (kidney profile)	From chart	X	X	–	–	X	–	–	X	–	–	X
Thyroxine	From chart	X	X	–	–	X	–	–	X	–	–	X
Ascorbate	X	X	X	X	X	X	X	X	X	X	X	X

[a] $N = 6$ subjects per group, males only.

Table 16. Effect of Vitamin C on Serum Lipid and Lipoprotein Concentrations in Hyper-β-Lipoproteinemic Patients[a]
Group B

	Period 0			Period 1			Period 2			Period 3		
Time Period	*1st week*	*2–3 weeks later*	*4th week (time zero)*	*End of 10th week*			*End of 16th week*			*End of 22nd week*		
Treatment	*No vitamin C or placebo (maintain regular diet)*			*Off vitamin C (placebo)*			*On vitamin C*			*Off vitamin C (placebo)*		
				2nd	*4th*	*6th*	*2nd*	*4th*	*6th*	*2nd*	*4th*	*6th*
Physical Exam	–	–	X	–	–	X	–	–	X	–	–	X
Dietary History	Briefing	–	X	–	–	X	–	–	X	–	–	X
Laboratory Tests												
(need blood)	–	–	–	–	–	–	–	–	–	–	–	–
Cholesterol	From chart	X	X	X	X	X	X	X	X	X	X	X
Triglyceride	From chart	X	X	X	X	X	X	X	X	X	X	X
Phospholipid	–	X	X	X	X	X	X	X	X	X	X	X
Lipoprotein electrophoresis	From chart	X	X	X	X	X	X	X	X	X	X	X
Total protein	From chart	X	X	–	–	X	–	–	X	–	–	X
Protein electrophoresis	From chart	X	X	–	–	X	–	–	X	–	–	X
SMA-12/60	From chart	X	X	–	–	X	–	–	X	–	–	X
SMA-6/60 (kidney profile)	From chart	–	X	–	–	X	–	–	X	–	–	X
Thyroxine	From chart	X	X	–	–	X	–	–	X	–	–	X
Ascorbate	X	X	X	X	X	X	X	X	X	X	X	X

[a] $N = 5$ subjects per group; males only.

Table 17. Group A Daily Food–Intake Data During Study Periods

Diet Components	*Baseline Period*	*Ascorbic Acid Period*	*Placebo Period*	*Ascorbic Acid Period*
Total calories	1993.2 ± 389.81	2191.9 ± 408.16	2083.6 ± 49.04	2939.3 ± 787.81
Calories from carbohydrate (%)	40.6 ± 5.69	42.3 ± 3.98	37.5 ± 1.84	37.6 ± 7.68
Calories from protein (%)	20.0 ± 3.74	19.6 ± 2.33	22.0 ± 5.19	15.4 ± 3.44
Calories from fat (%)	34.2 ± 7.15	31.8 ± 3.64	34.9 ± 8.63	35.4 ± 3.50
Calories from alcohol (%)	5.2 ± 4.23	6.3 ± 3.29	5.6 ± 8.69	11.6 ± 8.10
Ascorbic acid (mg)	138.2 ± 73.83	114.5 ± 30.29	86.5 ± 14.53	77.7 ± 27.08
Cholesterol (mg/dl)	328.4 ± 145.60	327.6 ± 164.55	366.4 ± 138.00	386.9 ± 89.27

Table 18. Group B Daily Food–Intake Data During Study Periods

Diet Components	*Baseline Period*	*Placebo Period*	*Ascorbic Acid Period*	*Placebo Period*
Total calories	1980.0 ± 392.11	1861.8 ± 277.37	2058.4 ± 267.74	1855.5 ± 277.48
Calories from carbohydrates (%)	39.2 ± 15.52	35.0 ± 14.94	33.6 ± 11.30	34.5 ± 10.29
Calories from protein (%)	19.9 ± 3.42	20.3 ± 3.55	18.9 ± 4.15	19.6 ± 3.81
Calories from fat (%)	32.4 ± 7.74	32.2 ± 7.27	35.4 ± 5.15	35.0 ± 3.50
Calories from alcohol (%)	9.5 ± 9.43	13.2 ± 14.35	12.8 ± 14.77	11.4 ± 11.38
Ascorbic acid (mg)	120.0 ± 39.54	105.6 ± 20.33	130.0 ± 91.06	108.4 ± 46.52
Cholesterol (mg)	293.5 ± 97.86	258.9 ± 79.72	294.6 ± 62.95	305.0 ± 63.44

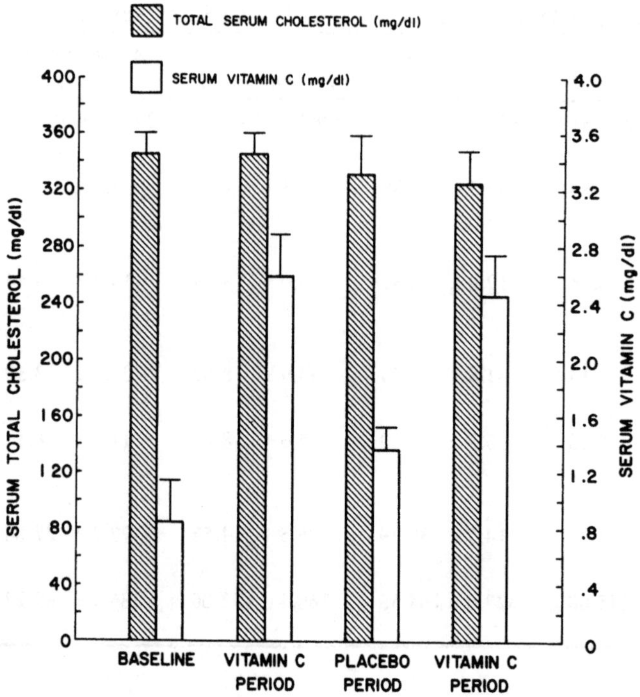

Fig. 4. Effect of vitamin C consumption on serum ascorbate and cholesterol levels in Group A patients.

vitamin C on the parameters measured. Since the participants were free-living, a dietary history was recorded by a dietitian by three-day detailed record-keeping each week. The composition of the dietary intake was calculated using tables from Feeley et al. (1972), Watt and Merrill (1963), and Church and Church (1977). The results are presented in Tables 17 and 18. The dietary intake study indicated that the caloric intake, percent of calories as carbohydrates, proteins, fat, alcohol, as well as the ascorbate (besides the vitamin C tablets) and cholesterol intake, during each of the four periods (baseline periods 1, 2, and 3) were not statistically different from each other in both Groups A and B. The low cholesterol intake is due to the low-cholesterol diet that the subjects were ingesting. The effect of 1 g of vitamin C per day on serum lipids is shown in Figs. 4–9. Despite a 2½ to threefold elevation in serum ascorbate levels during the vitamin C periods (compared to baseline), the serum cholesterol, triglyceride, and phospholipid concentrations did not change in either Group A or Group B. To ensure that all the participants consumed the placebo and vitamin C each day during the study, a pill count was made every two weeks when participants came in for bleeding and physical examination. Compliance on the pills was 98 percent in Group A

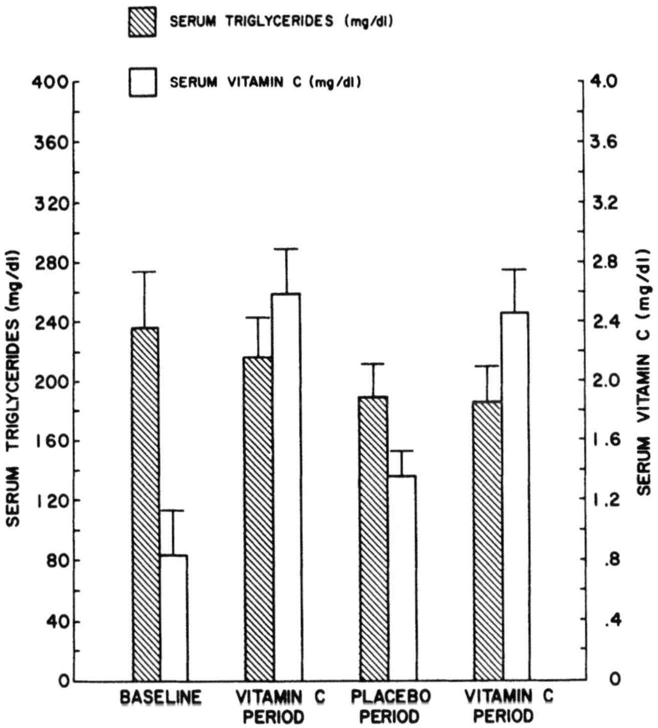

Fig. 5. Effect of vitamin C consumption on serum ascorbate and triglyceride levels in Group A patients.

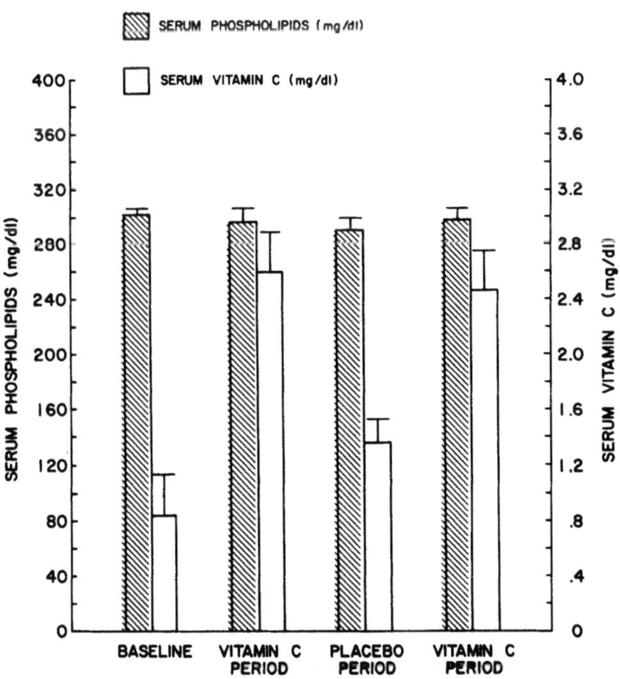

Fig. 6. Effect of vitamin C consumption on serum ascorbate and phospholipid levels in Group A patients.

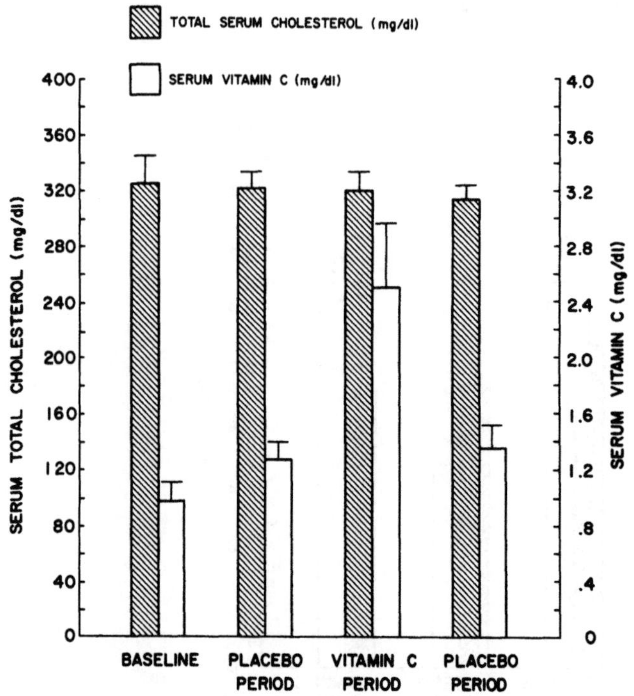

Fig. 7. Effect of vitamin C consumption on serum ascorbate and cholesterol levels in Group B patients.

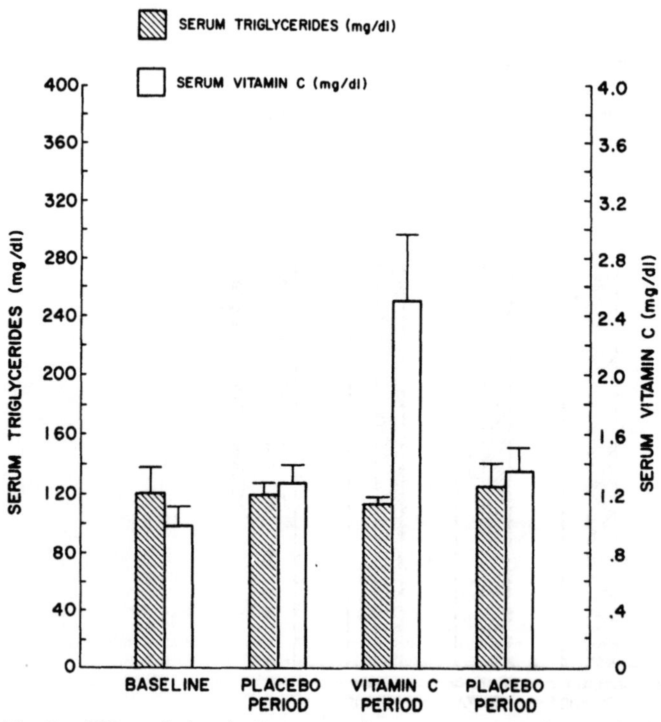

Fig. 8. Effect of vitamin C consumption on serum ascorbate and triglyceride levels in Group B patients.

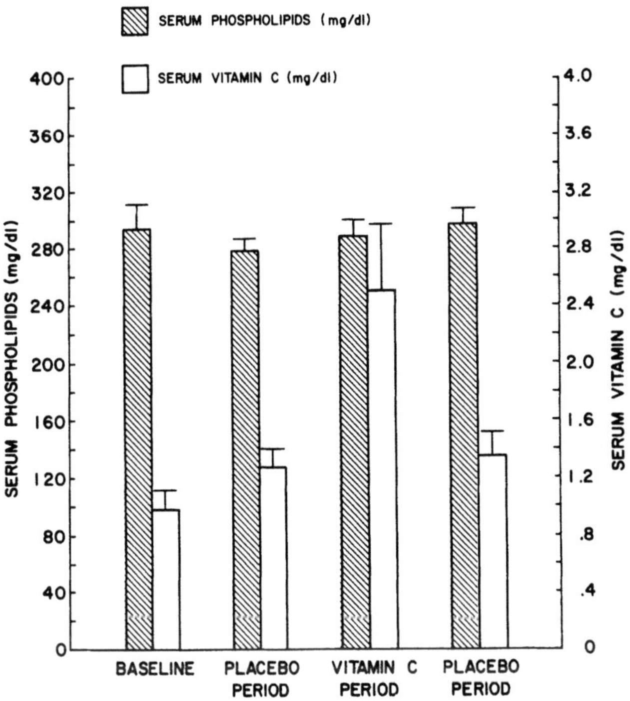

Fig. 9. Effect of vitamin C consumption on serum ascorbate and phospholipid levels in Group B patients.

and 99 percent in Group B during the entire study. Because high dosages of vitamin C intake can result in oxylate stone formation in the kidneys (Barness, 1975) and electrolyte imbalances (Lewin, 1974), 18 different analytes were monitored on the Technicon SMA 12/60 and 6/60 (Technicon AutoAnalyzer, 1974). The results (Tables 19 and 20) indicated that little change in the concentration of the various analytes occurred during the different experimental periods. In addition, there was no change in body weight, blood pressure, or thyroxine concentration (in either group) during the different periods. This study indicates that in adult male individuals with hyper-β-lipoproteinemia, large intake of vitamin C does not appear to be effective in lowering serum lipids.

Dietary Fiber and Lipid Metabolism

Current interest in the role of fiber in human disease is due mainly to the observations of Burkitt (1973) and Trowell (1972), who found that certain diseases which are prevalent in Western countries are almost unknown in

Table 19. Concentration of Various Serum Constituents of Group A Patients During Vitamin C Study

	T.P. (g/dl)	ALB. (g/dl)	Ca^{2+} (mg/dl)	Inorganic Phos. (mg/dl)	Cholesterol (mg/dl)	Glucose (mg/dl)	Uric Acid (mg/dl)	T. Bili. (mg/dl)	Alkaline Phos. (μl)	CPK (μl)	LDH (μl)	SGOT (μl)
Baseline	7.36 ± .07	4.54 ± .11	9.8 ± .2	3.30 ± .07	298 ± 11	102 ± 4	7.04 ± .26	0.78 ± .23	60 ± 7	128 ± 9	168 ± 12	28.6 ± 2.9
Period 1	7.34 ± .08	4.48 ± .05	9.5 ± .08	3.04 ± .19	301 ± 39	96 ± 5	6.7 ± .22	0.72 ± .22	58 ± 7	112 ± 10	162 ± 8	30 ± 2.7
Period 2	7.34 ± .03	4.42 ± .12	9.48 ± .19	3.16 ± .09	297 ± 20	99 ± 6	7.14 ± .22	0.84 ± .29	58 ± 10	130 ± 22	165 ± 11	28 ± 2.5
Period 3	7.4 ± .03	4.48 ± .09	9.58 ± .15	3.10 ± .18	297 ± 16	101 ± 4	6.66 ± .36	0.58 ± .09	57 ± 8	121 ± 12	164 ± 10	27.5 ± 3.2

	Na^+ (mEq/liter)	K^+ (mEq/liter)	Cl^- (mEq/liter)	CO_2 (mEq/liter)	BUN (mg/dl)	Creatinine (mg/dl)	T_4 [a] (%)
Baseline	141 ± .5	4.56 ± .16	100 ± .8	28 ± 1	19.6 ± 3.2	1.24 ± .07	0.94 ± .02
Period 1	143 ± .5	4.00 ± .27	106 ± 5	30 ± .9	21.3 ± 3.3	1.35 ± .06	0.91 ± .01
Period 2	142 ± 1	4.15 ± .17	101 ± 2	28 ± .5	22.0 ± 3.5	1.33 ± .1	0.92 ± .04
Period 3	142 ± .8	4.36 ± .1	102 ± 1	29 ± .9	20.6 ± 3.4	1.24 ± .04	0.93 ± .02

[a] Expressed as free-thyroxine index.

Table 20. Concentration of Various Serum Constituents of Group B Patients During Vitamin C Study

	T.P. *(g/dl)*	*ALB.* *(g/dl)*	Ca^{2+} *(mg/dl)*	*Inorganic Phos.* *(mg/dl)*	*Cholesterol* *(mg/dl)*	*Glucose* *(mg/dl)*	*Uric Acid* *(mg/dl)*	*T. Bili.* *(mg/dl)*	*Alkaline Phos.* *(μl)*	*CPK* *(μl)*	*LDH* *(μl)*	*SGOT* *(μl)*
Baseline	7.34	4.55	9.82	3.46	296	104	6.64	1.06	68	122	163	27
	± .17	± .13	± .11	± .05	± 11	± 4	± .67	± .14	± 5	± 36	± 8	± 2.5
Period 1	7.18	4.44	9.5	3.12	304	108	6.88	1.02	69	145	166	26
	± .22	± .81	± .13	± .14	± 5	± 6	± .61	± .24	± 3	± 24	± 12	± 3.3
Period 2	7.36	4.48	9.82	3.28	300	106	6.64	1.12	69	155	165	30
	± .11	± .15	± .25	± .19	± 13	± 8	± .62	± .26	± 5	± 46	± 11	± 2.7
Period 3	7.26	4.5	9.58	3.30	296	106	6.96	0.84	67	122	167	37
	± .15	± .13	± .14	± .09	± 15	± 7	± .41	± .18	± 3	± 14	± 7	± 4.4

	Na^+ *(mEq/liter)*	K^+ *(mEq/liter)*	Cl^- *(mEq/liter)*	CO_2 *(mEq/liter)*	*BUN* *(mg/dl)*	*Creatinine* *(mg/dl)*	T_4[a] *(%)*
Baseline	142 ± .8	4.60 ± .09	103 ± .4	28 ± 1.1	17 ± 1.0	10.7 ± 3.9	0.88 ± .02
Period 1	142 ± .6	4.68 ± .34	102 ± 2	30 ± 1.4	19 ± 1.9	13 ± 5.1	0.91 ± .02
Period 2	143 ± 1	4.78 ± .47	103 ± 1	29 ± .8	19 ± 2.9	10.8 ± 6.0	0.89 ± .02
Period 3	141 ± .7	4.58 ± .24	101 ± 1	29 ± 1.0	18 ± 1.8	11.7 ± 4.6	0.92 ± .03

[a]Expressed as free-thyroxine index.

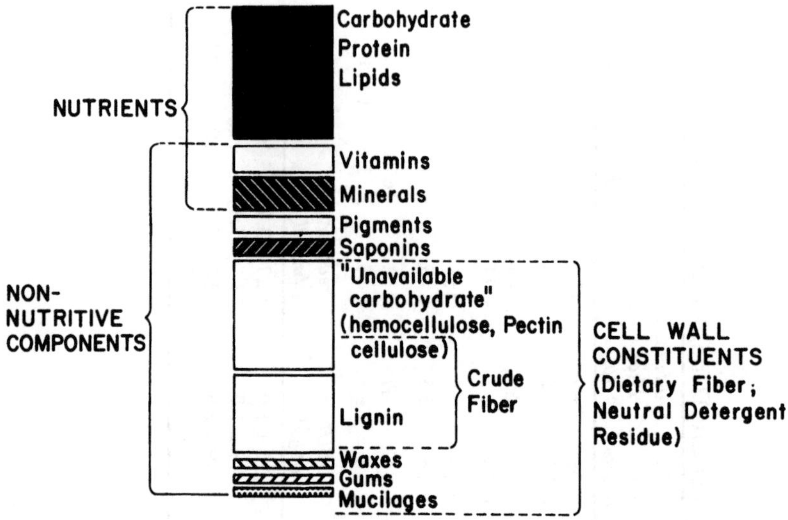

Fig. 10. Schematic diagram of the composition of fiber.

developing African countries. Earlier work by Walker and Arvidson (1934) suggested that fiber may play an important role in cancer and heart disease. Portman and Murphy found that when rats were fed a semipurified, fiber-free diet containing starch, they excreted 72 percent less cholic acid and 36 percent less neutral steroids than when fed rat chow. The half-life of cholic acid in these rats was increased by about 60 percent. Substitution of sucrose for starch caused further declines in excretion of cholic acid and neutral steroids and a further rise in cholic acid half-times.

It must be understood that there is no standard definition of the term *fiber.* The term *dietary fiber* was suggested, to apply to all the constituents derived from the plant cell wall in the diet that are nondigestible by the digestive enzymes (Walker and Arvidson, 1934). This term was chosen in order to distinguish between dietary fiber and fiber (or crude fiber). The term *crude fiber* has been used for many years to denote an estimate of the indigestible matter in animal feeds. This distinction is necessary because crude fiber is an empirically determined fraction of a food product which gives an estimate of the cellulose and lignin content and does not include many of the cell wall polysaccharides that are not digested by humans. By the above definition, dietary fiber includes all of the unavailable carbohydrates and noncarbohydrate lignin (Fig. 10). This fiber is a complex matrix of substances, the proportions of which differ with the stage of maturity of the plant, plant part, soil composition, season, and species. All of these factors influence the physiologic role plant fiber plays in human and animal nutrition. More information on the chemistry of fiber can be obtained elsewhere (Cummings, 1976).

There is increasing evidence that the ingestion of certain types of fiber will lower serum cholesterol level (Story and Kritchevsky, 1976). Not all types of fiber seem to work. Bran is an example. Semipurified diets (whose cholesterol content varied from 34 to 120 mg/100 kcal) were fed to adult cynomolgus monkeys (*Macaca fascicularis*) for 9 months (Malinow et al., 1975, 1976b). The diet had a fat content similar to that of the typical American diet. The intake of dietary fiber was increased from 0 g intake in the control animals to 35 g per animal per day through the addition of wheat, rice, or soya brans. The monkeys were stratified according to their cholesterol values and only animals between 346 and 421 mg/dl were selected and assigned to one of five groups. There were six monkeys in each of the following groups: (1) control; (2) wheat bran; (3) rice bran; (4) soya bran; and (5) cholestyramine. None of the brans reduced plasma levels of cholesterol, whereas cholestyramine produced marked hypocholesterolemic effects. Serum triglycerides increased with higher cholesterol intake, but no additional changes were induced by any of the experimental diets. The failure of bran to lower serum cholesterol may be due to a high proportion of the fiber as cellulose, which has been reported to have a poor ability to bind bile acids (Kritchevsky and Story, 1974; Story, 1980), and/or due to a low amount of saponins which have been shown to bind cholesterol (Malinow et al., 1977a,b; 1978). Bran itself is not homogenous and is not entirely of fiber. By definition, bran is the outer layer of wheat grain, which consists of the pericarp, seed coat, and aleurone layer (Cummings, 1976). It is composed of 21 percent cellulose, 20 to 26 percent pentosan, 7 to 9 percent starch, 11 to 15 percent protein, 5 to 10 percent fat, 5 to 9 percent ash, and 14 percent water (Cummings, 1976). Studies by Story and Kritchevsky (1976b) show that lignin and alfalfa have higher binding capacity to various bile acids than cellulose or bran. Their study shows that cellulose bound taurocholate almost 30 percent less than did bran, which found significantly less than did alfalfa (Kritchevsky and Story, 1976). The binding capacity of alfalfa was striking. Balmer and Zilversmit (1974) compared the binding of taurocholate, in vitro, to several types of grains and grain products. Cellulose bound no bile acid under their conditions, and lignin bound 2.1 times as much taurocholate as did the stock diet. The lack of effect of bran could also be attributed to a low lignin content. Among the natural materials, lignin appears to have the highest binding capacity for bile salts.

Leveille and Sauberlich (1966) reported a large increase in bile acids, but not in neutral sterol excretion in rats fed pectin with 1 percent cholesterol. Kay and Truswell (1977) found that when citrus pectin was added for three weeks to metabolically controlled diets in nine subjects, plasma cholesterol decreased by 13 percent and fecal fat excretion increased by 44 percent. Neutral steroids and fecal bile acid excretions were elevated by 17 percent and 33 percent, respectively. Plasma triglyceride levels did not change.

Again, in studying dietary effects, one must be continually aware of the interactions among all dietary components. A minor point that is often neglected in human studies is the influence of various spices in the diet. Story and Kritchevsky (1975) found that many condiments and foodstuffs (curry powder, cloves, dried parsley, oregano, chili powder, thyme, paprika, red pepper, cinnamon, etc.) bind an appreciable quantity of sodium taurocholate.

Since our previous study (Malinow et al., 1976) suggested that alfalfa was hypocholesterolemic, we evaluated the effect on atherosclerosis in the aorta and coronary arteries of monkeys. Two hundred sixty-three adult cynomolgus monkeys were fed a semipurified diet containing 1.2 mg of cholesterol/cal for 30 days (Malinow et al., 1978b). Only the normo-responders were selected, eliminating the hypo- and hyper-responders to cholesterol feeding to avoid wide ranges within groups. The diet represented a semipurified diet similar to a typical American diet. Subsequently, the animals were ranked according to the average serum total cholesterol concentration and stratified into similar cholesterolemic intervals prior to being assigned to different control and experimental groups. One group (Group A) was placed on a regression diet (monkey chow diet) for 24 months after the short one-month induction period to allow minimal atherosclerosis to develop. After five more months on the induction diet, the rest of the animals were once again ranked, stratified, and randomly assigned to groups of 18 animals each, at which time the regression period began for an additional 18 months by feeding a 0.34 mg cholesterol per calorie diet to produce moderate hypercholesterolemia. One group of monkeys was sacrificed at the end of the 6-month induction period (Group B). Of the three groups that continued in the regression period, one group (Group C) was fed the cholesterol diet (0.34 mg/cal), another was fed the cholesterol plus alfalfa diet (Group D); the last group (Group E) continued to be fed a cholesterol-free diet. The lower-cholesterol diet (0.35 mg/cal) was fed to maintain a moderate cholesterol level of about 300 mg/dl, a level that is often seen in Type II hyperlipoproteinemic subjects. The serum cholesterol levels were 138 ± 9, 701 ± 51, 287 ± 23, 163 ± 7, and 139 ± 4 mg/dl for Groups A to E, respectively. The degree of aortic atherosclerosis was evaluated on a scale of +1 to +5, and was found to be 1.4 ± 0.1, 3.0 ± 0.3, 3.7 ± 0.3, 1.8 ± 0.2, and 1.8 ± 0.2 for Groups A to E, respectively. Coronary artery atherosclerosis was evaluated by the degree of lumenal encroachment, and was found to be 1.4 ± 0.2, 23.0 ± 5.1, 14.6 ± 2.9, 5.4 ± 1.3, and 7.6 ± 1.9 percent for Groups A to E, respectively. Encroachment on the lumen due to coronary atherosclerosis was significant in Groups B and C. When the 0.34 mg/cal regression diet was supplemented with 50 percent alfalfa meal and made isocaloric (Group D),

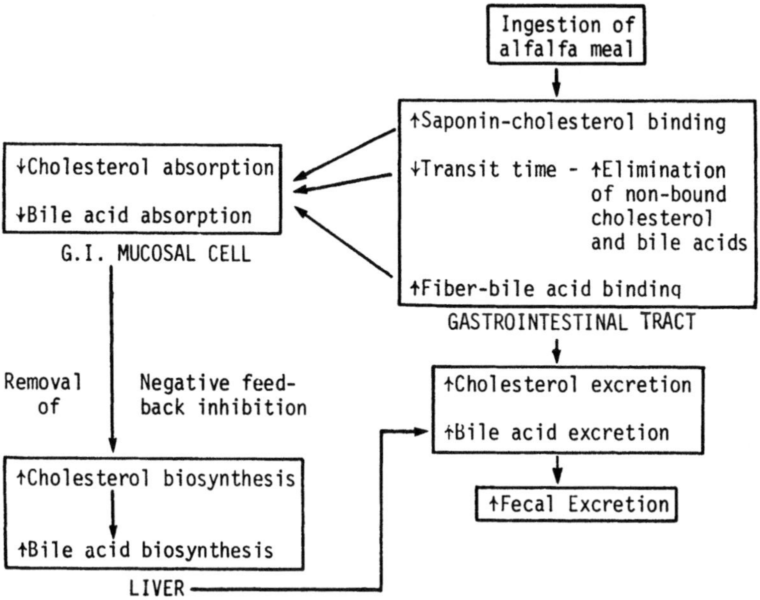

Fig. 11. Schematic diagram showing the possible mechanisms of the hypocholesterolemic effect of fiber.

the serum cholesterol levels were normalized to control levels, and the aorta showed 50 percent less atherosclerosis than the group without the addition of alfalfa in the diet (Group C). The coronary artery showed signs of regression. The intima was not thickened and no foam cells were observed in the intima or media. The internal elastic lamina was intact and not reduplicated. The occasional lesions observed consisted of minimal thickening of the intima or subintima with scanty mucropolysaccharides and no evidence of collagen.

The mechanism involved in the beneficial effects of alfalfa are not completely understood. Malinow et al. (1977a, b) have shown that alfalfa saponins prevent intestinal absorption of cholesterol in rats, as well as the expected rise in plasma cholesterol associated in monkeys with the ingestion of diets containing butter and cholesterol. Digitonin, a saponin, binds cholesterol in vitro (Malinow et al., 1978). Malinow et al. (1977a, b; 1978) also demonstrated that when digitonin or saponins extracted from alfalfa were mixed in the diet for rats and monkeys, it prevented the expected rise in plasma cholesterol in monkeys fed a diet containing butter and cholesterol. Since it has been reported that there are many different types of saponins in alfalfa (Morris et al., 1961; Djerassi et al., 1957; Walter et al., 1954) the

Table 21. Nutritional Factors Which Can Influence Serum Lipoproteins

Nutritional Factors	*VLDL*	*LDL*	*HDL*
Total calories	↑[a]	(↑)	(↓)
Total Fat	↑	↑	↓[b]
Saturated	↔[c]	↑	(↓)
Monounsaturated	↔	↔	↔
Polyunsaturated	↔	↓	(↑)
Cholesterol	(↑)	↑	(↑)
Phytosterols	↔	↓	↔
Protein			
Vegetable	?	↓	(↑)
Animal	?	↑	↔
Carbohydrates			
Simple	↑	↔	↓
Complex	↔	↓	↔
Alcohol	↑	(↑)	↑
Vitamin C	↔	↔	↔

[a] ↑ = Increased concentration.
[b] ↓ = Decreased concentration
[c] ↔ = No change.

question arises as to which of the saponins have the greatest cholesterol-binding activity. This is particularly important, since not all saponins have hypocholesterolemic effect. Saponins are widely distributed in nature, and there are well over 300 different forms of saponins (McIlroy, 1951). It is also possible that the hypocholesterolemic effect of alfalfa may be due to the binding of bile salts by the dietary fiber content, decreased transit time, and/or increased denudation of the endothelium of the gastrointestinal tract. Recent work from Dr. Malinow's laboratory suggests that the hypocholesterolemic effect of alfalfa is primarily due to the saponin effect rather than the fiber effect (Malinow et al., 1977). This is not to say that all types of plants containing saponins lower cholesterol mainly by the saponin effect rather than by the fiber effect or both (Fig. 11). Until the chemical nature of fiber derived from alfalfa is characterized more thoroughly, the mechanism of action of this dietary fiber on plasma lipids cannot be ascertained.

In summary, the relationship of serum lipids and lipoproteins to CHD has been reviewed. The effect of specific nutritional components in the diet on serum lipid and lipoprotein concentrations has been discussed (Table 21 provides a summary). An approach to dietary management of hyperlipidemic and hyperlipoproteinemic conditions was provided as a basis for future dietary trials. Finally, two topics of current interest, vitamin C and fiber, were discussed in greater detail, and recent data from our laboratory were included in this discussion.

REFERENCES

Anderson, T.W., Reid, D.E., and Beaton, G.H. Vitamin C and the common cold: A double blind trial. *Cand. Med. Assoc. J.* 107, 503-508 (1972).

Balmer, J. and Zilversmit, D.B. Effects of dietary roughage on cholesterol absorption, cholesterol turnover and steroid excretion in the rat. *J. Nut.* 104, 1319-1328 (1974).

Banerjee, S. and Singh, H.D. Cholesterol metabolism in scorbutic guinea pigs. *J. Biol. Chem.* 233, 336-342 (1958).

Barnes, M.J., Constable, B.J., Morton, L.F., and Kodicek, E.K. Studies in vivo on the biosynthesis of collagen and elastin in ascorbic acid-deficient guinea pigs. Evidence for the formation and degredation of a partially hydroxylated collagen. *Biochem. J.* 119, 575-585 (1970).

Barness, L.A. Safety considerations with high ascorbic acid dosage. *Ann. N.Y. Acad. Sci.* 258, 523-528 (1975).

Barr, D.P., Russ, E.M., and Eder, H.A. Protein-lipid relationships in human plasma. II. In atherosclerosis and related conditions. *Am. J. Med.* 11, 480-493 (1951).

Blackburn, H. Progress in the epidemiology and prevention of coronary heart disease, in *Progress in Cardiology*. P. Yu and J. Goodman, eds. Philadelphia: Lea and Febinger (1974), pp. 1-36.

Bondjer, G. and Bjokerud, S. Arterial repair and atherosclerosis after mechanical injury. *Atherosclerosis* 18, 235-255 (1974).

Bouchier, I.A. and Dawson, A.M. The effects of infusions of ethanol on the plasma free fatty acids in man. *Clin. Sci.* 26, 47-54 (1964).

Brown, H.B. Food patterns that lower blood lipids in man. *J. Am. Diet. Assoc.* 58, 303-311 (1971).

Brown, H.B., Lewis, L.A., and Page, I.H. Mixed hyperlipemia a sixth type of hyperlipoproteinemia. *Atherosclerosis* 17, 181-196 (1973).

Brunner, D., Altman, S., Lobl, K., and Schwartz, S. Alpha-cholesterol percentages in coronary patients with and without increased total serum cholesterol levels and in healthy controls. *J. Athero. Res.* 2, 424-428 (1962).

Burkitt, D.P. Some diseases characteristic of modern western civilization. *Br. Med. J.* 1, 274-278 (1973).

Carew, T.E., Hayes, S.B., Koschivsky, T., and Steinberg, D. A mechanism by which high-density lipoproteins may slow the atherogenic process. *Lancet* 1, 1315-1317 (1976).

Carlson, L.A. and Bottliger, L.E. Ischemic heart disease in relation to fasting values of plasma triglycerides and cholesterol. Stockholm prospective study. *Lancet* 1, 865-868 (1972).

Castelli, W.P., Doyle, J.T., Gordon, T., Hames, C.G., Hjortland, M.C., Hulley, S.D., Kagan, A., and Zukel, W.J. HDL-cholesterol and other lipids in coronary heart disease. *Circulation* 55, 767-772 (1977).

Church, C.F. and Church, N.H. *Food Values of Portions Commonly Used,* 12th ed. Philadelphia: J.B. Lippincott Company (1977), p. 1.

The Cleveland Clinic Foundation Diet Manual: A Key to Nutritional Care. The Cleveland Clinic Foundation, Cleveland, OH (1978) p. F4.

Connor, W.E. and Connor, S.L. The key role of nutritional factors in the prevention of coronary heart disease. *Prev. Med.* 1, 49-83 (1972).

Connor, W.E. and Connor, S.L. Dietary treatment of hyperlipidemia, in *Hyperlipidemia: Diagnosis and Therapy.* B.M. Rifkind and R.I. Levy, eds. New York: Grune and Stratton (1977), pp. 246-283.

Connor, W.E., Brown, H.B., Fredrickson, D.S., Steinberg, D., Connor, S.L., and Bickel, J.H. *A maximal approach to the dietary treatment of the hyperlipidemias.* Subcommittee on diet and hyperlipidemia, Council on Atherosclerosis. American Heart Association, New York (1973), pp. 1-27.

Corday, E. and Corday, S.R. Prevention of heart disease by control of risk factors: The time has come to face the facts. *Am. J. Card.* 35, 33-333 (1975).

Cox, G.E., Taylor, C.B., Cox, L.G., and Counts, M.A. Atherosclerosis in rhesus monkeys. *Arch. Path.* 66, 32-37 (1958).

Cummings, J.H. What is fiber? in *Fiber in Human Nutrition.* G.A. Speller and R.J. Amen, eds. New York: Plenum Press (1976), pp. 1-43.

Davis, C.E. and Havlik, R.J. Clinical trials of lipid lowering and coronary artery disease prevention, in *Hyperlipidemia: Diagnosis and Therapy.* B.M. Rifkind and R.I. Levy, eds. New York: Grune and Stratton (1977), pp. 79-92.

Dayton, S., Pearce, M.L., Hashimoto, S., Dixon, W.J., and Tomijarsu, U. A controlled clinical trial of a diet in unsaturated fat–in preventing complications of atherosclerosis. *Circulation* 39 and 40 (Suppl. 2).

Dietary Goals for the United States, 2nd ed. Select Committee on Nutrition and Human Needs. Washington, D.C.: Government Printing Office (1977), pp. 1-79.

Dietschy, J.M. and Wilson, J.D. Regulation of cholesterol metabolism. *N. Eng. J. Med.* 282, 1128-1241 (1970).

Djerassi, C., Thomas, D.B., Livingston, A.L., and Thompson, C.R. Terpenoids. XXXI. The structure and stereochemistry of medicagenic acid. *J. Am. Chem. Soc.* 79, 5292-5297 (1957).

Eades, C.H., Jr. Coronary atherosclerosis in renal hypertensive meat fed rats. *Trans. N.Y. Acad. Sci.* 28, 860-871 (1966).

Esterly, J.A. and Glagov, S. Altered permeability of the renal artery of the hypertensive rat: An electron microscopic study. *Am. J. Path.* 43, 619-638 (1963).

Feeley, R.M., Criner, P.E., and Walt, B.K. Cholesterol content of foods. *J. Am. Diet. Assoc.* 61, 134-149 (1972).

Feigle, J. Neve Untersuchungen zur Chemie des Blutes bie akuter Alkoholintoxikation und bie chronischen Alkoholismos mit besonderer Berücksichtigung von Fetten und Lipolden. *Biochem. Ztschr.* 92, 282-317 (1918).

Fillius, L.C. and Mann, G.V. The importance of sex in the variability of the cholesterolemic response of rabbits fed cholesterol. *Circ. Res.* 4, 406-411 (1956).

Fischer-Dzoga, K. and Wissler, R.W. Stimulation of proliferation in stationary primary cultures of monkey aortic smooth muscle cells. Part 2. Effect of varying concentrations of hypertipemic serum and low density lipoproteins of varying dietary fat origins. *Atherosclerosis* 24, 515-525 (1976).

Flores, H., Sierralta, W., and Monckeberg, F. Triglyceride transport in protein-depleted rats. *J. Nut.* 100, 375-379 (1970).

Food and Nutrition Board, National Academy of Sciences National Research Council on Foods and Nutrition, American Medical Association, Diet and Coronary Heart Disease, a joint statement. *Nut. Rev.* 30, 223-225 (1972).

Frantz, I.D., Dawson, E.A., Kuba, K., Brewer, E.R., Gatewood, L.C., and Bartsch, G.E. The Minnesota Coronary Survey: Effect of Diet on Cardiovascular Events and Deaths. *Circulation* 52 (Suppl. II), II, 4-9 (1975).

Fredrickson, D.S. and Levy, R.I. Familial hyperlipoproteinemia; in *The Metabolic Basis of Inherited Disease.* J.B. Stanburg, J.B. Wyngaarden, and D.S. Fredrickson, eds. New York: McGraw-Hill (1972), pp. 545-614.

Fredrickson, D.S., Levy, R.I., and Lees, R.S. Fat transport in lipoproteins–an integrated approach to mechanism and disorders. *N. Eng. J. Med.* 276, 34-42, 94-103, 148-156, 215-225, 273-281 (1967).

Fredrickson, D.S., Levy, R.I., Bonnell, M., and Ernst, N. *Dietary Management of Hyperlipoproteinemia: A Handbook for Physicians and Dietitians.* Department of Health, Education and Welfare. Publication No. (NIH) 75-110. Bethesda, Maryland: Heart and Lung Institute (1974).

Friedman, M. and Byers, S.O. Endothelial permeability in atherosclerosis. *Arch. Path.* 76, 99–105 (1963).

Galen, R.S. The normal range. A concept in transition. *Arch. Path. Lab. Med.* 101, 561–565 (1977).

Giese, J. Acute hypertensive vascular disease. 1. Relationship between blood pressure changes and vascular lesions in different forms of acute hypertension. *Acta Path. Microbiol. Scand.* 62, 481–496 (1964).

Ginter, E. Ascorbic acid in cholesterol and bile acid metabolism. *Ann. N.Y. Acad. Sci.* 258, 410–421 (1975).

Ginter, E. and Ondreicka, R. Liver cholesterol esters composition in guinea pigs with chronic ascorbic acid deficiency. *Nut. Metab.* 13, 321–330 (1971).

Ginter, E., Bobek, P., Kopec, Z., Ovecko, M., and Cerey, K. Metabolic disorders in guinea pigs with chronic vitamin C hyposaturation. *Versuchskierk* 9, 228–235 (1967).

Ginter, E., Kajaba, I., and Nizner, O. The effect of ascorbic acid on cholesterolemia in healthy subjects with seasonal deficit on vitamin C. *Nut. Metab.* 12, 76–86 (1970).

Ginter, E., Cerven, J., Nemec, R., and Mikus, L. Lowered cholesterol catabolism in guinea pigs with chronic ascorbic acid deficiency. *Am. J. Clin. Nut.* 24, 1238–1245 (1971).

Glomset, J.A. The plasma lecithins: Cholesterol acyltransferase. *J. Lipid. Res.* 9, 155–167 (1968).

Glomset, J.A. and Norum, K.R. The metabolic role of lecithin: cholesterol acyltransferase: perspectives from pathology. *Adv. Lipid Res.* 11, 1–65 (1973).

Glueck, C.J. and Conner, W.E. Diet-coronary heart disease relationships reconnoitered. *Am. J. Clin. Nut.* 31, 727–737 (1977).

Glueck, C.J., Gartside, P., Fallat, R.W., Sielski, J., and Steiner, P.M. Longevity syndromes: familial hypobeta and familial hyperalpha lipoproteinemia. *J. Lab. Clin. Med.* 88, 941–957 (1976).

Gordon, T., Garcia-Palmieri, M.R., Kagan, A., Kannel, W.B., and Schiffman, J. Differences in coronary heart disease in Framingham, Honolulu and Puerto Rico. *J. Chron. Dis.* 27, 329–344 (1974).

Gordon, T., Castelli, W.P., Hjortland, M.C., and Kannel, W.B. The prediction of coronary heart disease by high-density and other lipoproteins: An historical perspective, in *Hyperlipidemia: Diagnosis and Therapy.* B.M. Rifkind and R.I. Levy, eds. New York: Grune and Stratton (1977), pp. 71–78.

Gore, I. and Stefanovic, V. The relation of permeability of rabbit aorta to dietary induced lipid accumulation. *Fed. Proc.* 26, 431–433 (1967).

Gould, B.S. Ascorbid acid-independent and ascorbic acid-dependent collagen-forming mechanism. *Ann. N.Y. Acad. Sci.* 92, 168–174 (1961).

Grundy, S.M. Treatment of hypercholesterolemia. *Am. J. Clin. Nut.* 30, 985–992 (1977).

Grundy, S.M., Ahrens, E.H., and Davignon, J. The interaction of cholesterol absorption and cholesterol synthesis in man. *J. Lipid Res.* 10, 304–315 (1969).

Harman, D. Atherosclerosis; inhibiting effect of an antihistaminic drug, chlorpheniramine. *Circ. Res.* 11, 277–282 (1962).

Hegsted, D.M., McGrady, R.B., Meyers, M.L., and Stare, F.J. Quantitative effects of dietary fat on serum cholesterol in man. *Am. J. Clin. Nut.* 17, 281–295 (1965).

Holzbach, R.T., Corbusier, C., Marsh, M., and Naito, H.K. The process of cholesterol cholelithiasis induced by diet in the prairie dog: A physiocochemical characterization. *J. Lab. Clin. Med.* 87, 987–998 (1976).

Imai, Y. and Matsumara, H. Genetic studies on induced and spontaneous hypercholesterolemia in rats. *Atherosclerosis* 18, 59–64 (1973).

Imai, H., Werthessen, N.T., Taylor, C.B., and Lee, K.T. Angiotoxicity and arteriosclerosis due to contaminants of USP-grade cholesterol. *Arch. Path. Lab. Med.* 100, 565–572 (1976).

Jackson, R.L., Morrisett, J.D., and Gotta, A.M. Lipoprotein structure and metabolism. *Phys. Rev.* 56, 259–316 (1976).

Johnson, K.G., Yano, K., and Kato, H. Coronary heart disease in Hiroshima, Japan: A report of a six-year period of surveillance, 1958–1964. *Am. J. Pub. Health* 58, 1355–1367 (1968).

Kannel, W.B., Castille, W.P., Gordon, T., and McNamara, P.M. Serum cholesterol, lipoproteins and the risk of coronary heart disease. *Ann. Int. Med.* 74, 1–12 (1971).

Kay, R.M. and Truswell, A.S. Effect of citris pectin on blood lipids and fecal steroid excretion in man. *Am. J. Clin. Nut.* 30, 171–175 (1977).

King, C.G. and Waugh, W.A. Chemical nature of vitamin C. *Science* 75, 357–358 (1932).

Koletsky, S., Rivera, J.M., and Pritchard, W.A. Production of hypertension and vascular disease by angiotension. *Arch. Path.* 82, 99–106 (1966).

Kritchevsky, D. and Story, J.A. Binding of bile salts in vitro by nonnutritive fiber. *J. Nut.* 104, 458–462 (1974).

Kritchevsky, D., Kolman, R.R., Gottmacher, R.M., and Forbes, M. Serum cholesterol levels in germ-free chicks. *Arch. Biochem. Biophys.* 85, 444–453 (1959).

Kummerow, K.H. Neutrition-imbalance and angiotoxins as dietary risk factors in coronary heart disease. *Am. J. Clin. Nut.* 32, 58–83 (1979).

Kummerow, F.A., Cho, B.H.S., Huang, W.Y-T., Imai, H., Kamio, A., Duetsch, M.J., and Hooper, W.M. Additive risk factors in atherosclerosis. *Am. J. Clin. Nut.* 29, 579–584 (1976).

Kummerow, F.A., Kim, Y., Hull, M., Pollard, J., Ilinov, P., Dorossiev, D.L., and Valek, J. The influence of egg consumption on the serum cholesterol level in human subjects. *Am. J. Clin. Nut.* 30, 664–673 (1977).

Lauer, R.M., Connor, W.E., and Laverton, P.E. Coronary heart disease risk factors in school children: The Muscatine study. *J. Ped.* 86, 697–706 (1975).

Leren, P. The effect of plasma cholesterol lowering diet in male survivors of myocardial infarction. *Acta Med. Scand.* suppl. 466, 1–12 (1966).

Lee, R.E. Ascorbic acid and the peripheral vascular system. *Ann. N.Y. Acad. Sci.* 92, 295–301 (1961).

Lieber, C.S., Leevy, C.M., Stein, S.W., George, W.S., Cherrick, G.R., Abelmann, W.H., and Davidson, C.S. Effect of ethanol on plasma-free fatty acids in man. *J. Lab. Clin. Med.* 59, 826–832 (1962).

Lieber, C.S. Effects of ethanol upon lipid metabolism. *Lipids* 9, 103–116 (1974).

Leveille, G.A. and Fisher, H. Plasma cholesterol in growing chicken as influenced by dietary protein and fat. *Proc. Soc. Exp. Biol. Med.* 98, 630–642 (1958).

Leveille, G.A. and Sauberlich, H.E. Mechanism of the cholesterol-depressing effect of pectin in the cholesterol-fed rat. *J. Nut.* 88, 209–214 (1966).

Lewin, S. Evaluation of potential effects of high intake of ascorbic acid. *Comp. Biochem. Physiol.* 47, 681–695 (1974).

Lifton, L. and Scheig, R. Ethanol-induced hypertriglyceridemia. Prevalence and contributing factors. *Am. J. Clin. Nut.* 31, 614–618 (1978).

Lofland, H.B., Jr., Clarkson, T.B., St. Clair, R.W., and Lehner, N.D.M. Studies on the regulation of plasma cholesterol levels in squirrel monkeys of two genotypes. *J. Lipid Res.* 13, 39–47 (1972).

Losowsky, M.S., Jones, D.P., Davidson, C.S., and Lieber, C.S. Studies of alcoholic hyperlipemia and its mechanism. *Am. J. Med.* 35, 794–803 (1963).

McCullagh, E.P. and Lewis, L.A. A study of diet, blood lipids and vascular disease in trappists monks. *N. Eng. J. Med.* 263, 569–574 (1960).

McIlroy, R.J. *The Plant Glycosides.* London: Edward Arnold (1951).

Mahley, R.W., Weisgraber, K.H., and Innerarity, T. Canine lipoproteins and atherosclerosis. *Circ. Res.* 35, 722–733 (1974).

Malinow, R., McLaughlin, P., Papworth, L., Naito, H.K., and Lewis, L. Failure of bran to effect plasma lipids in cholesterol free monkeys. *Circulation* (suppl. II), II–83 (1975).

Malinow, M.R., McLaughlin, P., Papworth, L., Naito, H.K., Lewis, L., and McNulty, W.P. A model for therapeutic interventions on established coronary atherosclerosis in a non-human primate, in *Advances in Experimental Medicine and Biology: Atherosclerosis Drug Discovery.* C.E. Day, ed. New York: Plenum Press (1976a), pp. 3–31.

Malinow, R., McLaughlin, P., Papworth, L., Naito, H.K., and Lewis, L. Effect of bran and cholestyramine on plasma lipids in monkeys. *Am. J. Clin. Nut.* 29, 905–911 (1976b).

Malinow, M.R., McLaughlin, P., Kohler, G.O., and Livingston, A.L. Prevention of elevated cholesterolemia in monkeys. *Steroids* 29, 105–110 (1977).

Malinow, M.R., McLaughlin, P., Papworth, L., Strafford, C., Kohler, G.O., Livingston, A.L., and Cheeke, P.R. Effect of alfalfa saponins on intestinal cholesterol absorption in rats. *Am. J. Clin. Nut.* 30, 2061–2067 (1977).

Malinow, M.R., McLaughlin, P., and Stafford, C. Prevention of hypercholesterolemia in monkeys (Macaca fascicularis) by digitonin. *Am. J. Clin. Nut.* 31, 814–818 (1978).

Malinow, M.R., McLaughlin, P., Naito, H.K., Lewis, L.A., and McNulty, W.P. Effect of alfalfa meal on shrinkage (regression) of atherosclerotic plaques during cholesterol feeding in monkeys. *Atherosclerosis* 30, 27–43 (1978b).

Mattson, F.H., Erickson, B.A., and Kligman, A.M. Effect of dietary cholesterol on serum cholesterol in man. *Am. J. Clin. Nut.* 25, 589–594 (1972).

Mattson, F.H., Volpenhein, K.A., and Erickson, B.A. Effect of plant sterol esters on the absorption of dietary cholesterol. *J. Nut.* 107, 1139–1146 (1977).

Medalie, J.H., Kahn, H.A., Newfeld, H.N., Riss, E., and Goldbourt, V. Five year myocardial infarction incidence–II. Association of single variables to age and birthplace. *J. Chron. Dis.* 26, 329–349 (1973).

Meeker, D.R. and Kesten, H.D. Experimental atherosclerosis and high protein diets. *Proc. Soc. Exp. Biol. Med.* 45, 543–545 (1940).

Miettinen, M., Turpeinen, O., Karvonen, M.J., Elosuo, R., and Paavilainen, E. Effect of cholesterol lowering diet on mortality from coronary heart disease and other causes. *Lancet* 2, 835–838 (1972).

Miller, N.E., Førde, O.H., Thelle, D.S., and Mjøs, O.D. The Tromsø heart study. High-density lipoprotein and coronary heart disease: A prospective case control study. *Lancet* 1, 8019–8025 (1977).

Minamisano, T., Wada, M., Akamatsu, A., Okabe, M., Handa, J., Morita, T., Asagami, C., Naito, H.K., Nakamoto, S., Lewis, L.A., and Mise, J. Dislipoproteinemia (a remnant lipoprotein disease) in uremic patients on hemodialysis. *J. Clin. Chim. Acta* 84, 163–172 (1978).

Mistius, S.P. and Ockner, R. Effects of ethanol on endogenous lipid and lipoprotein metabolism in small intestine. *J. Lab. Clin. Med.* 80, 34–46 (1972).

Mjøs, O.D., Thelle, D.S., Førde, O.H., and Vik-Mo, H. Family study of density lipoprotein cholesterol and the relation of age and sex. The Tromsø heart study. *Acta Med. Scand.* 201, 323–329 (1977).

Morris, R.J., Dye, W.B., and Gisler, P.S. Isolation, purification and structural identity of an alfalfa root saponin. *J. Organic Chem.* 26, 1241–1243 (1961).

Naito, H.K. and Gerrity, R.G. Unusual resistance of the ground squirrel to the development of dietary-induced hypercholesterolemia and atherosclerosis. *Exp. Mol. Path.* 31, 452–467 (1979).

Naito, H.K., Holzbach, R.T., and Corbusier, C. Characterization of serum lipids and lipoproteins of prairie dogs fed a chow diet or cholesterol supplemented diet. *Exp. Mol. Path.* 27, 81–92 (1977).

National Diet-Heart Research Group; The national diet-heart study final report. *Circulation* 38 (Suppl. I), 428 (1968).

Newburg, L.H. and Squire, T.L. High protein diets and arteriosclerosis in rabbits: A preliminary report. *Arch. Intern. Med.* 26, 38–40 (1920).

Nichols, A.B., Ravenscroft, C., Lamphier, D.E., and Ostrander, L.D. Daily nutritional intake and serum lipid levels. The Tecumseh study. *Am. J. Clin. Nut.* 29, 1384–1392 (1977).

Nicolosi, R.J., Hojnacki, J.L., Llansa, N., and Hayes, K.C. Diet and lipoprotein influence on primate atherosclerosis. *Proc. Soc. Exp. Biol. Med.* 156, 1–7 (1977).

Nikkila, E. Studies on lipid-protein relationships in normal and pathological sera and effect of heparin on serum lipoproteins. *Scand. J. Clin. Lab. Invest.* 5 (Suppl. 8), 1–12 (1953).

Nishida, T.F., Takenaka, F., and Kummerow, F.A. Effect of dietary protein and heated fat on serum cholesterol and beta-lipoportein levels and on the incidence of experimental atherosclerosis in chicks. *Circ. Res.* 6, 194–201 (1958).

Onitiri, A.C. and Boyo, A.E. Serum lipids and lipoproteins in children with kwashiorkor. *Br. Med. J.* 3, 630–631 (1975).

Osborne, J.C. and Brewer, B., Jr. The plasma lipoproteins. *Adv. Proc. Chem.* 31, 253–337 (1977).

Page, I.H. The Lewis A. Connor Memorial Lecture: Atherosclerosis. An Introduction. *Circulation* 10, 1–27 (1954).

Peng, S.K., Taylor, C.B., Tham, P., Werthessen, N.T., and Mikkelson, B. Effect of auto-oxidation products from cholesterol on aortic smooth muscle cells. *Arch. Path. Lab. Med.* 102, 57–61 (1978).

Peterson, V.E., Ceapo, P.A., Weininger, J., Ginsbers, H., and Olefsky, J. Quantification of plasma cholesterol and triglyceride levels in hypercholesterolemic subjects receiving ascorbic acid supplements. *Am. J. Clin. Nut.* 28, 584–587 (1975).

Reid, M.E. and Briggs, G.M. Development of semi-synthetic diet for young guinea pigs. *J. Nut.* 51, 341–354 (1953).

Rhoads, G.G., Gulbrandsen, C.L., and Kagan, A. Serum lipoproteins and coronary heart disease in a population study of Hawaii Japanese men. *N. Eng. J. Med.* 294, 293–300 (1976).

Robertson, A.L., and Khairallah, P.A. Angiotension II: Rapid localization in nuclei of smooth and cardiac muscle. *Science* 172, 1138–1139 (1971).

Robertson, A.L. and Khairallah, P.A. Arterial endothelial permeability and vascular disease. The "trap door" effect. *Exp. Mol. Path.* 18, 241–260 (1973).

Robertson, W. and Van, B. The biochemical role of ascorbic acid in connective tissue. *Ann. N.Y. Acad. Sci.* 92, 159–167 (1961).

Roe, J.H. and Kuether, C.A. The determination of ascorbic acid in whole blood and urine through the 2,4-Dinitrophenylhydrazine derivative of dehydroascorbic acid. *J. Biol. Chem.* 147, 399–407 (1943).

Ross, J.H. and Glomset, J.A. Atherosclerosis and the arterial smooth muscle cell: Proliferation of smooth muscle cell is a key event in the genesis of the lesion of atherosclerosis. *Science* 180, 1332–1339 (1973).

Schapiro, R.H., Scheig, R.L., Drummey, G.D., Mendelson. J.H., and Isselbacher, K.J. Effect of prolonged ethanol injestion on the transport and metabolsim of lipids in man. *N. Eng. J. Med.* 272, 610–615 (1965).

Shimamoto, T., Numano, F., and Fjuta, T. Atherosclerosis-inhibiting effect on an anti-bradykinin agent, pyridinolcarbamate. *Am. Heart J.* 71, 216–227 (1966).

Sokoloff, B., Hori, M., Saelhof, C., McConnell, B., and Imai, T. Effect of ascorbic acid on certain blood fat metabolism factors in animals and man. *J. Nut.* 91, 107–118 (1967).

Spittle, C.R. Atherosclerosis and vitamin C. *Lancet* 2, 1280–1281 (1972).

Stanhope, J.M., Sampson, V.M., and Clarkson, P.M. High-density-lipoprotein cholesterol and other serum lipids in a New Zealand biracial adolescent sample. The Wairoa College survey. *Lancet* 1, 968–970 (1977).

Stein, Y., Glangeaul, M.C., Fainaru, M., and Stein, O. The removal of cholesterol from aortic smooth muscle cells in culture and Landschutz ascites cells by fractions of human high density apolipoprotein. *Biochim. Biophys. Acta* 380, 106–118 (1975).

Stein, O., Vanderhoek, J., and Stein, Y. Cholesterol content and sterol synthesis in human skin fibroblasts and rat aortic smooth muscle cells exposed to lipoprotein-depleted serum and high density apolipoprotein/phospholipid mixtures. *Biochim. Biophys. Acta.* 431, 347–358 (1976).

Stone, N.J. and Levy, R.I. Hyperlipoproteinemia and coronary heart disease. *Prog. Card. Dis.* 14, 341–359 (1972).

Story, J.A. and Kritchevsky, D. Binding of sodium tavrocholate by various foodstuffs. *Nut. Rep. Int.* II, 161–163 (1975).

Story, J.A. and Kritchevsky, D. Dietary fiber and lipid metabolism, in *Fiber in Human Nutrition.* G.A. Spiller and R.J. Amen, eds. New York: Plenum Press (1976a), pp. 171–184.

Story, J.A. and Kritchevsky, D. Comparison of the binding of various bile acids and bile salts in vitro by several types of fiber. *J. Nut.* 106, 1292–1294 (1976).

Story, J.A. Dietary fiber disease, in *Nutritional Elements and Clinical Biochemistry.* M.A. Brewster and H.K. Naito, eds. New York: Plenum Press (1980), pp. 383–396.

Taura, M., Taura, S., Tokuhasu, K., Cho, B.H.S., and Kummerow, F.A. Untrastructural changes in the coronary artery induced by hypervitaminosis. *J. Am. Oil Chem. Soc.* 55, 237A (1978).

Technicon AutoAnalyzer 12/60 and 6/60. Technicon Instruments Corp., Tarrytown, N.Y. (1974).

Trowell, H.C. Ischemic heart disease and dietary fiber. *Am. J. Clin. Nut.* 25, 926–932 (1972).

Van die Redaskie. Coronary heart disease in China. *S. Afr. Med. J.* 47, 1485–1491 (1973).

Veressy, B., Balint, A., Kocz, A., and Jellinek, H. Increasing aortic permeability by atherogenic diet. *Atherosclerosis* 11, 369–371 (1970).

Walker, A.R.P. and Arvidsson, V.B. Fat intake, serum cholesterol concentration, and atherosclerosis in the South African Bantu. Part I. Low fat intake and the age trend of serum cholesterol concentration in the South African Bantu. *J. Clin. Invest.* 33, 1358–1365 (1954).

Walter, E.D., Van atta, G.R., Thompson, C.R., and Maclay, W.D. Alfalfa saponin. *J. Am. Chem. Soc.* 76, 2271–2273 (1954).

Watt, B.K., and Merrill, A.L. *Composition of Foods.* U.S. Department of Agriculture Handbook No. 8. Washington, D.C.: U.S. Government Printing Office (1963).

Wiener, J., Lattes, R.G., Meltzer, B.G., and Spiro, D. The cellular pathology of experimental hypertension. *Am. J. Path.* 54, 187–208 (1969).

Wilhelmsen, L., Wedel, H., and Tibblin, G. Multivariate analysis of risk factors for coronary heart disease. *Circulation* 48, 950–958 (1973).

Willis, G.C. An experimental study of the intimal ground substance in atherosclerosis. *Canad. Med. Assoc. J.* 69, 17–24 (1953).

Willis, G.C., and Fishman, S. Ascorbic Acid content of human arterial tissue. *Canad. Med. Assoc. J.* 72, 500–502 (1955).

Yeh, Y.Y., and Leveille, G.A. Effect of dietary protein and hepatic lipogenesis in the growing chick. *J. Nut.* 98, 356–366 (1969).

13

Dietary Approach to Treatment of Hyperlipidemia: The Prudent Polyunsaturated Fat Diet

DONNA B. ROSENSTOCK
FRAN HOERRMANN
HERBERT K. NAITO

INTRODUCTION

The purpose of this chapter is to discuss the rationale for implementing a prudent low-fat diet, the parameters of the diet and additional benefits which may result from controlling other nutritional risk factors associated with coronary heart disease (CHD).

CHD and other forms of atherosclerosis are still the main cause of death of affluent cultures. The United States ranks second in the world on the incidence of deaths due to CHD (Table 1).

Change in CHD incidence, diet, and blood lipid levels are occurring. For instance, the following countries have experienced a significant decrease in annual reported CHD mortality rates between 1968 and 1976 (Ahrens, 1980):

United States
Canada
Australia
Finland
United Kingdom
Belgium
Israel
Japan
Norway

The following countries have experienced no apparent change:

Czechoslovakia
New Zealand
Italy
Netherlands
Austria
Federal Republic of Germany
Switzerland

Table 1. Coronary Heart Disease Mortality Rates[a,b]

Country	*Men*	*Women*
Eastern Finland	872	262
U.S.A.	793	318
New Zealand	740	311
Ireland	672	288
Australia	787	311
United Kingdom	702	254
Canada	663	247
Norway	581	173
Netherlands	502	168
Israel	625	352
Denmark	606	225
Belgium	463	163
Federal Republic of Germany	457	150
Sweden	588	214
Austria	435	164
Venezuela	323	189
Switzerland	279	90
Italy	309	127
France	205	72
Japan	115	61

[a]Rate per 100,000 people.
[b]From Stamler (1979).

The following countries appear to have experienced an increase in CHD deaths:

Sweden	Romania
Denmark	Bulgaria
France	Hungary
Poland	Republic of Ireland
Yugoslavia	Northern Ireland

The decreasing U.S. cardiovascular mortality trend is established for every age group, sex, race, and type of cardiovascular event. Thus, there appears to be no group impermeable to preventive influences. There is growing evidence that risk factor and risk behavior changes may precede or accompany changes in CHD mortality (Table 2).

The habitual diet of a population largely determines the wide variation in population means and distribution of blood lipid and lipoprotein concentrations which are, in turn, accompanied by widely varying rates of atherosclerotic disease. This epidemiologic evidence, widely recognized and accepted in the scientific community, is congruent with clinical and experimental findings on the etiology of atherosclerosis. Substantial changes are now occurring

Table 2. Primary and Secondary CHD Risk Factors[a]

Primary	*Secondary*
Heredity	Age
Elevated blood lipids	Male sex
Elevated blood pressure	Overweight
Cigarette smoking	Lack of exercise
	Endocrine disorders
	Oral contraceptive agents
	Stress
	Thrombogenic disorders
	Hemodynamics
	Toxic agents
	Nutrition

[a]From Stamler (1979).

in the eating patterns of many cultures; these changes appear to have an effect on the population means and distribution of blood lipid and lipoprotein levels (McGandy, 1975).

In recent years, changing trends can be seen in the American lifestyle. There is reason to believe that these lifestyle changes have played a role in reducing the incidence of CHD in the United States. People are becoming more concerned with ways in which they can improve their health. Several trends that have had a positive effect on these lifestyle changes are:

1. Increased interest in physical fitness
2. Preventative medical practices
3. Increased consumer awareness
4. Better health education
5. Changes in dietary habits

Regarding the fifth category, changes in food habits are occurring in the United States' population (as compared to the turn of the century) and are seen in Table 3. This has resulted in a change in the composition of the average American daily dietary intake, as shown in Table 4.

Although the lipid hypothesis is still controversial, human metabolic studies have been consistent in regard to the relationships between saturated and polyunsaturated fats and their effect on plasma cholesterol concentration. Ahrens (1954), Keys et al. (1957), and Hegsted (1965) have demonstrated that increases in saturated fats in the diet will elevate serum cholesterol con-concentrations, whereas polyunsaturated fats will decrease the serum cholesterol level.

Western populations show a positive relationship between the mean intake of saturated fats, blood lipids, and incidence of CHD (Glueck and

Table 3. Changes in Dietary Consumption by the American Public[a,b]

↓	Egg
↓	Whole milk
↓	Butter
↓	Cream
↓	Pork fat
↑	Vegetable oils and fat
↑	Grains
↑	Ice cream
↑	Beef
↑	Cheese
↑	Alcohol

[a]From Stamler (1979).
[b]↓ = decrease; ↑ = increase.

Table 4. U.S. Dietary Intake[a,b]

↓	Cholesterol
↓	Saturated fat
↑	Polyunsaturated fat
↑	Fiber

[a]From Stamler (1979).
[b]↓ = decrease; ↑ = increase.

Connor, 1979). Conversely, vegetable-protein diets, such as those of the Seventh Day Adventists, or of vegetarians, have resulted in a low incidence of CHD. Migrants who have changed their food habits from a low to a high cholesterol diet have developed higher serum cholesterol levels and a higher incidence of CHD.

Numerous diet plans have been suggested by physicians, associations, and expert committees over the past 20 years to decrease CHD risk. No less than 20 expert scientific committees have recommended dietary modification as a means for controlling blood lipid levels and reducing the risk of CHD. Table 5 summarizes their recommendations. These committees, as well as the Select Committee on Nutrition and Human Needs, recommend changes in the food habits of the U.S. population. These changes are a decreased intake of cholesterol and saturated fats, and a relative increase in polyunsaturated fats. These dietary changes are also necessary for the treatment of the high-risk individual for CHD.

Atherosclerosis appears to be a constituent of the natural aging process and appears to take about 30 to 40 years to develop in most individuals. Accordingly, accelerated atherosclerosis leading to premature CHD does not manifest its symptoms until the fourth or fifth decade of life. Thus, one means of reducing lipid risk factors in high-risk persons via dietary regimens

Table 5. Recommendations of Expert Committees on Moderate Dietary Change to Reduce Risk of Coronary Heart Disease[a]

Country and Organization of Origin	For General Populations or High-risk Groups	As Percentage of Total Calories: Fat	PUFA[b]	SFA[c]	Cholesterol (mg/day)	Decrease Sugar
Scandinavian countries, 1968 Official collective recommendation	GP[d]	25–35	Increase	Decrease	–	Yes
United States, 1972 Inter-Society Commission for Heart Disease Resources	GP HR[e]	<35	Up to 10	<10	<300	–
United States, 1972 American Health Foundation	GP	<35	10–12	10–12	<300	Yes
United States, 1972 American Medical Association and National Academy of Sciences	HR	Substantial decrease in saturated fat	Substitute PUFA for SFA	Decrease	Reduce	–
United States, 1973 International Society of Cardiology	HR	<30	–	Decrease	<300	Yes
Netherlands, 1973 Nutrition Council	GP	30–35 Ideally 33	10–13	Decrease substantially	250–300	Yes
Australia, 1974 National Heart Foundation	GP HR	30–35	Increase	Decrease	<300	Yes
United Kingdom, 1974 Dept. of Health and Social Security	GP	Reduce	–	Reduce	–	–

Table 5. (Continued)

Country and Organization of Origin	For General Populations or High-risk Groups	As Percentage of Total Calories			Cholesterol (mg/day)	Decrease Sugar
		Fat	PUFA[b]	SFA[c]		
Germany, 1975 Federal Health Office	GP	20–25	10–15	Reduce	300	–
New Zealand, 1976 National Heart Foundation	GP	35	Substitute PUFA for SFA	Decrease	300–600	Yes
United Kingdom, 1976 Royal College of Physicians and British Cardiac Society	GP	Toward 35	Substitute PUFA for SFA	Reduce	Reduce	Yes
Norway, 1976 Ministry of Agriculture	GP	<35	Increase	Decrease	–	Yes
Canada, 1977 Dept. of National Health and Welfare	GP	30–35	Substitute PUFA for SFA	Decrease substantially	<400	Yes
Ireland, 1977 An Foras Taluntais	GP	Reduce	–	–	–	–
United States, 1977 Dietary Goals	GP	30	Up to 20	<10	<300	Yes

Table 5. (Continued)

Country and Organization of Origin	*For General Populations or High-risk Groups*	*As Percentage of Total Calories*			*Cholesterol (mg/day)*	*Decrease Sugar*
		Fat	*PUFA*[b]	*SFA*[c]		
United States, 1978 American Heart Association	GP	30–35	Up to 10	<10	<300	–
European Society of Cardiology, 1978	HR	Toward 30	Substitute PUFA for SFA	10	<300	Yes
Food and Agriculture Organization and World Health Organization, 1978	GP	30–35	10–12	Decrease substantially	<300	Yes

[a]From Bieber (1979).
[b]PUFA = polyunsaturated fatty acids.
[c]SFA = saturated fatty acids.
[d] GP = general population
[e]HR = high-risk groups.

should be initiated during adolescence, which may then result in the greatest effect in reducing the mortality and morbidity due to CHD (Kwiterovich, 1977). The Pediatric Lipid Clinic at the Cleveland Clinic Foundation, Cleveland, Ohio, follows children from family members who are at high risk for CHD. The pediatric dietitian is primarily responsible for the childrens' diets, which is separate from the adult population. Since our experience is limited with this population, further comment and recommendations will be out of context in this discussion.

It is generally recognized that CHD is caused by a combination of factors. Several of the known risk factors for CHD are high concentrations of blood lipids, hypertension, smoking, overweight, imbalanced diet, diabetes mellitus, gout, and renal disease (Hoerrmann et al., 1980). Many of the CHD risk factors can be manipulated or controlled by changing certain dietary habits. These dietary modifications include a reduction to ideal body weight, decreased consumption of foods high in cholesterol and saturated fats, increased intake of polyunsaturated fats, and limited intake of refined simple sugars, salt, and alcohol. A dietary regimen that is low in saturated fats and cholesterol will cause the greatest reduction in serum cholesterol in obese individuals who are hypercholesterolemic and reduce to ideal body weight.

RATIONALE OF THE DIET PARAMETERS

The initial dietary treatment for hyperlipidemia should meet the following criteria for maximum effectiveness:

1. Reduce cholesterol intake to $\leqslant$ 300 mg/day.
2. Increase polyunsaturated fat to saturated fat (P/S) ratio to 1.0 to 1.3.
3. Reduce total fat intake to 80 to 100 g/day (35 to 40 percent of total kilocalories).
4. Maintain caloric intake between 1800 to 2500 kcal/day.
5. Limit sodium intake to 4 to 6 g/day.
6. Decrease consumption of simple sugars.

The Cleveland Clinic Foundation's Prudent Polyunsaturated Fat Diet (PPFD) was developed by manipulating the saturated fat, polyunsaturated fat, and cholesterol content of meat products, dairy products, margarines, and oils (Table 6).

Table 6. Prudent Polyunsaturated-Fat Diet Calculations

	Fat (g)	*Saturated Fatty Acid (g)*	*Polyunsaturated Fatty Acid (g)*	*Cholesterol (mg)*
7 oz. lean beef (7 X 3 g)	21	9[a]	1.2[a]	196[b]
2 cups 1% milk (2 X 2.5 g)	5	3.1[c]	0.2[c]	14[d]
4 tsp tub margarine (4 X 4 g)	16	2.4[e]	4.8[e]	–
4 tsp corn oil (4 X 5 g)	20	2.6[f]	11.6[f]	–
Total	62	17.1	17.8	210
Calories	558	153.9	160.2	–
Percentage of total calories based on 1800 calories	31	8.5	8.8	–
Total P/S ratio			1.0	

Adapted from Brown, 1976.
[a]Beef fat saturated fat = 43 percent; polyunsaturated fat = 6 percent.
[b]Beef cholesterol = 28 mg/oz.
[c]Butter fat saturated fat = 62 percent; polyunsaturated fat = 4 percent.
[d]1 percent milk = 7 mg cholesterol.
[e]Tub margarine saturated fat = 15 percent; polyunsaturated fat = 30 percent.
[f]Corn oil saturated fat = 13 percent; polyunsaturated fat = 5.8 percent.

PPFD FAT-MODIFIED DIET

The Cleveland Clinic Foundation's PPFD was designed as a therapeutic regimen for hypercholesterolemia and concentrates on Brown's (1976) Master Food Plan, which is based on lean meat, fish and poultry, low-fat or skim milk diary products, and the use of polyunsaturated oils and margarines (see Table 7).

The PPFD is a nutritionally adequate diet with respect to calories, carbohydrate, protein, fat, vitamins, and minerals (Christakis and Rinzler, 1969; Inter-Society Commission for Heart Disease Resources, 1970, 1972; Anderson and Grande et al., 1973; Blackburn, 1978). The dietary regimen meets all presently known nutrient requirements for maintenance of good health.

ADDITIONAL BENEFITS OF A FAT-MODIFIED DIET

It should be emphasized that although the primary goal of the PPFD is to reduce serum cholesterol, secondary benefits also seem to occur. Diabetes

Table 7. Master Food Patterns[a,b,c]

Food Pattern	*Fat (% Calories)*	*Carbohydrate*[d] *(% Calories)*	*Saturated Fatty Acid*[d] *(% Calories)*	*Polyunsaturated Fatty Acid*[d] *(% Calories)*
Basic low fat	12	73	5	1
Moderate low fat	20	65	5	8
Moderate fat	33	52	7	12
Customary fat	38	47	10	15

[a]From Brown (1976).
[b]Mean daily protein intake: 15 percent of total calories (range = 15–20 percent).
[c]Mean daily cholesterol intake: 300 mg (range = 75 to 300 mg).
[d]Carbohydrate, saturated fatty acids, and polyunsaturated fatty acids.

mellitus and obesity are also known risk factors for CHD. Obesity is correlated to the high consumption of refined simple sugars, alcohol, and an excessive caloric intake. Therefore, it seems prudent to design a diet that can limit the intake of simple sugars and alcohol, yet provide adequate (but not excessive) calories. For people who are above their ideal body weight or have diabetes mellitus, we use a modified version of the American Diabetes Association's Exchange Lists (1976) for meal planning which incorporates the parameters of the PPFD, or part of the fat-modified diet plan. Further specific details of the PPFD is provided in the section of this chapter on diet development. It has been documented that diabetic patients following a fat-modified diet demonstrated better control of blood glucose levels and a decreased need for oral hypoglycemic drugs or insulin (Houtsmuller, 1975; Farinaro et al., 1977; Anderson and Ward, 1978; Hockaday et al., 1978).

Often a reduction in dietary cholesterol and saturated fat results in a deficit of calories. For individuals who are at their ideal body weight, this deficit is supplemented with an increased intake of complex carbohydrates, such as starches, fruits, vegetables, and vegetable proteins.

The amount of salt and high-sodium foods can affect the control of hypertension. By adding a salt (sodium) restriction to the PPFD, a simultaneous reduction in two risk factors for premature CHD, hypertension, and hypercholesterolemia will result. The average American diet contains approximately 7 to 15 g of sodium per day (Select Committee on Nutrition and Human Needs, 1977). However, these figures will vary depending on the quantity of convenience food items used in the diet. The sodium content of these foods is available in a handbook published by the West Suburban Dietetic Association (Rezabek, 1979).

DIET DEVELOPMENT

One apparent question is: What tools are available to the dietitian when planning a therapeutic diet? Diet histories and a 24-hour recall (Fig. 1–3) are

THE CLEVELAND CLINIC FOUNDATION
NUTRITION PROFILE FORM

Name:______________________ Age:____Height:____Weight:________

Address:____________________ Occupation:____________________

____________________ Scheduled Work Hours:______________

Phone:(home)__________________

(work)__________ __________ Date:____________________

1. List other household members:

	NAME	RELATION	AGE	SPECIAL DIET FOLLOWED
a.				
b.				
c.				
d.				
e.				

2. Do you now or have you ever followed a "special diet"? Yes____No____
If yes, what type of diet?____________________
How long did you follow the diet?____________________
For what reason did you follow the diet?____________________
From what source did you recieve the information about your diet?
Physician____Dietitian____Book or Magazine____Title____________
Special diet of health food store____Other____________________
3. Do you take vitamin/mineral/diet supplements? Yes____No____
If yes, list:____________________
4. Who is responsible for home food preparation?____________________
5. Who is responsible for food purchasing?____________________
6. Which meals are most often eaten away from home:____________________
Breakfast____Lunch____Dinner____Snacks____
7. Do you have trouble chewing or swallowing food Yes____No____
If yes, explain:____________________
8. Do you have any food allergies? Yes____No____
If yes, explain:____________________

Fig. 1 The Cleveland Clinic Foundation Nutrition Profile Form.

used in obtaining food preferences and identifying the particularities of an individual's eating pattern. Setting up a patient's profile containing this information will aid the dietitian in planning a therapeutic diet that is adaptable to lifestyle, needs, and preferences. This information will ensure optimal nutritional care, enhance patient dietary adherence, and provide a base for individual instructions. Reliable nutrient information can be obtained from food composition handbooks such as that of Church and Church (1975), and the United States Department of Agriculture (USDA) Handbook No. 456

NUTRITION PROFILE FORM - Page 2

9. Do you have frequent occurrences of the following?

	Yes	No		Yes	No
a. indigestion	____	____	d. diarrhea	____	____
b. nausea	____	____	e. constipation	____	____
c. vomiting	____	____			

10. Have you had any change in weight within the: a) past 3 months? b) past year? c) past 2 years? d) past 5 years? (please circle).
If yes, explain:____________________

____

____

11. Do you exercise or participate in athletic activities? Yes____ No____
If yes, what type?____________________
How often?____________________

12. What do you usually eat? Please list all foods that you usually eat between the time that you get up in the morning and the time you to to bed at night. Remember, everything you eat or drink is food. Cookies, nuts, sweets, salad dressings, gravy, cocktails, highballs, beer and soft drinks are food items just as are meat and potatoes. Indicate how the foods are prepared, such as broiled, baked, fried, boiled, etc.

At Breakfast	At Lunch	At Dinner
Mid-Morning Snack	Mid-Afternoon Snack	Before Bed Snack

During the night:____________________

____

Fig. 2 The Cleveland Clinic Foundation Nutrition Profile Form.

NUTRITION PROFILE FORM - Page 3

Please indicate below how often you eat or drink the following items.
Include amount and where indicated, circle the type of food eaten.
Example Milk: whole skim low-fat.

FOOD ITEM

Milk: whole skim low-fat chocolate: __________
Cheese buttermilk yogurt: __________
Pudding cottage cheese custard ice cream: __________
Beef lamb pork: baked broiled fried: __________
Chicken Turkey veal: baked broiled fried __________
Fish shellfish: baked broiled fried __________
Bacon sausage luncheon meat hot dogs: __________
Liver organ meats (kidney, tongue, etc.): __________
Eggs egg substitutes: __________
Dried beans peas legumes: __________
Peanut butter nuts seeds: __________
Cereals: whole grain sugar-coated other: __________
Breads: whole grain white other __________
Potatoes: baked mashed fried __________
Rice macaroni noodles spaghetti: __________
Dark green or yellow vegetables: __________
Other vegetables (including lettuce): __________
Citrus fruit or juice (not fruit drink): __________
Other fruit or juice: sweetened unsweetened __________
Cake cookies doughnuts pastries pie "Jello": __________
Sugar jelly syrup honey hard candy chocolate candy: __________
Pretzels potato chips peanuts salty snack foods: __________
Soups: cream other __________
Butter lard shortening bacon fat: __________
Margarine vegetable oil (list brand names): __________
Salad dressings mayonnaise: __________
Gravy cream sauces: __________
Alcoholic beverages: Type beer/wine other alcohol: __________
Kool-Aid fruit drinks lemonade punch: __________
Soft drinks ("pop") Diet soft drinks: __________
Coffee tea decaf. coffee Postum: __________

Which of the following do you add to your coffee or tea? Indicate amount per cup:

Nothing____ Cream____ Nondairy Cream____ Sugar____

Saccharin____ Honey____ Other____

Fig. 3 The Cleveland Clinic Foundation Nutrition Profile Form.

(Adams, 1975), or from USDA Handbook No. 8 (Watt and Merrill, 1963), or a nutrient data bank. Food values are listed in either grams or in common household measurements. Accessibility to a nutrient data bank greatly facilitates the dietitian's work load when developing individually tailored diets.

The HVH-CWRU Nutrient data base at Case Western Reserve University, Cleveland, Ohio is a computerized food table data storage facility that contains more than 2300 food items and recipes. The food items, including brand-name items, in the data base have been selected as a result of analysis of several thousand 24-hour intake records from several areas of the United

States. For each food item, there is a storage space for 71 nutrients. The nutrient composition of foods is derived from a variety of sources (Mattice, 1950; Toepfer et al., 1951; Orr and Watt, 1957; Leverton and Odell, 1958; Hardinge, 1961; Leung, 1961; Diem and Lenter, 1962; Watt and Merrill, 1963; Dicks, 1965; Umbarger, 1965; Eheart and Mason, 1967; Fetcher, 1967; McCarthy, 1968; Zook and Lehman, 1968; Orr, 1969; Feeley and Watt, 1970; Gormican, 1970; Nutrient Composition of Common Sizes and Measures of Foods, 1970; Streiff, 1971; Feeley et al., 1972; Sturdevant et al., 1973; Adams, 1975; American Home Economics Association, 1975; Anderson et al., 1975; Fristrom et al., 1975; Matthews and Garrison, 1975; Murphy, 1975; Posati et al., 1975; Posati et al., 1975; Anderson, 1976; Brignoli et al., 1976; Exler and Weihrauch, 1976; Fristrom and Weihrauch, 1976; Posati and Orr, 1976; Weihrauch et al., 1976; Anderson et al., 1977; Exler and Avena, 1977; Exler and Weihrauch, 1977; Consumer and Food Economics Institute, 1977; Perloff and Butrum, 1977; Dunbar and Stunkard, 1979; National Research Council, 1980). Needless to say, this type of facility greatly adds to the speed and convenience of analyzing an individual's dietary intake with great precision. This information has been carefully evaluated for methodology and reliability before incorporation into the data base. It must be recognized that for some nutrients, that is, vitamin D, vitamin B_6, iodine, copper, biotin, and pantothenic acid, only a limited amount of reliable food composition data are available. All nutrient data for food items are calculated on the basis of 100-g portions. However, analysis for all food items may be retrieved in a variety of weights (that is, from grams to ounces or pounds and, for many items, analysis may be retrieved for volume equivalents and for descriptive terms). An example of a computer printout is illustrated in Figs. 4 and 5.

The use of two egg yolks per week was calculated on a weekly basis (71 mg cholesterol/day). To achieve the indicated P/S ratio, special consideration was placed on margarines. The PPFD recommends using margarines that list either liquid safflower, liquid sunflower, or liquid corn oil as the first ingredient and that the ratio of polyunsaturated fat to saturated fat is $\geqslant 2.0$. The meats allowed in the diet have an average cholesterol content of 30 mg or less per ounce. This includes the use of Brown's (1976) recommendations of low- and medium-fat meats such as lean beef, pork, ham, Canadian bacon, lamb, veal, fish, and poultry without the skin. The meat group is limited to a total intake of 7 oz/day or 210 mg cholesterol.

Skim milk and foods made with skim milk may be used as desired. If 2 percent milk is preferred, 8 oz may be incorporated into the daily meal plan or 16 oz of 1 percent milk may be substituted.

The desired P/S ratio is achieved by using 2 to 3 tablespoons of margarine or acceptable oils each day. The acceptable oils are liquid safflower,

NUTRIENT ANALYSIS SUMMARY
NAME:
HVH-CWRU NUTRIENT DATA BASE **DATE: Friday, November 30, 1979** **ID: CC 002 05**

			Kcal	T-Prc (g)	T-Fat (g)	T-CHO (g)	Chol (mg)	PUFA (g)	SFA (g)	Fiber (g)
Breakfast										
6	Vol (Oz)	ORANGE JUICE UNSW, CANNED	90	1.5	0.4	20.9	–	–	–	.1867
1	Large	EGG WHOLE, POACHED	79	6.0	5.6	0.6	273	.72	1.665	0
2	Wt (Oz)	CANADIAN BACON, BROILED OR FRIED, DRAINED, SERVING WT	157	15.7	9.9	0.2	50	1.527	3.365	0
1	Slice	WHOLE WHEAT TOAST	55	2.4	0.7	10.8	–	–	.1121	.361
2	Teasp	MARGARINE REGULAR, FLEISCHMANN	68	0.1	7.6	0.0	0	2.026	1.231	–
Lunch										
2	Wt (Oz)	BEEF ROUND RUMP ROAST BONELESS LM ROASTED, SERVING WT	118	16.5	5.3	0.0	52	.681	2.213	0
2	Slice	WHOLE WHEAT BREAD	112	4.8	1.4	21.9	–	–	.2714	.736
.5	Cup	PINEAPPLE CHUNKS, CANNED, SOLIDS & LIQUIDS, JUICE PACK	71	0.5	0.1	18.6	–	–	–	.369
8	Vol (Oz)	SKIM MILK	86	8.4	0.4	11.9	5	.0171	.2867	0
.33	Cup	SUGAR GRANULATED, WHITE	244	0.0	0.0	63.0	0	0	0	0
.167	Teasp	CINNAMON, GROUND	1	0.0	0.0	0.3	0	.0020	.0024	.0921
.5	Cup	WALNUTS ENGLISH (HALVES)	326	7.5	32.0	7.9	0	21	3.47	1.05

Fig. 4 Case Western Reserve University Nutrient Analysis Summary.

			Kcal	T-Pro (g)	T-Fat (g)	T-CHO (g)	Chol (mg)	PUFA (g)	SFA (g)	Fiber (g)
Dinner										
4	Vol (oz)	APRICOT NECTAR, VITAMIN C ADDED	72	0.4	0.1	18.3	–	–	–	.251
3	Wt (oz)	FLOUNDER BAKED, SERVING WT	119	25.5	1.1	0.0	43	.5022	.2384	0
.5	Cup	POTATO PARED, BOILED & DICED OR SLICED	50	1.5	0.1	11.2	–	–	–	.3875
.5	Cup	WHITE SAUCE (MEDIUM)	203	4.9	15.6	11.0	16	–	8.75	–
.75	Cup	BEANS GREEN, CUT STYLE CANNED, DRAINED SOLIDS	24	1.4	0.2	5.3	–	–	–	1.013
1	Slice	WHOLE WHEAT BREAD	56	2.4	0.7	11.0	–	–	.1357	.368
.5	Cup	CABBAGE RAW COARSELY SHREDDED OR SLICED	8	0.5	0.1	1.9	–	–	–	.28
2	Teasp	MAYONNAISE	67	0.1	7.5	0.2	7	–	1.307	–
2	Teasp	MARGARINE REGULAR, FLEISCHMANN	68	0.1	7.6	0.0	0	2.026	1.231	–
Evening Snack										
1	Cup	SKIM MILK	86	8.4	0.4	11.9	5	.0171	.2867	0
.5	Medium	BANANA YELLOW RAW, EP	51	0.7	0.1	13.2	–	–	–	.2975
6	Number	STRAWBERRIES, WHOLE FRESH UNSW	41	0.8	0.6	9.4	–	–	–	1.453

Fig. 5 Case Western Reserve University Nutrient Analysis Summary.

Table 8. Fatty Acid Composition of Various Oils (Percentage of Distribution)[a]

Fatty Acid	*Coconut Oil*	*Palm Oil*	*Olive Oil*	*Corn Oil*	*Safflower Oil*
$C_{8:0}$	5.40	–	–	–	–
$C_{10:0}$	8.40	–	–	–	–
$C_{12:0}$	45.42	0.13	–	–	–
$C_{14:0}$	18.10	0.91	0.08	–	–
$C_{16:0}$	10.53	38.42	11.91	13.1	–
$C_{16:1}$	0.40	–	1.05	–	0.90
$C_{18:0}$	2.30	4.57	2.48	4.07	–
$C_{18:1}$	7.51	42.44	73.24	29.01	17.30
$C_{18:2}$	–	12.42	9.07	54.00	79.00
$C_{18:3}$	–	0.71	1.01	–	0.13
Other	1.94	0.40	1.16	–	2.67

[a]From H.K. Naito (unpublished report, determined by gas-liquid chromatography).

liquid soybean, liquid corn, liquid cottonseed, liquid sesame seed, and liquid sunflower seed oil.

The PPFD excludes the use of various convenience food items such as luncheon meats, frozen dinners and bakery products. The reasons that they are excluded are twofold. The first reason is the higher saturated fat content of these foods, and/or their cholesterol content, which is greater than 30 mg per ounce. The second reason is the lack of nutrient information regarding the total fat, saturated fat, and cholesterol content of commercially prepared convenience food items.

ADDITIONAL CONSIDERATIONS OF THE PPFD DIET

Age, socioeconomic conditions, number of meals eaten away from home, and any physical limitations are considerations which may necessitate additional dietary modification. Diet adherence is increased when information on label reading, food preparation, and dining out is provided by the clinician and dietitian when instituting dietary change.

By law, ingredients are listed on the label in descending order by weight. Many items, such as breads and cereals, contain small amounts of saturated fats. Such produces are allowed if the saturated fat is not listed as one of the first five ingredients.

When purchasing margarines and salad dressings, the degree of hydrogenation should be noted. Hydrogenation changes the chemical structure of an unsaturated fat to a saturated fat. If a vegetable oil is solid at room temperature or lists a partially hardened or hydrogenated oil as the first word on the list of ingredients, it should be avoided. All vegetable oils are not high in polyunsaturated fats (Table 8). Safflower oil is the highest in polyunsaturated fats, while coconut and palm oils are low. Most nondairy creamers and whipped toppings are made from coconut oil or palm oil which are saturated fats. Labels of products that state either "vegetable fat" or "vegetable oil" are usually one of these two oils and should be avoided.

With the elimination of many convenience food items, meal preparation will become more time consuming. Soups, casseroles, and baked goods must be homemade with acceptable ingredients. The amount of counseling and cooking suggestions given by the dietitian will vary, depending on the person's previous eating pattern. Several low-cholesterol cookbooks are available that will aid in the variety of the diet (Brown, 1968; American Heart Association, 1973; Jones, 1975).

Dining out in restaurants is an important part of the American lifestyle. Most restaurants and cafeterias offer a variety of foods from which to select a meal correctly. In many instances the frequency of meals eaten in restaurants may need to be reduced, but not omitted totally from the dietary protocol.

PATIENT ADHERENCE

Long-term adherence to any type of dietary protocol is a very difficult behavior modification to instill. Fat-modified diets are no exception. It is generally recognized that ongoing dietary follow-up protocols increase patient adherence and success with dietary changes. Although the Cleveland Clinic Foundation lacks rigid structure and consistency on the follow-up program, we feel that the PPFD has been effective. A preliminary study (see discussion below) indicates that patient adherence to the PPFD appears to be high.

A retrospective study was done on 59 males and 4 females ranging in age from 34 to 66 years, returning to the Cleveland Clinic Foundation for their six-week postoperative checkup during January and February 1979. All had attended the Prudent Polyunsaturated Fat Diet class prior to hospital discharge. During the postoperative checkup, a diet survey was distributed to the patients. Questions included a 24-hour recall designed to assess dietary adherence to the PPFD. Eighty-one percent admitted that the diet was a change from their previous eating habits. Seventy-two percent stated they did not have trouble following the diet and sixty-eight percent did not find the diet too restrictive. It was reported by eighty percent that the meat consumption was 7 oz or less per day. Sixty-three percent said that they could not reduce their meat consumption below the 7-oz allowance. Twenty-two percent avoided egg yolks in their diets completely and sixty-four percent ate one to two egg yolks per week. Fifty-two percent reported using skim milk as a beverage or in cooking and thirty-six percent indicated using 2 percent milk. Sixty-one percent used the recommended amounts of polyunsaturated oils and margarines per day.

Table 9. U.S. Dietary Goals

Dietary Constituents	*Current Diet (%)*	*Dietary Goals (%)*
Fat	42	30
Saturated	16	10
Poly- and monounsaturated	26	30
Protein	12	12
Carbohydrate	46	58
Simple	24	15
Complex	22	43

LONG-TERM GOALS

During the twentieth century, the composition of the average American diet has changed radically. Complex carbohydrates, which were once the mainstay of the American diet, now play a minor role. At the same time, the consumption of simple carbohydrates and fats has risen to a point where these two nutritional components alone now comprise at least sixty percent of the total caloric intake, up fifty percent from the turn of the century (Select Committee on Nutrition and Human Needs, 1977).

While we have discussed dietary modification as a therapeutic means of controlling the risk for CHD, one should develop dietary habits that evolve around the concept of preventive medicine, namely good nutrition. The Select Committee on Nutrition and Human Needs has set up guidelines for the consideration of the general public to adopt dietary goals (Table 9).

Adoption of these guidelines would mean that Americans would have to:

1. Increase carbohydrate consumption to account for 55 to 60 percent of total energy (caloric) intake.
2. Reduce overall fat consumption from approximately 40 to 30 percent of total energy intake.
3. Reduce saturated fat consumption to account for about 10 percent of total energy intake; and balance that with polyunsaturated and monounsaturated fats, which should each account for about 10 percent of total energy intake.
4. Reduce cholesterol consumption to about 300 mg per day.
5. Reduce sugar consumption by about 40 percent, so that it accounts for about 15 percent of total energy intake.
6. Reduce salt consumption by about 50 to 85 percent to approximately 3 g per day.

In terms of changes in food selection and preparation this would mean:

1. Increased consumption of fruits, vegetables, and whole grains.
2. Decreased consumption of meat and increased consumption of poultry and fish.
3. Decreased consumption of foods high in fat; and partial substitution of polyunsaturated fat for saturated fat.
4. Substitution of nonfat milk for whole milk.
5. Decreased consumption of butterfat, eggs, and other high-cholesterol foods.
6. Decreased consumption of sugar and foods high in sugar content.
7. Decreased consumption of salt and foods high in salt content.

While the adoption of these dietary goals by the general public for the practical prevention of diseases has not been established, it would seem like an excellent alternative approach to achieving good health in an affluent society such as ours. The real problem is implementing these guidelines on a national scale for a prolonged period.

CONCLUSION

The development and progression of CHD appears to have many contributing factors such as heredity, environment, and lifestyle. There is, at the time of writing, substantial evidence that the diet recommended here will aid in the control of certain known dietary risk factors for CHD. The most important criteria of the therapeutic success in the use of this diet are the long-term serum lipid and lipoprotein responses obtained in the individual patient. Once hypercholesterolemia is detected, dietary intervention will partially or completely reduce this lipid to within the normal range (in most individuals), and reduce the risk of premature myocardial infarcts. Ideally, dietary intervention should commence long before clinical symptoms of CHD are detected. Nutrient and calorie requirements are a primary consideration when designing a dietary protocol for the various age groups. It should be mentioned that any additional dietary risk factors, such as obesity, diabetes mellitus, and hypertension are just as critical to control as elevated serum lipids. Ongoing nutrition education will enhance dietary adherence, and contribute to the decline in the morbidity and mortality of CHD.

ACKNOWLEDGMENTS

We would like to acknowledge Mrs. Charlene B. Krejci, M.S., R.D., Mrs. Patricia Daniel, and the Cleveland Clinic Foundation's Department of

Nutritional Services for their assistance in the preparation of this manuscript. We would also like to express our gratitude to Phyllis Pittman and Jeannette Goodman for typing this manuscript. This work presented in this chapter was supported by Grant No. CRP 400 from the Cleveland Clinic Foundation, Grant No. HL-6835 from National Heart, Lung, and Blood Institute, and Grant No. 8557 from the Bleeksma Fund of the Cleveland Clinic Foundation.

APPENDIX

The following is a seven-day menu cycle illustrating the parameters of the Prudent Polyunsaturated Fat Diet. Each day's menu does not exceed 300 mg cholesterol, has a P/S ratio of 1.0 to 1.3, with a minimum caloric level of 2000 calories. The menus were analyzed at the Case Western Reserve University Data Bank and meet the Recommended Daily Allowances for protein, vitamins, and minerals for the reference male.

Day 1

Breakfast	Serving Size
Pineapple juice	6 oz
Omelet[a]	½ cup
Rye toast	2 slices
Margarine	3 tsp
Skim milk	8 oz
Lunch	
Cottage cheese fresh fruit plate	½ cup (low-fat cheese)
Melba toast	8 slices
Whole wheat cupcake[b]	2 cupcakes
Dinner	
Veal Italian style	6 oz
Noodles	1 cup
Zucchini	1 cup
Fresh spinach salad	1 cup
French dressing	3 tsp
Kaiser roll	2 rolls
Margarine	2 tsp
Fresh fruit cup	1 cup

[a]Made with low-cholesterol egg substitute.
[b]Reprinted with permission of American Heart Association (1973a).

Day 2

Breakfast	Serving Size
Orange juice	6 oz
Low-cholesterol egg substitute	½ cup
Whole wheat toast	2 slices
Margarine	3 tsp
Lunch	
Roast beef sandwich (on whole wheat bread)	1 (with 3 oz meat)
Pineapple chunks	¾ cup
Cinnamon Nuts[a]	1 cup
Skim milk	8 oz
Dinner	
Apricot nectar	6 oz
Baked fillet of flounder	4 oz
Delmonico potatoes[b]	1 cup
Green beans	¾ cup
Coleslaw	¾ cup
Whole wheat bread	2 tsp
Margarine	3 tsp
Evening Snack	
Banana–strawberry milkshake[c]	

[a]Reprinted with permission of American Heart Association (1973a).
[b]Made with acceptable ingredients.
[c]Made with skim milk.

Day 3

Breakfast	Serving Size
Grapefruit sections	½ cup
Oatmeal with raisins	1 cup (with ¼ cup raisins)
Bagel	1
Margarine	2 tsp
Skim milk	8 oz

Lunch	
Tuna salad sandwich (on whole wheat bread)	1 (2 oz tuna)
Mayonnaise	2 tsp
Fresh fruit cup	½ cup
Angel food cake	1½-inch slice
Skim milk	8 oz

Dinner	
Roast pork	5 oz
Mashed potatoes	1 cup
Broccoli	½ cup
Marinated beet and onion salad	¾ cup
Whole wheat bread	1 slice
Margarine	3 tsp
Pudding[a]	½ cup

Evening Snack	
Popcorn, popped	2 cups
Iced tea	12 oz

[a]Made with skim milk.

Day 4

Breakfast	Serving Size
Orange juice	6 oz
40% bran flakes	1 cup
Low-cholesterol egg substitute	¼ cup
Whole wheat toast	2 slices
Margarine	3 tsp
Skim milk	1 cup

Lunch	
Roast turkey sandwich (on whole wheat bread)	1 (3 oz meat)
Mayonnaise	2 tsp
Carrot and celery sticks	10 sticks
Apple	1 fruit

Dinner	
Broiled steak	4 oz
Baked potato	1 large (7 oz)
Asparagus	½ cup
Tossed salad	1 cup
Oil and vinegar dressing	2 tsp
French bread	One 1-inch slice
Margarine	3 tsp
Strawberries	1 cup

Day 5

Breakfast	Serving Size
Banana	1 medium
Special K cereal	1 cup
French toast[a]	2 slices
Margarine	3 tsp
Skim milk	8 oz

Lunch	
Baked perch	4 oz
Herb rice	1 cup
Parslied carrots	½ cup
Rye roll	2
Margarine	2 tsp
Skim milk	8 oz

Dinner	
Spaghetti with meat sauce	2 cups (with 3 oz meat)
Tossed salad	1 cup
Italian dressing	3 tsp
Garlic bread[b]	Two 1-inch slices
Melon	1 cup

[a]Made with low-cholesterol egg substitute and wheat bread.
[b]Made with acceptable ingredients.

Day 6

Breakfast	Serving Size
Cranapple juice	6 oz
Western omelet[a]	1
English muffin	1
Margarine	3 tsp

Lunch	
Chicken salad sandwich (on whole wheat bread)	1 (with 2 oz meat)
Mayonnaise	2 tsp
Carrot sticks	
Apple	1 large fruit
Skim Milk	8 oz

Dinner	
Roast beef	5 oz
Mashed potatoes	1 cup
Corn	¾ cup
Whole wheat bread	2 slices
Margarine	3 tsp
Pink lemonade pie[b]	1/8 pie
Skim milk	8 oz

[a]Made with acceptable ingredients.
[b]Reprinted with permission of American Heart Association (1973a).

Day 7

Breakfast	Serving Size
Orange juice	6 oz
Life cereal	1 cup
Low-cholesterol egg substitute	¼ cup
English muffin	1 muffin
Margarine	3 tsp
Skim milk	8 oz

Lunch

Hamburger on bun	One 3-oz pattie
Lettuce and tomato slices	1 each
Grapes	20 grapes
Iced tea	12 oz

Dinner

Pork chop	4 oz
Sweet potatoes	1 cup
Cauliflower	¾ cup
Biscuit[a]	3 biscuits
Lettuce wedge	2 tsp
French dressing	3 tsp
Skim milk	8 oz

[a]Homemade with acceptable ingredients.

REFERENCES

Adams, C. *Nutritive Value of American Foods in Common Units.* USDA Handbook No. 456. United States Department of Agriculture, Washington, D.C. (1975).

Ahrens, E.H., Jr. Evaluation of the evidence relating national dietary patterns to disease, in *Atherosclerosis V.* A.M. Gotto, Jr., L.C. Smith, and B. Allen, eds. Springer-Verlag, New York (1980), pp. 219–234.

Ahrens, E.H., Jr., Blankenhorn, D.H., and Tsaltas, T.T. Effect on human serum lipids of substituting plant for animal fat in diet. *Proc. Soc. Exp. Biol. Med.* 86, 872–878 (1954).

American Heart Association. *American Heart Association Cookbook.* David McKay, New York (1973a).

American Heart Association. *Diet and Coronary Heart Disease.* American Heart Association, New York (1973b).

American Home Economics Association. *Handbook of Food Preparation,* 7th ed. American Home Economics Association, Washington, D.C. (1975).

Anderson, B. VII. Pork products: Comprehensive evaluation of fatty acids in foods. *J. Am. Diet. Assoc.* 69, 44–49 (1976).

Anderson, B., Fristrom, G., and Weihrauch, J. X. Lamb and veal: Comprehensive evaluation of fatty acids in foods. *J. Am. Diet. Assoc.* 70, 53–58 (1977).

Anderson, B., Kinsella, J., and Watt, B. II. Beef products: Comprehensive evaluation of fatty acids in foods. *J. Am. Diet. Assoc.* 67, 35–41 (1975).

Anderson, J.T., Grande, F., and Keys, A. Cholesterol lowering diets. *J. Am. Diet. Assoc.* 62, 133–142 (1973).

Anderson, J.W., and Ward, K. Long term effects of high carbohydrate, high fiber diets on glucose and lipid metabolism; A preliminary report on patients with diabetes. *Diabetes Care* 1, 77–82 (1978).

Bieber, M.A. *Atherosclerosis Update: Emphasis on Diet.* Best Foods, Englewood Cliffs, New Jersey (1979).

Blackburn, H. How nutrition influences mass hyperlipidemia and atherosclerosis. *Geriatrics* 33, 42–46 (1978).

Brignoli, C., Kinsella, J., and Weihrauch, J. V. Unhydrogenated fats and oils: Comprehensive evaluation of fatty acids in foods. *J. Am. Diet. Assoc.* 68, 224–229 (1976).

Brown, H.B. *Low Fat Vegetable Oil Recipes.* Cleveland Clinic Research Division. Cleveland Clinic Foundation, Cleveland, Ohio (1968).

Brown, H.B. Diet Management of Hyperlipidemia. *Prac. Card.* 2 (4), 19–27 (1976).

Christakis, G., and Rinzler, S.H. Diet, in *Atherosclerosis.* F.G. Schettler and G.S. Boyd, eds. Elsevier, New York (1969), pp. 823–854.

Church, C., and Church, H. *Food Values of Portions Commonly Used,* 12th ed. J.B. Lippincott, Philadelphia (1975).

Consumer and Food Economics Institute. *Composition of Foods: Spices and Herbs–Raw, Processed, Prepared.* Consumer and Food Economics Institute. USDA Handbook No. 8-2. United States Department of Agriculture, Washington, D.C. (1977).

Dicks, M. *Vitamin E Content of Foods and Foods for Human and Animal Consumption.* Bulletin No. 435, Agricultural Experimental Station, University of Wyoming. Division of Biochemistry, Laramie, Wyoming (1965).

Diem, K., and Lentner, C., eds. *Documenta Geigy, Scientific Tables,* 6th ed. Ciba-Geigy, Ardsley, New York (1962).

Dietary Goals for the United States, 2nd ed. Government Printing Office, Washington, D.C. (1979).

Dunbar, J., and Stunkard, A. Adherence to medical regimen, in *Nutrition, Lipids and Coronary Heart Disease.* R. Levy, B. Rifkind, B. Dennis, and N. Ernst, eds. Raven Press, New York (1979), pp. 391–423.

Eheart, J., and Mason, B. Sugar and acid in the edible portion of fruits. *J. Am. Diet. Assoc.* 50, 130–132 (1967).

Exchange USB for Meal Planning. The American Dietetic Association, American Diabetes Association Inc. (1976).

Exler, J., and Weihrauch, J. VIII. Finfish: Comprehensive evaluation of fatty acids in foods. *J. Am. Diet. Assoc.* 69, 243–248 (1976).

Exler, J., and Weihrauch, J. XII. Shellfish: Comprehensive evaluation of fatty acids in foods. *J. Am. Diet. Assoc.* 71, 518–521 (1977).

Exler, J., Avena, R., and Weihrauch, J. XI. Leguminous seeds: Comprehensive evaluation of fatty acids in foods. *J. Am. Diet. Assoc.* 71, 412–415 (1979).

Farinaro, E., Stamler, J., Upton, M., Mojonnies, L., Hall, Y., Moss, D., and Berkson, D. Plasma glucose levels: Long term effect of diet in Chicago Coronary Prevention Evaluation Program. *Ann. Int. Med.* 86, 147–154 (1977).

Fetcher, E., Foster, N., and Anderson, J. Quantitative estimation of diets to control serum cholesterol. *Am. J. Clin. Nut.* 20, 475–492 (1967).

Feeley, F., Criner, P., and Watt, B. Cholesterol content of foods. *J. Am. Diet. Assoc.* 61, 134–149 (1972).

Feeley, R., and Watt, B. Nutritive value of foods distributed under U.S.D.A. Food Assistance Programs. *J. Am. Diet. Assoc.* 57, 528–547 (1970).

Fristrom, G., and Weihrauch, J. IX. Fowl: Comprehensive evaluation of fatty acids in foods. *J. Am. Diet. Assoc.* 69, 517–522 (1976).

Fristrom, G., Stewart, B., Weihrauch, J., and Posati, L. IV. Nuts, peanuts and soups: Comprehensive evaluation of fatty acids in foods. *J. Am. Diet. Assoc.* 67, 351–355 (1975).

Glueck, C.J., and Connor, W.E. Diet-coronary heart disease relationships reconnoitered. *Am. J. Clin. Nut.* 31, 727–734 (1979).

Gormican, A. Inorganic elements in foods used in hospital menus. *J. Am. Diet. Assoc.* 56, 397–403 (1970).

Hardinge, M. Lesser known vitamins in foods. *J. Am. Diet. Assoc.* 38, 240–245 (1961).

Hegsted, D.M., McGandy, R.B., Myers, M.L., and Stare, F.J. Quantitative effects of dietary fat on serum cholesterol in man. *Am. J. Clin. Nut.* 17, 281–295 (1965).

Hockaday, T.D.R., Hockaday, J.M., Mann, J.I., and Turner, R.C. Prospective comparison of modified fat high carbohydrate with standard low carbohydrate dietary advise in the treatment of diabetes: one year follow-up study. *Br. J. Nut.* 39, 357–362 (1978).

Hoerrmann, F.M., Rosenstock, D.B., and Naito, H.K. Dietary management of hyperlipidemia, in *Nutritional Elements and Clinical Biochemistry.* M. Brewster and H.K. Naito, eds. Plenum Press, New York (1980), pp. 317–356.

Houtsmiller, A.J. The role of fat in the treatment of diabetes mellitus, in *The Role of Fats in Human Nutrition.* A.J. Vergroesen, ed. Academic Press, New York (1975), pp. 231–302.

HVH-CWRU Nutrient Data Base. Department of Biometry, School of Medicine, Case Western Reserve University, Cleveland, Ohio (1980).

Inter-Society Commission for Heart Disease Resources. Atherosclerosis study group and epidemiology study group. Primary prevention of the atherosclerotic diseases. *Circulation* 42, 55A–59A (1970). (Revised 1972).

Jones, J. *Diet for a Happy Heart.* 101 Productions, San Francisco (1975).

Keys, A., Anderson, J.T., and Grande, F. Essential fatty acids, degree of unsaturation, and effect of corn (maize) oil on the serum cholesterol level in man. *Lancet* 2, 66–68 (1957).

Kwiterovich, P.O. Pediatric aspects of hyperlipoproteinemia, in *Hyperlipidemia Diagnosis and Therapy.* B.M. Rifkind and R.I. Levy, eds. Grune & Stratton, New York (1977), pp. 249–279.

Leung, W. *Food Composition Table for Use in Latin America.* Institute of Nutrition of Central America and Panama, and National Institutes of Health, Bethesda, Maryland (1961).

Leverton, R., and Odell, G. *The Nutritive Value of Cooked Meat.* Agricultural Experimental Station, Oklahoma State University, Publication No. MP-49. Oklahoma Agricultural Experimental Station, Stillwater, Oklahoma (1959).

Matthews, R., and Garrison, Y. *Food Yields Summarized by Different Stages of Preparation.* Consumer and Food Economics Institute, Northeastern Region, Agricultural Research Service. U.S.D.A. Handbook No. 102. United States Department of Agriculture, Washington, D.C. (1975).

Mattice, M. *Bridges' Food and Beverage Analyses,* 3rd ed. Lea and Febiger, Philadelphia (1950).

McCarthy, M. Phenylalaine and tyrosine in vegetables and fruits. *J. Am. Diet. Assoc.* 52, 130–134 (1968).

McGandy, R.B., and Hegsted, D.M. Quantitative effects of dietary fat and cholesterol on serum cholesterol in man, in *The Role of Fats in Human Nutrition.* A.J. Vergroesen, ed. Academic Press, London (1975), pp. 211–230.

Murphy, E., Willis, B., and Watt, B. Provisional tables on the zinc content of foods. *J. Am. Diet. Assoc.* 66, 345–355 (1975).

National Research Council. *Recommended Dietary Allowances,* 9th ed. Food and Nutrition Board, Committee on Dietary Allowances, National Academy of Sciences, Washington, D.C. (1980).

Orr, M. *Pantothenic Acid, Vitamin B6 and Vitamin B12 in Foods.* Home Economics Research Report No. 36. Consumer and Food Economics Research Division. Agricultural Research Service, USDA. United States Department of Agriculture, Washington, D.C. (1969).

Orr, M., and Watt, B. *Amino Acid Content of Foods.* Home Economics Research Report No. 4. United States Department of Agriculture, Washington, D.C. (1957).

Perloff, B., and Butrum, R. Folacin in selected foods. *J. Am. Diet. Assoc.* 70, 161–172 (1977).

Posati, L., Kinsella, J., and Watt, B. I. Dairy products: Comprehensive evaluation of fatty acids in foods. *J. Am. Diet. Assoc.* 66, 482–488 (1975).

Posati, L., Kinsella, J., and Watt, B. Eggs and egg products: Comprehensive evaluation of fatty acids in foods. *J. Am. Diet. Assoc.* 67, 111–115 (1975).

Posati, L., and Orr, M. *Composition of Foods: Dairy and Egg Products–Raw, Processed, Prepared.* Consumer and Food Economics Institute, USDA Handbook No. 8-1, United States Department of Agriculture, Washington, D.C. (1976).

Rezabek, K. *Nutritive Value of Convenience Foods,* 2nd ed. West Suburban Dietetic Association, Chicago, Illinois (1979).

Select Committee on Nutrition and Human Needs. *Dietary Goals for the United States,* 2nd ed. United States Senate. U.S. Government Printing Office, Washington, D.C. (1977).

Stamler, J. Population studies, in *Nutrition, Lipids, and Coronary Heart Disease.* R.I. Levy, B.M. Rifkind, B.H. Dennis, and N.D. Ernst, eds. Raven Press, New York (1979), pp. 25–88.

Streiff, R. Folate levels in citrus and other juices. *Am. J. Clin. Nut.* 24, 1390–1392 (1971).

Sturderant, R.A., Pearce, M.L., and Dayton, S. Increased prevalance of cholelithiasis in men ingesting a serum cholesterol-lowering diet. *N. Eng. J. Med.* 288 (1), 24–27 (1973).

Toepfer, E., Zook, E., Orr, M., and Richardson, L. *Folic Acid Content of Foods.* USDA Handbook No. 29. United States Department of Agriculture, Washington, D.C. (1951).

Umbarger, B. *Phenylalanine Content of Foods.* Children's Hospital Research Foundation and the University of Cincinnati College of Medicine, Cincinnati, Ohio (1965).

Watt, B., and Merrill, A. *Composition of Foods–Raw, Processed, Prepared.* USDA Agriculture Handbook No. 8. United States Department of Agriculture, Washington, D.C. (1963).

Weihrauch, J., Kinsella, J., and Watt, B. VI. Cereal products: Comprehensive evaluation of fatty acids in food. *J. Am. Diet. Assoc.* 68, 335–340 (1976).

Zook, E., and Lehmann, J. Mineral composition of fruits. *J. Am. Diet. Assoc.* 52, 225–231 (1968).

14

Management of Hypercholesterolemia by Partial Ileal Bypass

HENRY BUCHWALD
RICHARD L. VARCO

INTRODUCTION

The assumption has been made that if elevated lipid levels (mainly cholesterol) are lowered, the atherosclerosis risk rate will be decreased as well. Though eminently logical, this lipid-atherosclerosis hypothesis still requires rigorous, statistically sound proof. To this end, several large national and international clinical intervention trials have been funded. One, a secondary intervention trial, utilizes the partial ileal bypass operation as the means for cholesterol lowering. Until the lipid-atherosclerosis hypothesis is confirmed or denied by clinical trial, we believe judicious and rational hyperlipidemia management is indicated, in the light of current knowledge.

One method in the hyperlipidemia management armamentarius is the partial ileal bypass operation, a technique tested by our research group since 1962 and first performed in a human patient in May 1963. This procedure is (1) highly effective, (2) lasting, (3) safe, and (4) obligatory, that is, free of the need for continuous patient cooperation.

LABORATORY ANTECEDENTS AND CONCURRENT RESEARCH

In 1963–1964, we published the preliminary experiments on the rationale for partial ileal bypass management of the hyperlipidemias, and a clinical report of the first four cases (Buchwald, 1963a, b; 1964). We postulated that a partial ileal bypass operation should result in a significant cholesterol reduction by a twofold mode of action: (1) interference with the enterohepatic cholesterol cycle, thereby effecting a direct drain on the body cholesterol pool; and (2) interference with the enterohepatic bile acid cycle, resulting in a marked increase in bile acid synthesis from cholesterol, thereby effecting an indirect drain on the body cholesterol pool.

We demonstrated that bypass of the distal one-third to one-half of the small intestine of the New Zealand white rabbit resulted in a decrease of 85 percent in cholesterol-absorptive capacity and a decrease of 28 percent in circulating whole-blood cholesterol ($p < .005$). Comparable results were found in the pig. After demonstration of an extremely low plasma cholesterol concentration in a retrospective study of humans after resection of the distal ileum, we initiated our clinical study.

Subsequently, numerous animal experiments have been conducted in our laboratory, and in laboratories of other investigators, to elucidate further the enterohepatic cholesterol and bile acid mechanisms and the effect on the atherosclerotic process of interference with these mechanisms. We demonstrated that the entire small intestine of the rabbit is capable of cholesterol absorption, and that there was no unique focus for localization of the active process of cholesterol absorption (Buchwald, 1964; Gebhard and Buchwald, 1970). With normal bowel continuity, however, preferential cholesterol absorption occurs in the distal half of the small bowel, since the first part of intestinal passage is primarily concerned with the emulsification of cholesterol and the formation of micelles in preparation for the absorptive process. Similarly, we demonstrated that bile acids are preferentially absorbed in the distal small intestine (Buchwald and Gebhard, 1968). Thus, our data seem to confirm the postulate we proposed for the action of this metabolic operation.

Utilizing the rabbit as an atherosclerosis model, we were able, by feeding a diet rich in cholesterol content, to create a preparation with a reliable 50 percent myocardial infarction rate (Buchwald, 1965b). In both the mature and the infant rabbit, we demonstrated that ileal bypass will prevent hypercholesterolemia and atherosclerosis in animals placed on a severely atherogenic 2 percent cholesterol diet for four months; that ileal bypass in rabbits with established hypercholesterolemia and atherosclerosis will reverse the hypercholesterolemia and reduce cholesterol deposits, despite continuation of the 2 percent cholesterol diet; and that ileal bypass in rabbits will arrest the atherosclerotic process, with an accompanying evolvement of plaque lesions from a proliferative to a healing phase (Buchwald, 1965a; Buchwald et al., 1972).

Scott and co-workers (1966) studied the effect of ileal bypass in hypercholesterolemic dogs, and found that a 40 percent distal small intestinal bypass uniformly protected them from the development of hypercholesterolemia and atherosclerosis; indeed, blood-cholesterol concentration following bypass was significantly lower than that of the control animals. This group of investigators also demonstrated that the cholesterol-lowering effect of the bypass operation protected dogs (Frost et al., 1970) and monkeys (Shepard et al., 1968) from atherosclerotic lesions, and seemed to reverse established atherosclerotic plaque deposition. They also showed that ileal bypass afforded twice the cholesterol reduction of cholestyramine in their primate preparation (Younger et al., 1969). Utilizing the White Carneau pigeon, a species with naturally occurring atherosclerosis, Gomes and co-workers demonstrated that ileal bypass did reverse aortic atherosclerosis, without interfering with animals' growth or weight (Gomes et al., 1971).

Currently, in order to inhibit the markedly enhanced cholesterol synthesis induced by the ileal bypass operation and, thereby, to augment the cholesterol-lowering effect of the procedure, our work has turned to methods of interfering with hepatic cholesterol synthesis following partial ileal bypass. Feedback inhibitors of hepatic cholesterol synthesis are thought to be cholesterol itself and its metabolic end product, bile acids. However, the infusion of glycodeoxycholic acid, the predominant bile acid in the rabbit, into an isolated ileal segment resulted in increased hepatic cholesterol synthesis, rather than in the expected reduction in synthesis (Coyle, 1976). In an experiment currently in progress, we are testing for a humoral, or blood-borne, factor in cholesterol synthesis control. Using pairs of rats surviving aortic cross-circulation, with one member of each pair having had a previous partial ileal bypass, we are measuring the circulating cholesterol concentration in each member of the pair prior to cross-circulation and in the common circulation after cross-circulation, as well as the relative cholesterol synthesis in the livers of these animals. Our preliminary data show that a synthesis stimulator, or inhibitor, from the liver of one animal in such a pair influences hepatic cholesterol metabolism in the other.

CLINICAL METABOLIC DATA

In 1964 we published a method for measuring the cholesterol-absorptive capacity from the blood radioactivity levels following a standard oral test dose of ^{14}C-4-cholesterol in butter (Buchwald and Gebhart, 1964). In 30 patients studied before and at three months after partial ileal bypass, the cholesterol-absorptive capacity was reduced an average of 60 percent (range 37 to 95 percent) (Buchwald and Varco, 1967; Moore et al., 1970). This reduction in cholesterol-absorptive capacity has been retested in certain of these patients for as long as ten years, and has been shown to be maintained.

Fecal steroid excretion has been measured in selected patients before and after partial ileal bypass, using an isotope-balance technique following a single intravenous injection of ^{14}C-4-cholesterol (Moore et al., 1969; Buchwald et al., 1975). Following operation there was a 3.8-fold increase in total fecal steroid excretion, with a much greater increase in bile acids (4.9-fold) than in neutral steroids (2.7-fold). Similar magnitudes of steroid excretion were observed in two patients studied at one year after operation, demonstrating the apparent permanent effect of ileal bypass on fecal steroid excretion.

We have used an in vivo method for estimating cholesterol biosynthesis, based on the incorporation of tritium from body water into the serum cholesterol (Moore et al., 1969; Buchwald et al., 1975). By this method, we have determined cholesterol synthesis in 15 patients before, and three months after, operation—and again at one year in six of these patients. This index of cholesterol biosynthesis was found to be significantly increased ($p < .001$) following ileal bypass. The magnitude of this postoperative increase was marked in each patient and the overall group response was 5.7-fold higher. The six patients restudied one year after surgery showed that this increase in the cholesterol synthesis was lasting.

We have also determined the isotopic cholesterol turnover rate, and the exchangeable pool sizes, from the disappearance curve of radioactively labeled serum cholesterol in partial ileal bypass patients (Moore et al., 1969; Buchwald et al., 1975). Partial ileal bypass resulted in a marked and persistent increase in cholesterol turnover. Calculating the sizes of the cholesterol pools, we found that they were larger in hypercholesterolemic subjects than in normals. One year after partial ileal bypass, there was a marked reduction in the exchangeable cholesterol pools in all patients studied to date. Indeed, there was a reduction of approximately one-third in the total miscible cholesterol pool. In each patient there was a relatively greater reduction in the slowly miscible pool than in the freely miscible pool, suggesting a loss of cholesterol from tissues other than the blood, liver, and gut mucosa; possibly, this loss came from the arteries.

OPERATIVE TECHNIQUE

Under general intubation anesthesia, entrance is gained into the abdominal cavity by right lower quadrant transverse incision some 2 cm below the umbilicus, unless a concomitant procedure (e.g., cholecystectomy) is planned. After abdominal exploration, the entire small intestine is measured along the mesenteric border with a piece of calibrated umbilical tape. In our experience, the intestinal length varies from 400 to 650 cm between the ileocecal valve and the ligament of Treitz. The bowel is transected 200 cm from the ileocecal valve, or one-third the length of the small bowel, whichever is larger. The upper segment is anastomosed, end-to-side, to the cecum on the anterior taenia just above the inverted appendiceal stump (the appendix is removed if present). The cecum is retained to maximize water-absorbing surface, and anastomosis distal to the ileocecal valve is carried out in order to minimize ileal retention and resorption of cholesterol and bile acids. The upper end of the bypassed distal bowel is closed and subsequently tacked down to the anterior taenia of the cecum, between the anastomosis and the appendiceal stump, to prevent future intussusception. A small divisional mesenteric defect and the large rotational mesenteric defect are carefully closed to prevent internal herniation. The abdomen is closed in layers and no drains are used.

OPERATIVE MORTALITY AND MORBIDITY

Only 1 patient out of 350 has died following partial ileal bypass. This individual died of a myocardial infarction on the fourth postoperative day; he had sustained three myocardial infarctions prior to operative intervention. No other operative death has been reported in the literature. Immediate in-hospital complications have been limited to rare (2 percent) and minor (wound, phlebitis, etc.) problems, seldom prolonging hospitalization. The diarrhea following this limited one-third intestinal bypass is transient and readily controlled with mild medications. The only lasting side effect of this procedure is the need for parenteral (1000 μg every two months) vitamin B_{12}. This operation is not associated with weight loss or the significant side effects and complications seen following jejunoileal bypass for obesity. It is essential to make this important distinction when considering partial ileal bypass for a given individual.

RESULTS

Cholesterol

To date, the average cholesterol-level reduction after partial ileal bypass, from the preoperative but postdietary baseline of 359 mg percent in our series, has been 41.4 percent (Buchwald et al., 1974, 1975). All patients have appropriate dietary therapy for at least three months before surgery; the operation has been effective in patients with poor or no response to diet and/or drug therapy. The cholesterol-lowering effect of this procedure has been long-lasting for the 14 years of our study. Over 80 percent of our patients, at one year, have cholesterol levels below 250 mg percent. Sixty-five percent of the patients have exceeded a 35 percent reduction, and 47 percent have had reductions greater than 40 percent from the postdietary cholesterol baseline.

In 24 heterozygous Type II patients with an average premanagement plasma cholesterol concentration of 423 mg percent, three months of judicious adherence to a stringent low-cholesterol, low-saturated-fat diet resulted in a cholesterol reduction of 11 percent. One year following partial ileal bypass, in this 24-patient cohort, the average plasma cholesterol level was 224 mg percent, representing an additional 42 percent lowering in cholesterol. Thus, the combination of dietary and partial ileal bypass management is capable of achieving what is essentially a halving of the cholesterol concentration.

A review of the literature shows that the experiences of others with partial ileal bypass are comparable to our own, namely, an average cholesterol lowering by this procedure of approximately 40 percent. The poorest results to date have been achieved in homozygous Type II children, though Balfour and Kim (1974) have reported excellent results in this group as well.

Triglycerides

The available triglyceride data are not as extensive as the cholesterol data; nevertheless, marked changes in the triglyceride concentration after partial ileal bypass have been recorded. The Type IV patients, or those individuals with genetic hypertriglyceridemia, sustained an average triglyceride reduction of 52.6 percent from the postdietary baseline one year after partial ileal bypass (Buchwald et al., 1974, 1975).

Xanthomata

We have noted a decrease in size and the disappearance of periorbital xanthelasma, subcutaneous xanthomata and even tendon xanthomata, following partial ileal bypass. This phenomenon has not been uniform or predictable (Buchwald et al., 1974, 1975).

Angina Pectoris

It has been documented by several investigators that partial ileal bypass patients volunteer that they have had a subjective improvement in their symptoms of angina pectoris, often with an increase in exercise capacity, after this operative procedure (Buchwald et al., 1974, 1975). Indeed, approximately 70 percent of our patients with preoperative angina testify to the fact that they have a reduction or a complete disappearance of their symptom complex after the bypass procedure. In some, an improvement in the time-graded exercise capacity on the treadmill electrocardiogram has been associated with reduction in symptoms; however, this pattern has not been persistent. We do not know the specific cause for this mitigation of myocardial ischemic symptoms. We believe, however, that this is a real finding, and suspect that the mechanism for this phenomenon resides with a change in blood rheology, or oxygen transport, brought about by a reduction in the cholesterol content of the red blood cell membrane.

Arteriography

Our associates in radiology have published reports on the serial appraisal of coronary angiograms in partial ileal bypass patients (Baltaxe et al., 1969; Knight, 1972). Approximately half of carefully documented sequential arteriograms showed no change in plaque lesions; 22.7 percent showed progression of disease; 9.0 percent showed questionable improvement; and 13.6 percent demonstrated true arteriographic evidence of disease regression on the basis of a decrease in size, or complete disappearance, of plaques.

CONCLUSIONS

We believe that there will be greater use of the partial ileal bypass operation in the future. Experience has clearly documented that diet and current drug therapy, singly or in combination, infrequently approach the lipid reduction feasible by partial ileal bypass. Contrary to the results of drug therapy, the cholesterol-lowering effect of partial ileal bypass is lasting; there has been no report of response escape. Clearly, this procedure is safe and, after 14 years of clinical experience, the reported side effects and complications associated with it have been minimal. Patients may or may not adhere to diet, may or may not take pills; but once the operation is performed, its therapeutic effects are lasting and obligatory. This is an important advantage, especially in the treatment of young, asymptomatic individuals. We believe that clinicians who become familiar with partial ileal bypass management will arrive at comparable conclusions.

REFERENCES

Balfour, J.F. and Kim, R. Homozygous type II hyperlipoproteinemia treatment, partial ileal bypass in two children. *JAMA* 227, 1145–1151 (1974).

Baltaxe, H., Amplatz, K., Varco, R.L., and Buchwald, H. Coronary arteriography in hypercholesterolemic patients. *Am. J. Roent.* 105, 784–790 (1969).

Buchwald, H. Localization of cholesterol absorption. *Circulation* 28 (suppl. 2), 649 (1963a).

Buchwald, H. Surgical operation to lower circulating cholesterol. *Circulation* 28 (suppl. 2), 649 (1963b).

Buchwald, H. Lowering of cholesterol absorption and blood levels by ileal exclusion: Experimental basis and preliminary clinical report. *Circulation* 29, 713–720 (1964).

Buchwald, H. The effect of ileal bypass on atherosclerosis and hypercholesterolemia in the rabbit. *Surgery* 58, 22–36 (1965a).

Buchwald, H. Myocardial infarction in rabbits induced solely by a hypercholesterolemic diet. *J. Atheroscler. Res.* 4, 407–419 (1965b).

Buchwald, H. and Gebhard, R. Effect of intestinal bypass on cholesterol absorption and blood levels in the rabbit. *Am. J. Physiol.* 207, 567–572 (1964).

Buchwald, H. and Gebhard, R.L. Localization of bile salt absorption in-vivo in the rabbit. *Ann. Surg.* 167, 191–198 (1968).

Buchwald, H. and Varco, R.L. Partial ileal bypass for hypercholesterolemia and atherosclerosis. *Surg. Gyn. Obst.* 124, 1231–1238 (1967).

Buchwald, H., Moore, R.B., and Varco, R.L. Surgical treatment of hyperlipidemia. *Circulation* 49 (suppl. 1), 1–35 (1974).

Buchwald, H., Moore, R.B., Bertish, J., and Varco, R.L. Effect of ileal bypass on cholesterol levels, atherosclerosis and growth in the infant rabbit. *Ann. Surg.* 175, 311–319 (1972).

Buchwald, H., Varco, R.L., Moore, R.B., and Schwartz, M.Z. Intestinal bypass procedures: Partial ileal bypass for hyperlipidemia and jejuno-ileal bypass for obesity. *Curr. Prob. Surg.*, April (1975), pp. 1–51.

Coyle, J.J., Varco, R.L., and Buchwald, H. Effect of bile acids on hepatic cholesterol synthesis in partial ileal bypass in rabbits. *Surg. Forum* 27, 447–448 (1976).

Frost, J.W., Finch, W.T., Younger, R., Butts, W.H., Scott, H.W., Jr. Pilot study of the therapeutic effects of ileal bypass in dogs with experimentally established hypercholesterolemia and atherosclerosis. *Surg. Forum* 21, 398–399 (1970).

Gebhard, R.L., and Buchwald, H. Cholesterol absorption after reversal of the upper and lower halves of the small intestine. *Surgery* 67, 474–477 (1970).

Gomes, M.M., Kottke, B.A., Bernatz, P., and Titus, J.L. Effect of ileal bypass on aortic atherosclerosis of White Carneau pigeons. *Surgery* 70, 353–358 (1971).

Knight, L., Scheibel, R., Amplatz, K., Varco, R.L., and Buchwald, H. A radiographic appraisal of the Minnesota partial ileal bypass study. *Surg. Forum* 23, 141–142 (1972).

Moore, R.B., Frantz, I.D., Jr., and Buchwald, H. Changes in cholesterol pool size, turnover rate, and fecal bile acid and sterol excretion after partial ileal bypass in hypercholesterolemic patients. *Surgery* 65, 98–108 (1969).

Moore, R.B., Frantz, I.D., Jr., Varco, R.L., and Buchwald, H. Cholesterol dynamics after partial ileal bypass, in *Proceedings of the Second International Symposium on Atherosclerosis.* R.J. Jones, ed. Springer-Verlag, New York (1970), pp. 295–300.

Scott, H.W., Jr., Stephenson, S.E., Jr., Younger, R., Carlisle, B.B., and Turney, S.W. Prevention of experimental atherosclerosis by ileal bypass: Twenty percent cholesterol diet and I^{131}-induced hypothyroidism in dogs. *Ann. Surg.* 163, 795–807 (1966).

Shepard, G.H., Wimberly, J.E., Younger, R., Stephenson, S.E., Jr., and Scott, H.W., Jr. Effects of bypass of the distal third of the small intestine on experimental hypercholesterolemia and atherosclerosis in rhesus monkeys. *Surg. Forum* 19, 302–303 (1968).

Younger, R., Shepard, G.H., Butts, W.H., and Scott, H.W., Jr. Comparison of the protective effects of cholestyramine and ileal bypass in Rhesus monkeys on an atherogenic regimen. *Surg. Forum* 20, 101–102 (1969).

15

Value of Magnesium Supplements During Open-Heart Surgery — A Double-Blind Trial

MICHAEL P. HOLDEN

In the daily routine of the vast practice of open-heart surgery throughout the world, it is widely accepted that it is essential to maintain the serum levels of potassium in the upper part of the normal range. By doing so the ventricles are made less irritable. It is also acknowledged that an infusion of calcium after open-heart surgery has a pronounced ionotropic effect, albeit short-lived (Heilbrunn and Wiercinski, 1947).

However, while magnesium is quantitatively the fourth most important cation in the body after sodium, potassium, and calcium, relatively little interest has been shown in its clinical changes and therapeutic applications in the cardiac field in spite of the interest stimulated by Szekely (1946) and Zwillinger (1935) with regard to the treatment of arrhythmias. Almost thirty years have elapsed since the changes in serum magnesium occurring during open-heart surgery were first investigated, even though many operations are bedeviled with troublesome, and often fatal, arrhythmias. Even today clinicians prefer to depress the myocardium with beta-blockers or local anesthetic derivatives rather than investigate or correct magnesium imbalance. This is partly due to the difficulty in obtaining reliable and speedy results, because, as well as having to perform atomic absorption spectrophotometry, a sympathetic laboratory staff is required.

Bearing in mind the disturbances of myocardial metabolism during anoxic arrest, ventricular fibrillation, and coronary perfusion (Moffit et al., 1965, 1969), and the known reciprocal function of the Ca^{2+} ions in sarcomere contraction, he investigated serum and urine magnesium changes in fifty

Table 1. Goals of Survey Conducted by Scheinmann (San Francisco, 1969–71) and Holden (United Kingdom, 1971), Given that Serum Magnesium Level Decreases During Open-Heart Surgery

1. To determine if serum magnesium levels can be restored and maintained
2. To assess by blind controlled randomized trial if administering parenteral magnesium will:
a. Reduce incidence of arrhythmias
b. Reduce incidence of arrhythmias associated with digoxin and pacing
c. Reduce psychoneurologic problems
d. Improve peripheral perfusion
e. Improve urinary output
f. Affect bleeding

Table 2. Preoperative Factors Creating the Unstable State of Open-Heart Surgery Patients

Malnutrition
Diuretics
Abnormal fluid distribution due to congestive heart failure
Disordered renal function

patients undergoing open-heart surgery (Holden et al., 1972). They were compared with a similar number of patients undergoing major surgery without the use of cardiopulmonary bypass.

We concluded that:

1. Patients with valvular heart disease who had been in congestive heart failure (CHF) and on diuretics were more likely to have lower serum magnesium levels on admission than were those patients not on diuretics.
2. Most patients with valvular heart disease, who had undergone replacement surgery on cardiopulmonary bypass, had lowered serum magnesium concentrations for the first two postoperative days, with diminished excretion of magnesium in the urine.
3. All patients who had undergone major surgery without cardiopulmonary bypass had lowered serum magnesium levels on the first postoperative day. This suggests that the reduction in serum magnesium levels in the open-heart group is due, in part, to the "metabolic response due to trauma."
4. Abnormalities in serum and urinary levels of magnesium had all resolves spontaneously (except in one case) by the time the patients were discharged from hospital on the twelfth day, although 90 percent of them were receiving diuretics again.

Table 3. Intraoperative Factors Creating the Unstable State of Open-Heart Surgery Patients

Anticoagulants
Anesthetic agents
Blood infusion
Crystalloid infusion
Osmolality changes
Temperature changes
pH changes
Protein denaturation
Disorganized perfusion of organs
Frank ischemia–cell membranes
Metabolic response to trauma
Cellular trauma of blood

Table 4. Postoperative Factors Creating the Unstable State of Open-Heart Surgery Patients

Blood transfusion
Anesthetic agents
Crystalloid infusion
Insulin/K^+/Dextrose infusion
Calcium per unit of blood
Diuretics
Poor perfusion (now pulsatile)
Gastric aspiration (20–30 mg/day)
Gut stasis
Malnutrition
Catabolism
Infection

Similar findings have been obtained by Scheinman et al. (1969, 1971), Paschen et al. (1972), and Khan et al. (1973).

Having demonstrated diminution of serum magnesium concentration and being aware of the known clinical manifestations of hypomagnesemia, it seemed logical to assess: (1) whether serum levels could be restored to normal; and (2) whether some of the problems occurring after open-heart surgery, such as arrhythmia, and psychoneurologic and hematologic abnormalities which mimic magnesium deficiency states, could be reduced or abolished. This clinical study was undertaken, and is presented in this chapter (see Table 1).

It should be emphasized that one of the almost insuperable problems involved when studying any parameter in patients undergoing open-heart surgery (particularly when the topic of investigation is a cation with a considerable flux across cell membranes, and which is normally in a state of equilibrium with a large body pool), is the fact that it is a multifactorial system with so many variables that are difficult to stabilize. This is illustrated in Tables 2, 3, and 4.

MATERIALS AND METHODS

Eighty patients undergoing mitral and/or aortic valve replacement were randomly selected by the pharmacy department to receive one of two solutions. One solution contained 100 mg $MgSO_4 \cdot 7H_2O$ (2 ml of a 5 percent solution = 0.8 meq). The placebo solution contained 2 ml normal saline. The patients received six doses of one solution commencing one hour after surgery, and thereafter at six hourly intervals intramuscularly. For a variety of reasons (mainly inadequacies in sampling techniques), only 70 patients were finally included in the series. Thirty-three individuals were found to have received the solution containing magnesium (referred to subsequently as Solution A) and 37 individuals received the placebo solution (referred to as Solution B).*

The solution code was changed at approximately four-week intervals to further blind the clinicians involved in the study.

Serum and 24-hour urine specimens for magnesium, calcium, sodium, chloride, potassium, and urea were measured on admission, and 1, 2, 3, 6, 12, 18, 24, 48, and 72 hours postoperatively. Albumin, pH and hematocrit were measured with each blood specimen.

This regime of magnesium infusion had been adopted following a pilot survey involving ten patients. Five patients received intravenous injections and five received intramuscular injections. Figures 1 and 2 show the mean levels of serum magnesium after two bolus doses of 100 mg $MgSO_4 \cdot 7H_2O$. It appears that the intramuscular route produced a slower rise in blood levels of magnesium, and surprisingly there was an earlier fall in these levels. It was initially considered safer to adopt this route of administration because there would be fewer problems with sudden hypermagnesaemia associated with oliguria. However, it has subsequently become apparent that the intravenous route is superior; it is less painful and avoids muscle pooling during low cardiac output states. Also, there has been a progressive improvement in renal function following open-heart surgery over the recent years, with the introduction of better perfusion techniques.

RESULTS

When all the data was collected and parameters set forth (see Table 1) the pharmacy then released the code. The patients' results were subsequently

---

*Composition of Groups A and B was as follows:
Group A females 20 patients: mean age 44 years (range 22 to 65)
Group A males 13 patients: mean age 51 years (range 27 to 65)
Group B females 25 patients: mean age 47 years (range 25 to 63)
Group B males 12 patients: mean age 42 years (range 29 to 61)

SERUM URINARY MAGNESIUM LEVELS FOLLOWING INFUSION OF $MgSO_4$ FOLLOWING OPEN HEART SURGERY

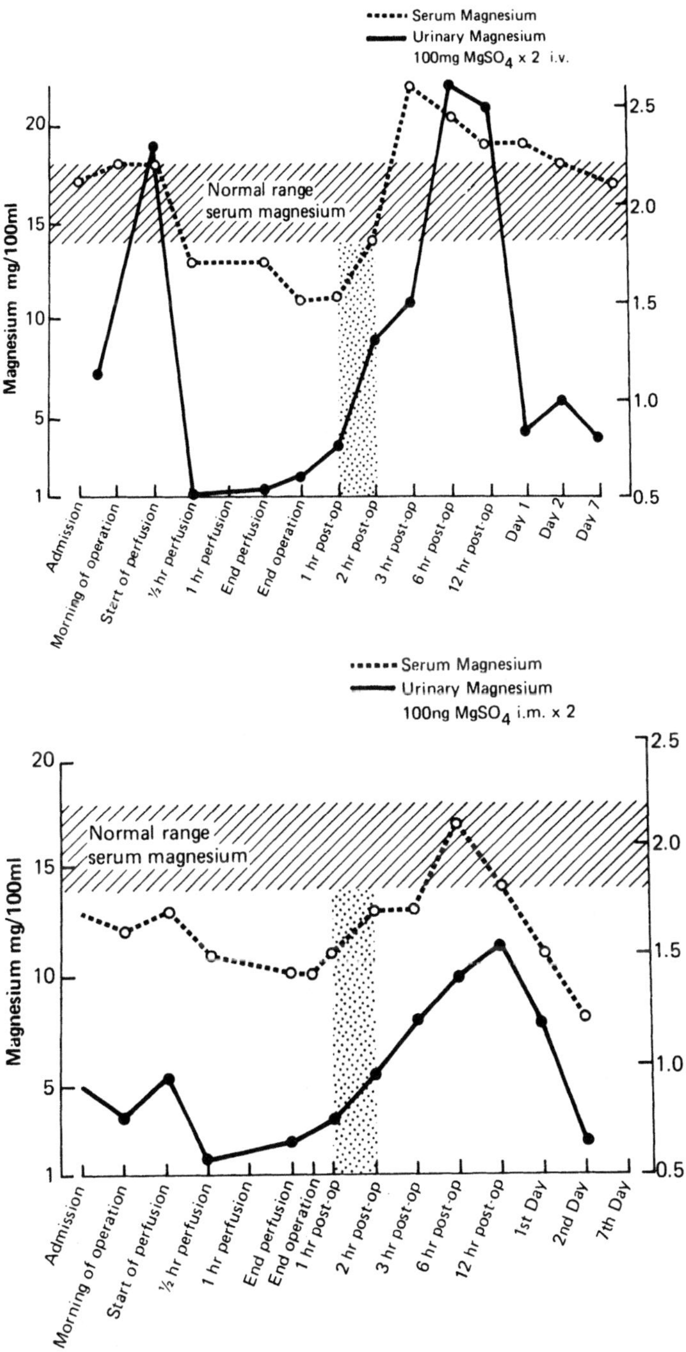

Fig. 1 and 2 Comparison of serum and urinary levels of magnesium in two groups of five patients each. One group received intravenous magnesium therapy; the other received magnesium intramuscularly.

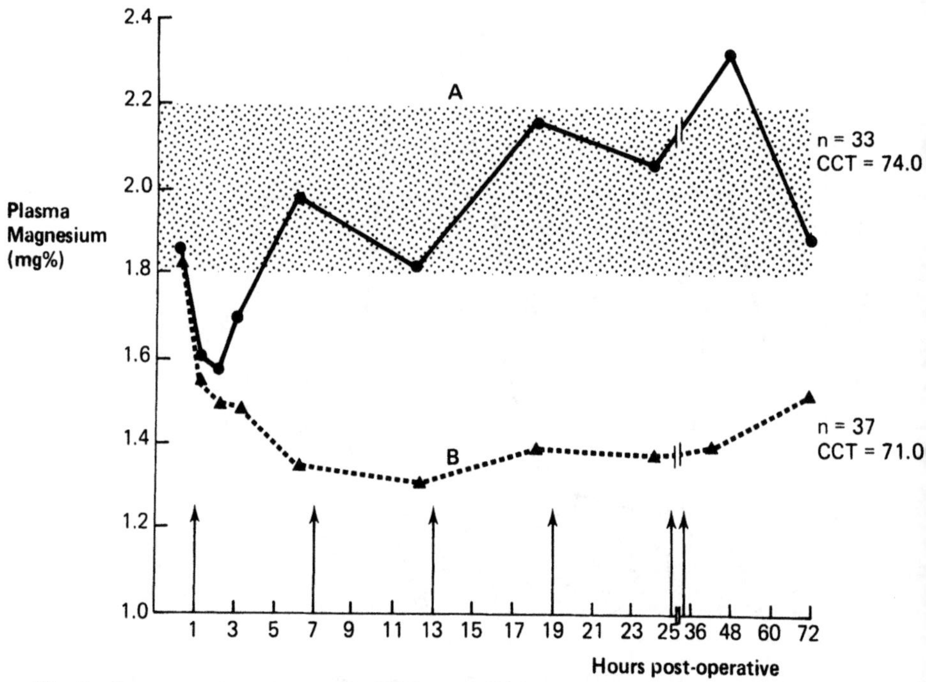

Fig. 3 Demonstration of the plasma levels of magnesium in the Groups A and B. The vertical arrows indicate the time of each dose of magnesium or placebo. The horizontal dotted band is the normal range. CCT = creatinine clearance test.

categorized into Group A (magnesium infusion) and Group B (placebo).

It can be seen from Fig. 3 that the regime of magnesium infusion is adequate in restoring serum levels to normal in the blood and maintaining them at that concentration. However, it is clear that the first dose should be given earlier or by the intravenous route to counteract the initial fall in serum levels of magnesium (Table 5). Of particular note is the incidence of arrhythmias and pacing problems occurring in Group A, mainly during this first hour, as shown by the number in parentheses in the first column of Table 5. After the first hour, when the serum magnesium levels were returned to the normal range, there were virtually no cardiac rhythm problems

Table 5. Postoperative Incidence of Clinical Problems

Clinical Problem	*Group A (33)*	*Group B (37)*
Pacing difficulties	0 (3)	8 (21%)
Arrhythmia	2 (7)	9 (24%)
Arrhythmia following Digoxin	0 (3)	3 (8%)
Mental problems	2	8 (22%)
Peripheral neurological problems	1	4 (11%)
Death	2	1 (3%)

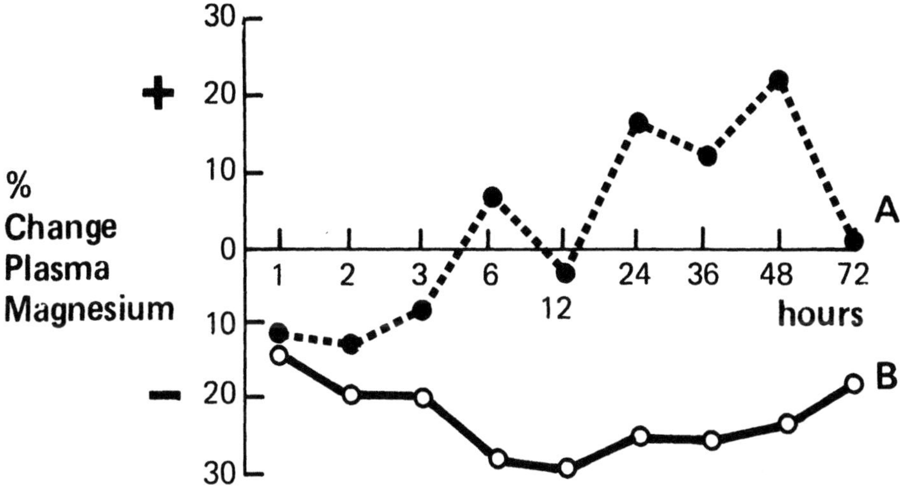

Fig. 4 Percentage change in plasma magnesium levels in Groups A and B, determined from their respective magnesium levels on admission.

with or without digoxin, and no pacing problems. However, the numbers are too small to be of statistical significance.

By the sixth hour postoperatively all the *mean levels of plasma magnesium* in Groups A and B were significantly different ($p < .001$), with high confidence limits (95 percent level). The percentage change in plasma magnesium levels is detailed graphically in Fig. 4.

There is a considerable increase in *urinary magnesium* content (Table 6), probably indicating that most of the infused magnesium is rapidly excreted by the kidneys.

There was no significant effect on *postoperative bleeding* or on *urinary output*, but it must be emphasized that each of these two parameters is influenced by many additional interrelated factors which are impossible to control independently.

There were less *mental and peripheral neurologic problems* in the group receiving magnesium, but the numbers were too small to achieve statistical significance with confidence.

Table 6. Comparison of Urine Magnesium Levels

	Mg/24 h		*Mg/100 ml*	
Time	*Group A*	*Group B*	*Group A*	*Group B*
Day of admission	71	81	7.2	6.6
Day 1	222	80	17.1	4.6
Day 2	317	90	19.6	4.8
Day 3	150	80	8.1	4.4

Table 7. Sinus Rhythm Versus Atrial Fibrillation

	Preoperative Status		*Postoperative Problems*		*No Postoperative Problems*	
	Group A	*Group B*	*Group A*	*Group B*	*Group A*	*Group B*
Atrial fibrillation	18	22	1	12	17	10
Sinus rhythm	15	15	1	4	14	19
	33	37				

There was no significant difference in *peripheral perfusion,* as assessed by the skin temperature on the dorsum of the foot. This was at variance with the findings of Browne (1971), and Frewth et al. (1971), who found clinical benefit by vasodilation of peripheral, coronary, and cerebral arteries—albeit working with more stable patients.

There were similar numbers of patients in each group experiencing atrial fibrillation and sinus rhythm preoperatively (Table 7). In addition, there were similar numbers in each group having no rhythm problems postoperatively. However, arrhythmias were more likely to occur in Group B patients if atrial fibrillation had been present preoperatively rather than sinus rhythm. Also, there were more arrhythmias in the sinus rhythm patients who had not received magnesium supplements, but numbers were not statistically significant ($p < .5$).

DISCUSSION

The results of this study on the effects of magnesium infusions on (1) peripheral perfusion, (2) postoperative bleeding, (3) urinary output, and (4) psychoneurologic problems were inconclusive.

One incidental finding from the study was the greater facility to electrically pace the myocardium when the plasma magnesium was in the normal range. All patients in the series had two temporary pacing wires placed 1 cm apart on the anterior aspect of the right ventricle, and were paced at 100 beats/minute. As can be seen from Table 5, there were more problems with pacing in Group B patients; it can also be seen that once magnesium in the blood was in the normal range there were no further pacing problems in Group A patients. The main problems were that the threshold of pacing required was too high, and that arrhythmias made it impossible to capture the heart rate by overdrive pacing.

In each group (Table 5) there were three patients with arrhythmias which occurred after digoxin was given for rapid atrial fibrillation. The

Table 8. Ventricular Fibrillation Group

11 patients: Nine postoperative; two preoperative
Mean plasma magnesium level during Ventricular Fibrillation = 1.79 mg%
Received: lignocaine; epanutin; β-blockers; correction acidosis; cardiac massage mean ½ hour; defibrillation shocks (mean 12)
All patients returned to sinus rhythm or atrial fibrillation within two minutes of intravenous $MgSO_4$ (2 ml 5%) = 0.81 mEq

arrhythmias in Group A patients were abolished after the first dose of magnesium sulphate.

The beneficial effects of magnesium on cardiac arrhythmia caused by digitalis have been known for some time (Szekely and Wynne, 1951), and the mechanism of action of magnesium has been partially elucidated by Seller (1971) and by Specter et al. (1975). By exclusion Specter et al. (1975) felt that magnesium had a direct effect on calcium and potassium fluxes across the myocardial cell membrane, because in their experiments it did not reactivate digitalis-inhibited Na^+,K^+–ATPases, or displace digoxin from the heart or the microsomal fraction containing Na^+,K^+–ATPases, nor did it appear to act as an antiarrhythmic agent because of its sympatholytic effects. This concept is in keeping with earlier experimental and clinical work by Szekely and Wynne (1963), who showed that reduction of serum calcium by the chelating agent disodium EDTA abolished digitalis-induced ventricular arrhythmia.

The value of magnesium salts on all forms of arrhythmias was emphasized by Szekely (1946) and again by Condorelli (1968), but their message was not accepted with much enthusiasm by the rest of the cardiologic profession, who preferred more complex durgs, such as local anesthetic derivatives and beta-blockers. Following open-heart surgery we had nine patients in Group B with troublesome arrhythmias, and seven in Group A. Five of these Group A patients were rapidly restored to normal rhythm after the first magnesium supplementation.

In addition to this series of patient studies, we have had 14 patients during the last six years who have had intractable ventricular fibrillation and who were treated in the conventional manner (Table 8) for one-half hour without success. These patients were presumed to be irretrievable until intravenous magnesium sulphate was given. All of the subjects were restored to sinus rhythm or atrial fibrillation, even though the mean plasma magnesium level during ventricular fibrillation was 1.79 mg percent.

It is not uncommon on the cardiac intensive-care ward to find patients with ventricular ectopic beats (Lockey et al., 1966) persisting after large doses of intravenous potassium chloride, and evidencing serum potassium levels at the upper range of normal, who are restored to normal rhythm after being given magnesium sulphate intravenously.

CONCLUSIONS AND SUMMARY

This limited study shows that parenteral $MgSO_4 \cdot 7H_2O$ given post-operatively plays a useful role following open-heart surgery in reducing the incidence of arrhythmias which may or may not be due to digitalis. It also suggests, incidentally, that raising the serum magnesium levels may improve the ability to electrically pace the heart.

It is possible to quickly and safely restore the lowered serum levels of magnesium to the normal range, but it is necessary to repeat the dose regularly to keep pace with increased urinary excretion. The intravenous route is probably superior in all aspects to the intramuscular route.

It was not possible to detect any improvement in peripheral perfusion or urinary output, or to produce a significant decrease in psychoneurologic problems. However, fortunately the latter is relatively infrequent now, due largely to improvement in cardiopulmonary bypass techniques. There was no apparent increase in bleeding problems.

If the clinician has the necessary facilities available for frequent blood sampling and rapid return of results, then a continuous infusion should be instituted as soon as cardiopulmonary bypass is terminated. This method will probably be the best system of administrating $MgSO_4 \cdot 7H_2O$, assuming that the patient has an adequate urinary output. Such a regime will supplement the magnesium content of the cardioplegic solution used during surgery. It is believed that magnesium is equally as important as potassium and calcium in the management of open-heart-surgery patients.

REFERENCES

Browne, S.E. Parenteral magnesium sulphate in arterial disease. *Practitioner* 192, 791–797 (1964).

Condorelli, L. L'azione degli ioni magnesio sulle turbe batmotrope del miocardio ventriculare. *Boll. Soc. Ital. Card.* XIII, 381–418 (1968).

Frewin, D.B., Teh, Y.F., and Whelan, R.F. Effect of magnesium sulphate on the blood vessels of the upper limb in man. *Austr. J. Exp. Biol. Med. Sci.* 49, 101–109 (1971).

Heilbrunn, L.V., and Wiercinski, F.J. The action of various cations on muscle protoplasm. *J. Cell. Comp. Physiol.* 29, 15 (1947).

Holden, M.P., Ionescu, M.I., and Wooler, G.H. Magnesium in patients undergoing open heart surgery. *Thorax* 27 (2), 212–218 (1972).

Khan, R.M.A., Hodge, J.S., and Basset, H.F.M. Magnesium in open heart surgery. *J. Thorac. Cardiovasc. Surg.* 66 (2), 185–191 (1975).

Lockey, E., Longmore, D.B., Ross, D.N., and Sturridge, M.F. Potassium and open heart surgery. *Lancet* 1, 671–675 (1966).

Moffit, E.A., Maher, F.T., and Kirklin, J.W. Effects of cardiopulmonary bypass and haemodilution on some constituents of the blood. *Canad. Anesthet. Soc. J.* 12, 458–464 (1965).

Moffit, E.A., Rosevear, J.W., and McGoon, D.C. Myocardial metabolism in open heart surgery; arterial levels of metabolites, electrolytes, oxygenation and acid-base balance. *Anaesthet. Analg.* 48, 633–641 (1969).

Paschen, K., Fuch, C., Hoffmeister, H.E., Regensburger, D., and Konez, J. Der Kalzium, Magnesium, und Kalium-Haushaft bei Operationen mit Kardio-pulmonalem Bypass. *Thoraxchirurgie* 20, 43–50 (1972).

Scheinman, M.M., Sulivan, R.W., and Hyatt, K.H. Magnesium metabolism in patients undergoing cardiopulmonary bypass. *Circulation* 39 (suppl. 1), 235–246 (1969).

Scheinman, M.M., Sulivan, R.W., Hutchinson, J.C., and Hyatt, K.H. Clinical significance of changes in serum magnesium in patients undergoing cardiopulmonary bypass. *J. Thorac. Cardiovasc. Surg.* 61, 135–140 (1971).

Seller, R.H. Role of magnesium in digitalis toxicity. *Am. Heart J.* 82, 551–556 (1971).

Specter, M.J., Schweizer, E., and Goldman, R.H. Studies on magnesium's mechanism of action in digitalis-induced arrhythmias. *Circulation* 52, 1001–1005 (1975).

Szekely, P. The action of magnesium on the heart. *Br. Heart J.* VIII (3), 115–123 (1946).

Szekely, P., and Wynne, N.A. The effects of magnesium on cardiac arrhythmias caused by digitalis. *Clin. Sci.* 10 (2), 241–247 (1951).

Szekely, P., and Wynne, N.A. Effects of calcium chelation on digitalis-induced cardiac arrhythmias. *Br. Heart J.* XXV (5), 589–594 (1963).

Zwillinger, L. Über die magnesiumwirkung auf das herz. *Klin. Wschr.* 14, 1429–1433 (1935).

16

Serum Lipids in Total Parenteral Nutrition

EZRA STEIGER
DAVID M. GRISCHKAN
HERBERT K. NAITO
RAYMOND J. SHAMBERGER

Intravenous hyperalimentation or total parenteral nutrition (TPN) is a technique of intravenous feeding designed to meet the nutritional requirements of patients when their gastrointestinal system does not adequately function to provide for these needs. There are a number of disease states in which the gastrointestinal tract is not functional in absorbing sufficient nutrients to provide for adequate nutrition. Some of these conditions include obstructing intestinal cancers, pyloric stenosis secondary to severe peptic ulcer disease, enterocutaneous fistulae, and severe inflammatory diseases of the intestine. Malnutrition often accompanies these processes and compounds the risk of necessary surgery. To provide for the patient's caloric intake and vitamin, mineral, and nitrogen requirements, a concentrated dextrose solution with crystalline amino acids, and added vitamins and minerals are infused through a large-bore central vein (Dudrick et al., 1970). For the usual patient, the daily infusion of approximately 3000 calories and 20 grams of nitrogen (in the form of crystalline amino acids) is delivered through a percutaneously placed subclavian catheter whose tip lies in the superior vena cava. This method allows for the achievement of positive nitrogen balance and weight gain. The techniques used in placing and caring for the catheter, assessing the patient's ability to tolerate the hypertonic sugar solution, and monitoring of the patient have been well documented. The nutrient solution used for TPN is a 25 percent dextrose solution formulated so that three liters of it per day will remain within the patient's tolerance for fluid while providing approximately 3000 calories per day. Dextrose remains the major source of calories in TPN. Essential fatty acid (EFA) deficiency syndromes have been reported to occur in patients on long-term TPN when fat emulsions were not used. Clinically, this syndrome is characterized by the appearance of a desquamating skin rash in which circular patches of skin start to peel from the periphery. These flakes of skin can often be seen on the arms and legs, as well as in the patient's bedsheets. In addition, hair growth will become sparse and alopecia can result.

Fats are found in tissues (particularly in adipose tissue), as well as in the blood as lipoproteins; they are also structural components of membranes. Fats also function as vehicles for absorption and transport of fat-soluble vitamins and as a source of mechanical protection and insulation. Linoleic acid cannot be synthesized by humans and is thus an essential fatty acid. Adults have two sources of linoleic acid. The prime source is from dietary fat, usually more than enough to meet the body's requirements. The second major source is from the rich adipose tissue stores, which are 8 to 10 percent linoleic acid and may amount to as much as 700 g or more. This is enough EFA to meet the body's requirements. In the starved patient receiving fat-free TPN, both sources of linoleic acid are cut off; firstly, because there is none in the parenteral fluid and, secondly, because the high insulin levels accompanying glucose infusions block the lipolysis of adipose tissue triglyceride stores.

With the increasing use of fat-free TPN, a number of reports have documented biochemical and clinical evidence of EFA deficiency. Hansen and co-workers (1947) were among the first to draw attention to fatty acid deficiencies. They reported that three-fourths of their pediatric patients with severe eczema and low levels of unsaturated serum lipids responded favorably to dietary supplements of corn oil or lard. Collins et al. (1971) characterized this EFA syndrome by the presence of eicosatrienoic acid, an abnormal fatty acid, in serum phospholipids, along with low levels of linoleic and arachidonic acids. The clinical manifestations included a dry, scaly skin rash and a refractory anemia not responsive to vitamin B_{12}, folate, or iron administration. With the infusion of a soybean oil fat emulsion providing 22.8 g/day of linoleic acid, marked improvement in clinical and biochemical abnormalities were noted.

More specific descriptions of the relationship between fat-free nutrition and the EFA deficiency syndrome are provided by Holman (1968), Wilmore et al. (1973), Richardson and Sgoutas (1975), Riella et al. (1975), Flemming et al. (1976), and O'Neill et al. (1977). These reports suggest that the syndrome is characterized by desquamative dermatitis, hair loss, thrombocytopenia, a triene (5,8,11-eicosatrienoic acid) to tetraene (arachidonic acid) ratio above 0.4 (a biochemical marker for EFA deficiency), and possibly poor wound healing, refractory anemia, elevated SGOT (serum glutamic oxalacetic transaminase), SGPT (serum glutamine pyruric transaminase), LDH, and CPK. Therapeutic correction of the biochemical abnormalities using daily infusions of 500 ml of a 10 percent fat emulsion requires one to three weeks, while the cutaneous manifestations take longer to resolve.

Wene et al. (1975), induced biochemical evidence of EFA deficiency in eight normal volunteers by two weeks of either intravenous or intragastric fat-free feedings. Then, using a tube-fed diet with 2.6 percent of the calories as linoleic acid, they were able to revert the serum fatty acid profile to normal after 13 days.

When they were first introduced in the 1950s, intravenous fat emulsions carried great promise because they offered a concentrated source of calories, 9 kcal/g, and could be given through a peripheral vein since they were not hypertonic. Unfortunately early experience with Lipomul® (Upjohn, Kalamazoo, Michigan), a cottonseed oil emulsion, was complicated by fever, jaundice, hemorrhage, and embolism. This was due to a nonextractable toxic substance in the cottonseed oil, and also to the emulsifying agent which damaged erythrocytes (Lawson, 1965).

Only recently has the soybean oil emulsion, Intralipid®, 10 percent (Cutter Laboratories, Berkeley, California), been approved for use as a calorie source in parenteral feeding in the United States.* It consists of 10 percent soybean oil, 1.2 percent egg yolk phospholipids, 2.25 percent glycerin, and water for injection. This provides 27 g linoleic acid, 13 g oleic acid, 4.5 g palmitic acid, and 4.0 g linolenic acid per each 500-ml bottle. The preparation is isotonic (280 m*M*/liter), provides 1.1 kcal/ml, and has proven to be very safe (Hallberg et al., 1967).

Intralipid® can be used clinically in one of two ways. In small amounts it can prevent and treat the EFA deficiency syndrome during periods of fat-free nutrition (Holman, 1968; Wilmore et al., 1973; Richardson and Sgoutas, 1975; Riella et al., 1975; Flemming et al., 1976; and O'Neill et al., 1977). Our policy at The Cleveland Clinic is to administer one 500-ml bottle every other day to each patient who is expected to receive TPN for two weeks or longer. This provides about 13.5 g of linoleic acid per day, which usually meets the patient's daily requirements to prevent the EFA deficiency syndrome. When clinical or biochemical evidence of EFA deficiency already exists, one 500-ml bottle of 10 percent Intralipid® is given daily. Fat emulsions given in large amounts can also be used as a major calorie source, and substituted for part of the dextrose calories in parenteral nutrition.

---

*Liposyn®, 10 percent (Abbott Laboratories, Chicago, Illinois) has also been commercially introduced as a parenteral fat emulsion.

Dietel and Kaminsky (1974) described the peripheral lipid system consisting of 10 percent Intralipid® and a 5 percent dextrose-5 percent amino acid solution to which appropriate vitamins and minerals have been added. These solutions were infused into a peripheral vein through separate lines that connected terminally into one by a Y-connector. In 23 patients so treated for 4 to 78 days, weight gain and wound healing was reported in all individuals. Specific advantages of this system included: (1) avoidance of subclavian vein catheterization and infusion and all its associated complications; (2) reduced possibility of hyperglycemia and hypertonic state; and (3) the technique is simple to institute. Similar success using the peripheral lipid system in 72 patients was reported by Silberman et al. (1977). In Silberman's study he observed positive nitrogen balance, weight gain, and closure of enteric fistulas. Other investigators, such as Hansen et al. (1970), Broviac et al. (1976), and Jeejeebhoy et al. (1976) have used variable proportions of lipid as a caloric source (either centrally or peripherally) and have reported excellent results.

The controversial question remains whether a fat calorie is as effective as a carbohydrate calorie in TPN across a wide span of clinical situations. According to Daniel et al. (1975) and Long et al. (1977), a fat calorie cannot be efficiently utilized in severe states of stress and malnutrition. Jeejeebhoy and co-workers (1976) showed that there is no appreciable difference between a fat and carbohydrate calorie in promoting positive nitrogen balance and weight gain. Zohrab et al. (1973), subjected 27 patients to a trial in which a constant nitrogen input was maintained and nonprotein calories rotated between 100 percent glucose, 83 percent lipid with 17 percent glucose, and 50 percent lipid with 50 percent glucose. The results indicated that the source of calories had no influence on nitrogen balance, demonstrating that a high lipid input is as effective as 100 percent glucose in protein sparing. In a subsequent study (Jeejeebhoy et al., 1976), similar comparisons were made in 24 patients using sequential infusion of glucose alone (glucose system) or 83 percent Intralipid® (lipid system), with each patient serving as his or her own control. Results of each system were comparable, again demonstrating the effectiveness of lipids. According to this group, studies comparing glucose and lipid calories must allow three to four days for a period of equilibration, otherwise inaccurate nitrogen balance data will be obtained.

Based on current data, it appears that a fat calorie is as good as a glucose calorie in most patients. The most optimal and physiologic formula for TPN may be a mixture of both lipid and glucose calories. Thus, one can tailor the nutritional therapy to the specific needs of the patients, utilizing either the lipid system, glucose system, or a mixture of both. Another major consideration, however, is that on a caloric basis fat emulsions are much more expensive than hypertonic dextrose solution.

Table 1. TPN Dietary Regimens (Formulation)

Composition	*Fat-free TPN Group II (ml)*	*TPN with Fat Group III (ml)*
Base solutions		
8.5% freamine	500	500
50% dextrose	500	300
Sterile water	109	–
10% Intralipid®	–	309
Additives		
10% Ca-gluconate	10 (4.6 mEq)	10 (4.6 mEq)
50% $MgSO_4$	0.2 (0.81 mEq)	0.2 (0.81 mEq)
14.9% KCl	35 (70 mEq)	35 (70 mEq)
23.4% NaCl	8 (32 mEq)	8 (32 mEq)
16.4% Na-acetate	9 (16 mEq)	8 (16 mEq)
MVI (multivitamin infusion)	5	5

At The Cleveland Clinic Foundation, a rat model developed by Steiger et al. (1972) has been extensively used to study surgical nutrition. This system uses a special harness and swivel assembly that allows the unrestrained rat to be fed exclusively by vein for weeks at a time.

In one such study, Steiger et al. (1977) investigated the utilization and efficacy of fat containing versus fat-free TPN in protein-malnourished rats. Forty male adult rats were assigned to one of three study groups. Group I (12 rats) was sacrificed immediately at the end of the six-week protein depletion phase, while Groups II and III underwent an additional seven days of TPN with one of two diets. Group II (15 rats) was repleted intravenously with a TPN solution that contained 100 percent of its calories in the form of dextrose for seven days prior to sacrifice, and Group III (15 rats) was given a TPN solution containing 40 percent of its calories in the form of the fat emulsion and 60 percent in the form of dextrose (see Table 1). The intravenous diets were isocaloric and isonitrogenous, and similar volumes were infused containing identical amounts of vitamins and minerals. The results indicated that there was no significant difference in weight gain or nitrogen balance between Groups II and III after seven days of TPN. Furthermore, liver triglyceride elevations noted in the Group I (protein-depleted) rat livers returned toward normal levels in both Groups II and III. Liver phospholipid and cholesterol content, however, became significantly elevated in Group III (lipid-treated) rats (see Table 2). The significance of these changes on liver composition over a long period of time remains to be elucidated.

In a subsequent study, Steiger et al. (1978) studied the effects of fat-free versus fat-containing TPN on serum lipid concentration in protein-

Table 2. Liver Composition (mg/100 g Liver Tissue)

Study Groups	*Total Cholesterol*	*Triglycerides*	*Phospholipids*
Normal	219 ± 23	394 ± 73	3247 ± 207
Group I (Protein-depleted)	461 ± 64	5840 ± 2764	2398 ± 144
Group II (Fat-free TPN)	304 ± 47	754 ± 591	3221 ± 178
	↑ $p < .005$ ↓	↑ N.S. ↓	↑ $p < .001$ ↓
Group III (TPN with Fat)	423 ± 61	1151 ± 277	3627 ± 62

P values represent comparison between Group I and Group II.

malnourished rats. The experimental group design was similar to the one just described. Results showed that the weight gain was similar for Group II and Group III rats at the end of the seven-day hyperalimentation period. While serum triglycerides showed no significant difference between any of the treatment groups, total cholesterol was slightly but significantly elevated in Group II (fat-free TPN), and markedly elevated in Group III (fat-containing TPN). The former group demonstrated a modest increase in the ester cholesterol fraction while the latter group showed a marked increase in free cholesterol. Serum phospholipids were also markedly elevated in the lipid-treated group (see Table 3).

Fat-free TPN has been found to significantly decrease serum cholesterol in malnourished patients as well as in normal human volunteers. DenBesten et al. (1973) studied the effects of a fat-free high carbohydrate diet on serum lipids in eight healthy volunteers. This involved feeding each subject a seven-day general diet followed by two 12-day periods of either a nasogastric or intravenously-fed fat-free high-carbohydrate diet and finally, again, a seven-day general diet. The data indicated that the fat-free high-carbohydrate diet

Table 3. Serum Lipids in TPN Concentration (mg/100 ml)

Study Groups	*Total Cholesterol*	*Ester Cholesterol*	*Free Cholesterol*	*Phospholipids*	*Triglycerides*
Group I (Protein-depleted)	68 ± 8	43 ± 20	25 ± 14	119 ± 20	42 ± 28
	$p < .01$	$p < .005$	$p < .005$	N.S.	N.S.
Group II (Fat-free TPN)	81 ± 12	73 ± 11	8 ± 6	125 ± 19	35 ± 11
	$p < .001$	N.S.	$p < .001$	$p < .001$	N.S.
Group III (TPN with fat)	276 ± 47	80 ± 20	125 ± 52	644 ± 143	55 ± 30
Normal rats	57 ± 6	53 ± 9	4 ± 1	96 ± 13	70 ± 32

consistently showed a decrease in serum cholesterol irrespective of the mode of feeding. On this same diet, the serum triglyceride level dropped with intravenous feeding and increased with oral feeding.

Abbott et al. (1976) studied the lipid profiles of 22 patients on fat-free TPN. As in DenBesten's study (DenBesten et al., 1973), serum cholesterol levels dramatically dropped from a mean of 190 mg/dl before therapy to 112 mg/dl by the twenty-first day of therapy. Serum triglyceride levels remained on the low side of normal.

The hypercholesterolemic effect noted in our laboratory in rats using fat-free TPN is in contrast to the documented hypocholesterolemic effect of fat-free TPN in humans noted in the above two reports. A possible explanation may be the difference in nitrogen content.

Olson et al. (1970) reported that diets containing essential amino acids plus glutamate significantly reduced cholesterol levels, whereas replacing the glutamate with glycine had no effect on the serum cholesterol levels. The protein hydrolysate used by DenBesten et al. (1973) and Abbott et al. (1976) contained glutamate, whereas the diets used in our laboratory contained glycine and no glutamate.

In addition, when charts of 54 consecutive patients receiving TPN with glutamate-free amino acids were reviewed at The Cleveland Clinic, a small but significant increase in blood cholesterol concentration was noted at about two weeks after the initiation of the TPN treatment.

Our studies with the fat-containing TPN solutions further confirm the findings of Koga et al. (1975) and Broviac et al. (1976), who found a marked increase in serum cholesterol when fat emulsions were used as the major calorie source. There are two possible explanations for the marked elevation in free cholesterol levels in Group III rats (lipid-containing TPN). First there may be a defect in the cholesterol-esterifying enzyme system, lecithin-cholesterol acyltransferase (LCAT), or the cholesterol present in the fat emulsion may not be readily accessible to the LCAT enzyme, thus resulting in an accumulation of free cholesterol in the blood. The TPN lipid emulsions used in our study contain a small amount of cholesterol (mostly free cholesterol), approximately 50 mg/100 ml. This source of exogenous free cholesterol may contribute, after a prolonged period, to the elevated blood cholesterol levels observed in these animals. The significance of the elevated serum cholesterol (both total and free) is presently under investigation. According to Small (1977) and Ross and Harker (unpublished data) chronic elevation of blood free cholesterol can enhance the development of arteriosclerotic lesions. Thus, our findings of the observed increased free-cholesterol levels in the rat studies may have important clinical implications.

In summary, parenteral fat emulsions are safe, and can be used to treat or prevent essential fatty acid deficiency states, as well as providing a major calorie source in total parenteral nutrition. While lipid emulsions have several advantages, their use should complement rather than replace hypertonic dextrose. Using a rat model, we have confirmed that a fat calorie appears to be identical to a dextrose calorie in terms of nitrogen balance and weight gain. We have noted marked elevations of liver and serum free cholesterol and phospholipids, when using lipid as a major caloric source in TPN; further investigation is required to determine whether this is endogenous or exogenous in origin, as well as its possible harmful effects.

REFERENCES

Abbott, W.M., Abel, R.M., and Fischer, J.F. The effects of total parenteral nutrition upon serum lipid levels. *Surg. Gyn. Ob.* 142, 565–568 (1976).

Broviac, J.W., Riella, M.C., and Scribner, B.H. The role of intralipid in prolonged parenteral nutrition; 1. As a caloric substitute for glucose. *Am. J. Clin. Nut.* 29, 255–257 (1976).

Collins, F.D., Sinclair, A.J., Royle, J.P., Coats, D.A., Maynard, A.T., and Leonard, R.F. Plasma lipids in human linoleic acid deficiency. *Nut. Metab.* 13, 150–157 (1971).

Daniel, A.M., Shizgal, H.M., and MacLean, L.J. Endogenous fuels in experimental shock. *Surg. Forum* 27, 32–33 (1976).

Deitel, M., and Kaminsky, V. Total nutrition by peripheral vein–the lipid system. *Canad. Med. Assoc. J.* 111, 152–154 (1974).

DenBesten, I., Reyna, R.H., Connor, W.E., and Stegink, L.D. The different effects on the serum lipids and fecal steroids of high carbohydrate diets given orally or intravenously. *J. Clin. Invest.* 52, 1384–1393 (1973).

Dudrick, S.J., Long, J.M., Steiger, E., and Rhoads, J.F. Intravenous hyperalimentation. *Med. Clin. N. Am.* 54, 577–589 (1970).

Flemming, C.R., Smith, L.M., and Hodges, R.E. Essential fatty acid deficiency in adults receiving total parenteral nutrition. *Am. J. Clin. Nut.* 29, 976–983 (1976).

Hallberg, D., Holm, I., Obel, A.L., Schuberth, O., and Wretlind, A. Fat emulsions for complete intravenous nutrition. *Postgrad. Med. J.* 43, 307–316 (1967).

Hansen, L.M., Hardie, W.R., and Hidalgo, J. Fat emulsion for intravenous administration: Clinical experience with intralipid 10 percent. *Ann. Surg.* 184, 80–88 (1970).

Hansen, A.E., Knott, E.M., McQuarrie, I., Shaperman, E., and Wiese, H.F. Eczema and essential fatty acids. *Am. J. Dis. Child.* 73, 1–18 (1947).

Holman, R.T. Essential fatty acid deficiency, in *Progress in the Chemistry of Fats and Other Lipids,* Vol. 9. E.E. Editor(s), ed(s). Elmsford Pergamon Press, Elmsford, N.Y. (1968), pp. 279–348.

Jeejeebhoy, K.N., Anderson, G.H., Nakhooda, A.F., Greenberg, G.R., Sanderson, I., and Marliss, E.B. Metabolic studies in total parenteral nutrition with lipid in man. *J. Clin. Invest.* 57, 125–136 (1976).

Koga, Y., Ikeda, K., and Inokuchi, K. Effect of complete parenteral nutrition using fat emulsion of liver. *Ann. Surg.* 181, 186–190 (1975).

Lawson, L.J. Parenteral nutrition in surgery. *Br. J. Surg.* 52, 795–900 (1965).

Long, J.M., Wilmore, D.W., and Mason, A.D. Effect of carbohydrate and fat intake on nitrogen excretion during total intravenous feeding. *Ann. Surg.* 185, 417–422 (1977).

Olson, R.E., Nichaman, M.Z., Nittka, J., and Eagles, J.A. Effect of amino acid diets upon serum lipids. *Am. J. Clin. Nut.* 23, 1614–1625 (1970).
O'Neill, J.A., Caldwell, M.D., and Meng, H.C. Essential fatty acid deficiency in surgical patients. *Ann. Surg.* 185, 535–542 (1977).
Richardson, T.J., and Sgoutas, D. Essential fatty acid deficiency in four adult patients during total parenteral nutrition. *Am. J. Clin. Nut.* 28, 258–263 (1975).
Riella, M.C., Broviac, J.W., Wells, M., and Scribner, B.H. Essential fatty acid deficiency in human adults during total parenteral nutrition. *Ann Int. Med.* 83, 786–789 (1975).
Silberman, H., Freehauf, M., Fong, G., and Rosenblatt, N. Parenteral nutrition with lipids. *JAMA* 238, 1380–1382 (1977).
Small, D.M. Cellular mechanisms for lipid deposition in atherosclerosis. *N. Eng. J. Med.* 297, 873–877 (1977).
Steiger, E., Naito, H., Cooperman, A., and O'Neill, M. Effect of lipid calories on weight gain, nitrogen balance, liver weight, and composition in total parenteral nutrition (TPN). *Surg. Forum* 28, 83–85 (1977).
Steiger, E., Naito, H.K., O'Neill, M., and Cooperman, A. Serum lipids in total parenteral nutrition (TPN): Effect of fat. *J. Surg. Res.* 24, 527–531 (1978).

17

Role of Magnesium in Pharmacology of Lithium and in Development of Fetal Cardiovascular Defects

NICHOLAS J. BIRCH

INTRODUCTION

Lithium carbonate has been successfully used in the preventative treatment of recurrent affective disorder (manic-depressive psychosis) (Schou and Thomsen, 1975). The scale of its usage is often underestimated: in Great Britain in 1975, 6700 kg of lithium carbonate was prescribed to an estimated one in 2000 individuals of the total adult population (Hullin, 1978). The therapeutic success rate is considered to be around 80 percent.

Despite such widespread use, no definitive mechanism of action has been demonstrated (Birch, 1978a). Early theories have implicated changes in monoamine metabolism (Murphy, 1976) or electrolyte metabolism (Jenner, 1973). Recently it has been proposed that since lithium (Li) is chemically similar to magnesium (Mg) and calcium (Ca) as a result of the "diagonal relationship" between these elements in the periodic table (Cotton and Wilkinson, 1972), a biochemical relationship might also exist (Birch, 1970). This hypothesis would also allow the explanation of a number of hitherto inexplicable effects of Li, and also could encompass aspects of the monoamine and electrolyte theories.

Many enzymes are Mg-dependent; some of these have been shown by various workers to be inhibited by Li (see Table 1). However, much of the Li literature is derived from studies at Li concentrations which are higher than the pharmacologically relevant range (less than 2 mmol/liter). One should extrapolate with caution from such studies, in which Li concentrations are frequently 150 mmol/liter or above.

Table 1. Enzyme Systems Whose Activity is Effected by Lithium[a]

In vivo	*In vitro*
Acetyl cholinesterase	ATPases, (Na^+, K^+), Mg^{2+}, Ca^{2+}
Acid phosphatase	Alkaline phosphatase
Aconitase	DNA polymerase
Alkaline phosphatase	Enolase
Aryl sulphatase	Fructose 1,6-diphosphatase
Cholinesterase	Hexokinase
Drug-metabolizing enzymes	Pyruvate kinase
Glucokinase	RNA synthetase
Hexokinase	
Pyruvate kinase	
RNA synthesis	
Succinic dehydrogenase	
Tryptophan oxygenase	
Tyrosine aminotransferase	

[a]For bibliographic details see Birch, 1978c.

Studies have been carried out on a number of Mg-dependent enzymes at pharmacologic Li concentrations. Early studies of rabbit muscle pyruvate kinase showed that Li did indeed inhibit the enzyme at concentrations as low as 2 mmol/liter (Birch, 1978b). The inhibition was not competitive with respect to Mg, although Li was competitive to Adenosine Diphosphate (ADP); this is significant, since it may be that the active substrate is a Mg-ADP complex. Further studies have provided preliminary evidence of a ternary Li-Mg-ADP complex which might act as a false substrate (Birch and Goulding, 1975). However, pyruvate kinase has at least three different isoenzymes, and these studies have therefore been extended to investigate purified rat brain pyruvate kinase, since it might be argued that rabbit muscle enzyme has little relevance to the brain of manic-depressive patients (Kajda et al., 1979). Brain pyruvate kinase had similar kinetics and inhibitory characteristics to the muscle enzyme and was inhibited to a slightly greater extent by lithium (Table 2).

It is clear that Li might have an effect on Mg-sensitive processes, particularly since it has been established that there is often a bell-shaped curve of Mg-dependency: slight decrease or increase of Mg activity results in disproportionate loss of function (Günther, 1977). For instance, if Li were to affect, by even a small amount, the various Mg-dependent enzymes on the glycolytic pathway, the cumulative effect would be large, since 8 of the 13 enzymes require Mg.

Conducting tissues require Mg not only in intermediary metabolism but also to stabilize membranes, in membrane pumps such as Na^+,K^+-ATPase, in the synthesis, storage, and release of transmitters, and also at receptor sites in the synthesis and breakdown of 3′,5′-cyclic AMP. It is not surprising,

Table 2. Inhibition of Pyruvate Kinase by Lithium

Substrate	*Rat Brain Pyruvate Kinase*	*Rabbit Muscle Pyruvate Kinase*
Mg^{2+}	n.c.[a]	n.c.
K^+	n.c.	n.c.
Phosphoenol pyruvate	n.c.	n.c.
ADP	comp.[b]	comp.
Inhibition at 2 mmol $liter^{-1}$ Li^+	7–12%	5–8%
Inhibition at 10 $mmol^2$ $liter^{-1}$ Li^+	25–32%	16–24%

[a]n.c. = noncompetitive inhibition.
[b]comp. = competitive inhibition.

therefore, that sporadic reports appear of Li effects on the heart, although these have received inadequate consideration. The most common effect seen is to be depression or inversion of the *T* wave of the electrocardiograph (ECG). (Demers and Heninger, 1971), although occasional reports of transmission defects occur (Jaffe, 1977). One such report is of particular interest, since a refractory cardiac arrhythmia was controlled by intravenous $MgSO_4$ administration (Worthley, 1974).

However, one most disturbing effect is that reported on the cardiovascular system of fetuses of mothers receiving Li for manic-depressive disorders. Because of fears of teratogenicity, a register has been maintained of babies born from mothers who received Li at some stage in their pregnancy (Weinstein and Goldfield, 1975). The results of this survey, recently updated (Schou and Weinstein, 1978, and personal communication), are shown in Table 3.

First, the number of defects reported is small, and must be weighed against the dangers to the mother and child of not continuing Li treatment for manic-depressive psychoses. It is clear, however, that not only is there a high preponderance of cardiovascular defects over all other nontrivial abnormalities (normally 12.5 percent; 72 percent in Li babies), but there is an excessive representation of Ebstein's anomaly compared with all congenital cardiovas-

Table 3. Lithium Babies Reported to *Lithium Register*[a,b]

Number of infants reported	217
Stillborn	7[b]
Down's syndrome	2
Malformed	25
Cardiovascular malformations	18
Ebstein's anomaly	6
Other malformations	7

[a]Data updated through October, 1978. See Schou and Weinstein, 1979.
[b]One of these was malformed, and is also included in that group.

cular defects. The normal incidence is 0.74 to 1.0 percent (Nadas and Fyler, 1972) or 1.25 percent (Schou and Weinstein, 1978); in Li babies it is 33.3 percent (Schou and Weinstein, 1978). The latter authors suggest that some degree of distortion of the true situation may have occurred, since serious anomalies are more assiduously reported than minor defects, and these again are more readily reported than totally normal births. However, it does seem that Ebstein's anomaly occurs more frequently in children born of mothers who received Li_2CO_3 during pregnancy.

The intriguing possibility now arises that perhaps such cardiovascular defects might be attributable to Li-induced Mg deficit. Previous studies have shown altered brain distribution of Mg following Li treatment (Birch and Jenner, 1973; Bond et al., 1975) and the divergent reports in changes in renal excretion of the element have been reviewed (Birch, 1978c). Mg deficit is associated with other pediatric cardiovascular disorders (Seelig, 1978, 1979; Seelig and Haddy [in press]). Cardiac defects occur in fetal alcohol syndrome following maternal alcoholism in pregnancy, in fetal abnormality following maternal anticonvulsant therapy during pregnancy, and in myocardial disorders in infants born of eclamptic mothers (Seelig; Chapter 3 of the present volume; Seelig, 1978, 1979). Hypervitaminosis D is known as a cause of cardiovascular defects, cardiofacies and mental retardation in association with Mg deficit (Seelig, 1969). There are presently no data on the incidence of Ebstein's anomaly in any of these groups and the possible role of Mg deficit in its etiology is a provocative speculation.

The increased incidence of Ebstein's anomaly, and indeed of all cardiovascular defects, in Li-treated fetuses may, therefore, be a further example of drug-induced Mg deficit which is exacerbated in the fetus by maternal Mg deficiency. The interpretation of the incidence data relies heavily on the accuracy of individual reports and is complicated by local variables, such as dietary differences in intake of vitamin D, Ca, Mg, P, and possibly other elements, such as the individual government's dietary supplementation policy and local cultural habits (e.g., high intakes of phosphated drinks in North America and of fish oils in Scandinavian countries).

It might, therefore, be considered desirable to provide routine dietary Mg supplements to pregnant women, especially those receiving Mg-depleting drugs, in order to provide protection for the fetus against Mg deficit. Such a course would be inexpensive and could have no deleterious effect, except in cases of advanced renal insufficiency where any increased solute load would be contraindicated. Presumably Mg salts could be incorporated into the iron-containing preparations which are already routinely prescribed in most centers.

The effects of Li on Mg metabolism are being revealed slowly. Such findings suggest that it is biochemically reasonable to speculate that the extensive congenital cardiovascular defects following maternal Li treatment might be related to induced Mg deficit. This biochemical speculation now requires interdisciplinary investigation in order for this hypothesis to be confirmed or denied.

ACKNOWLEDGMENTS

I wish to thank Dr. Mildred Seelig, whose correspondence provoked the ideas presented here. I also wish to extend my thanks to Professor Mogens Schou and to acknowledge the assistance of the late Dr. Morton Weinstein (who died in 1979) in providing the latest unpublished information from the lithium register.

REFERENCES

Birch, N.J. Effects of lithium on plasma magnesium. *Br. J. Psych.* 116, 461 (1970).

Birch, N.J. Lithium in medicine, in *New Trends in Bio-inorganic Chemistry.* R.J.P. Williams, and J.J.R.F. da Silva, eds. Academic Press, London (1978a), pp. 389–435.

Birch, N.J. Metabolic effects of lithium, in *Lithium in Medical Practice.* F.N. Johnson and S. Johnson, eds. M.T.P. Press, Lancaster, England (1978b), pp. 89–114.

Birch, N.J. Lithium and manic-depressive psychoses: inorganic perspectives in psychopharmacology. *Inorg. Perspec. Biol. Med.* 1, 173–215 (1978c).

Birch, N.J., and Goulding, I. Lithium-nucleotide interactions investigated by gel-filtration. *Anal. Biochem.* 66, 293–297 (1975).

Birch, N.J., and Jenner, F.A. The distribution of lithium and its effects on the distribution and excretion of other ions. *Br. J. Pharm.* 47, 586–594 (1973).

Bond, P.A., Brooks, B.A., and Judd, A. The distribution of lithium, sodium and magnesium in rat brain and plasma after various periods of administration of lithium in the diet. *Br. J. Pharm.* 53, 235–239 (1975).

Cotton, F.A., and Wilkinson, G. *Advanced Inorganic Chemistry.* Wiley-Interscience, New York (1972).

Demers, R.G., and Heninger, G.R. Electrocardiographic T-Wave changes during lithium carbonate treatment. *JAMA* 218, 381–386 (1971).

Günther, T. Stoffwechsel und Wirkungen des intrazellulären Magnesium. *J. Clin. Chem. Clin. Biochem.* 15, 433–438 (1977).

Hullin, R.P. The place of lithium in biological psychiatry, in *Lithium in Medical Practice.* F.N. Johnson and S. Johnson, eds. M.T.P. Press, Lancaster, England (1978), pp. 433–454.

Jaffe, C.M. First degree atrioventricular block during lithium carbonate treatment. *Am. J. Psych.* 134, 88–89 (1977).

Jenner, F.A. Lithium and affective psychoses, in *Biochemistry and Mental Illness.* L.L. Iverson and S.P. Rose, eds. Biochemical Society Special Publications No. 1. Biochemical Society, London (1973), pp. 101–111.

Kajda, P.K., Birch, N.J., O'Brien, M.J., and Hullins, R.P. Rat brain pyruvate kinase: purification and effects of lithium. *J. Inorgan. Biochem.* 11, 361–366 (1979).

Murphy, D.L. Effects of lithium on catecholamines and other brain neurotransmitters, in *The Neurobiology of Lithium.* W.E. Bunney and D.L. Murphy, eds. Neurosciences Research Program Bulletin, vol. 14. Neurosciences Research Program, Boston (1976), pp. 165–169.

Nadas, A.S., and Fyler, D.C. *Pediatric Cardiology,* 3rd ed. W.B. Saunders, Philadelphia (1972), pp. 597–607.

Schou, M., and Thomsen, K. Lithium prophylaxis of recurrent endogenous affective disorders, in *Lithium Research and Therapy.* F.N. Johnson, ed. Academic Press, London (1975), pp. 63–84.

Seelig, M.S. Vitamin D and cardiovascular, renal and brain damage in infancy and childhood. *Ann. N.Y. Acad. Sci.* 147, 537–582 (1969).

Seelig, M.S. Magnesium deficiency with phosphate and vitamin D excesses: Role in pediatric cardiovascular disease? *Card. Med.* 3, 637–650 (1978).

Seelig, M.S. *Magnesium in the Pathogenesis of Disease,* Vol. I. L.V. Avioli, ed. Plenum Press, New York (1979).

Seelig, M.S., and Haddy, F.J. Magnesium deficiency in arterial disease, in *Magnesium in Health and Disease.* Proceedings on 2nd International Symposium on Magnesium, Montreal, 1976. M. Cantin and M.S. Seelig, eds. SP Medical and Scientific Books, Jamaica, N.Y. (1981), pp. 000–000.

Weinstein, M.R., and Goldfield, M.D. Administration of lithium during pregnancy, in *Lithium Research and Therapy.* F.N. Johnson, ed. Academic Press, London (1975), pp. 237–264.

Weinstein, M.R. Lithium teratogenesis: the register of lithium babies, in *Lithium: Controversies and Unresolved Issues.* T.B. Cooper, S. Gershon, N.S. Kline, and M. Schou, eds. Excerpta Medica (1st Congress Series 478), Amsterdam (1979), pp. 432–446.

Worthley, L.I.G. Lithium toxicity and refractory cardiac arrhythmia treated with intravenous magnesium. *Anaesthest. Intens. Care* 4, 357–360 (1974).

18

ECG Abnormalities in Magnesium Abnormalities

H. ZUMKLEY
A. LISON
O. KNOLL
M. ERNST
R. MARTIN

INTRODUCTION

The nature and quality of electrocardiograph (ECG) alterations due to metabolic magnesium imbalance require resolution. Hypomagnesemia is believed to cause depression of the *ST*-segment and negative *T*-waves (Seller et al., 1970). Hypermagnesemia may induce ECG alterations similar to those induced by hyperkalemia; that is, increase of *T*-wave amplitude (Wacker and Vallee, 1957). We report here animal experiments and clinical investigations which may clarify the relation of Mg abnormalities to ECG alterations.

METHODS

Clinical Investigations

Six patients (one with and five without renal insufficiency) were treated for 10 days with oral doses of 1,2 g magnesium carbonate ($MgCO_3$). Plasma Mg concentrations were determined every 2 to 3 days; ECGs were recorded at the same time. Furthermore, plasma magnesium, sodium, potassium, and calcium, concentrations as well as red blood cell Mg, were also measured before, during, and after hemodialysis of 33 patients undergoing intermittent hemodialysis. ECGs were recorded simultaneously.

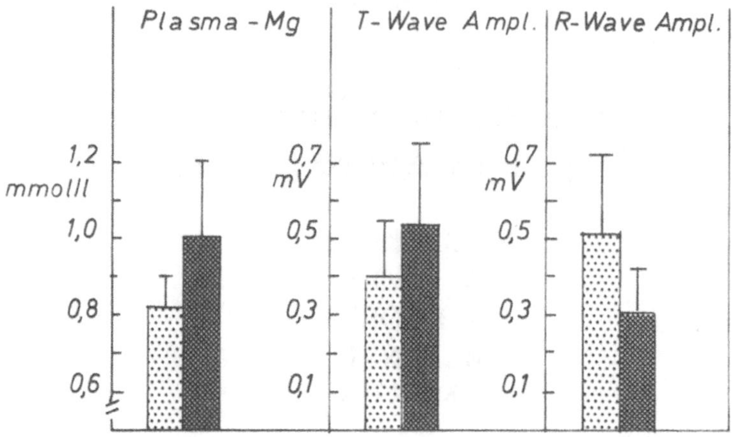

Fig. 1. Concentrations of plasma-magnesium, *T*- and *R*-wave amplitude in six patients before (dotted) and after (solid) treatment with magnesium carbonate. (error bar = S.D.)

Animal Experiments

To induce acute hypermagnesemia in the first experimental series, ten untreated rabbits were hemodialysed with a dialysate of high Mg concentration. Plasma Mg concentrations were determined before as well as 60, 90, and 120 minutes after hemodialysis had been started. ECGs were recorded at the same time.

In the second experimental series, ten rabbits pretreated with rauwolfia alkaloide (reserpine) were dialysed with a dialysate of high Mg concentration under standardized experimental conditions. Plasma Mg concentrations were measured before, as well as 60, 90, and 120 minutes after hemodialysis had been started. ECGs were recorded simultaneously.

Plasma Mg concentrations were measured by atomic absorption spectrometry. ECGs were recorded with a Siemens electrocardiograph. The following ECG parameters were analysed: (1) pulse rate, (2) *T*-wave amplitude, (3) *R*-wave amplitude, (4) PQ interval, (5) QT interval, and (6) QRS interval.

RESULTS

Figure 1 shows the reaction of plasma Mg concentration and *T*- and *R*-wave amplitudes of six patients before and after application of $MgCO_3$.

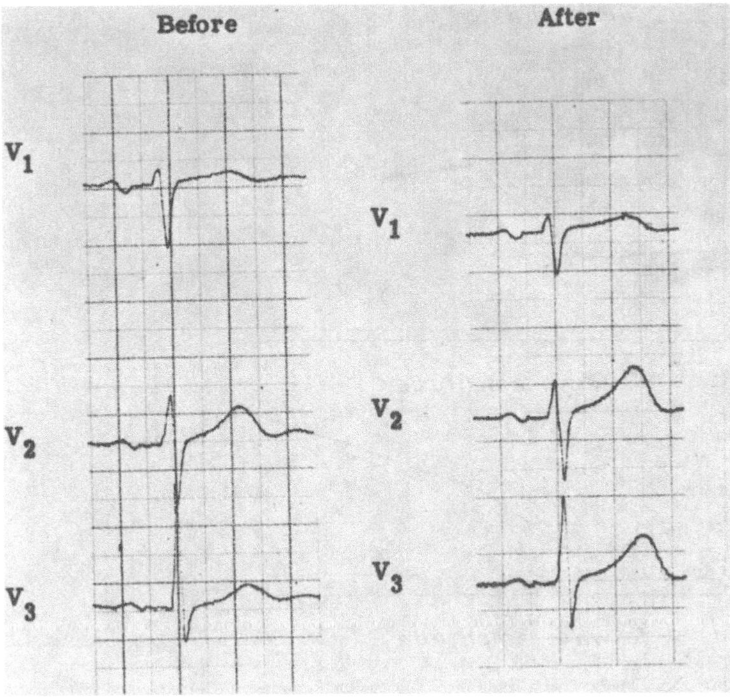

Fig. 2. ECG before and after treatment with magnesium carbonate.

The response of the ECG to administration of $MgCO_3$ is demonstrated in Fig. 2. After increase of the plasma Mg concentration, there was increased *T*-wave amplitude.

Figure 3 shows alterations of the ECG pattern and magnesium concentrations in the plasma of a patient after administration of $MgCO_3$. As the plasma Mg concentration increases, the amplitude of the *T*-wave increased and amplitude of the *R*-wave decreased.

Figure 4 shows the mean values of ECG parameters and plasma Mg concentrations in ten rabbits before, as well as 60, 90, and 120 minutes after hemodialysis with a dialysate of high Mg concentration (10 μmol/liter). The rabbits had been pretreated for ten days with rauwolfia alkaloids. Under hemodialysis there was a significant increase of plasma Mg concentration, combined with an increasing *T*-wave amplitude and decreasing *R*-wave ampli-

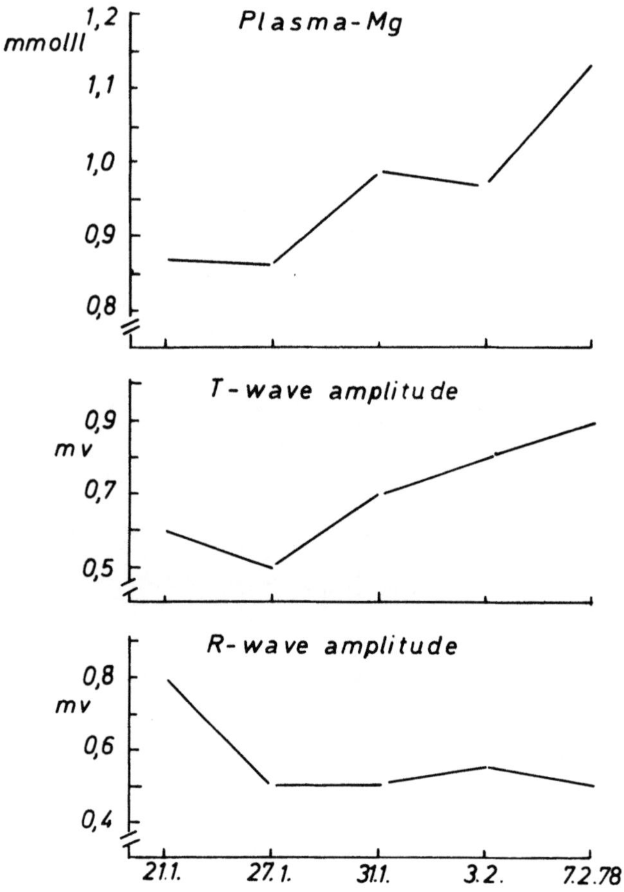

Fig. 3. Magnesium concentration, *T*- and *R*-wave amplitude in a patient without renal insufficiency after treatment with magnesium carbonate.

tude. PQ interval, QRS interval, and QT interval increased, whereas the pulse rate decreased.

As the mean plasma Mg concentrations rose in ten rabbits during hemodialysis with a dialysate of high Mg concentration from values before and 60, 90, and 120 minutes after hemodialysis. At the same time there was a decrease of the *R*- and *T*-wave amplitudes (Fig. 5).

Among 33 chronically hemodialyzed patients as the mean values of plasma levels decreased from values before dialyses in the course of the hemodialysis, the *T*-wave amplitudes decreased (Fig. 6).

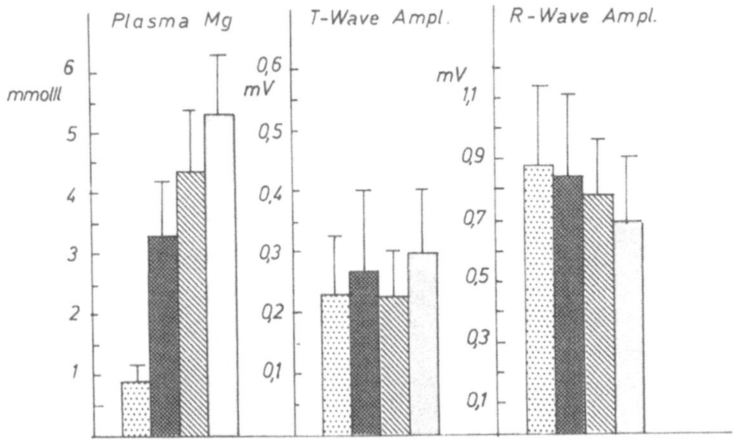

Fig. 4. Magnesium concentrations in plasma, *T*- and *R*-wave amplitude in pretreated rabbits with Reserpine before (░), 60 minutes (■), 90 minutes (▧), and 120 minutes (□) after hemodialysis against high magnesium concentration. (┬ = S.D.)

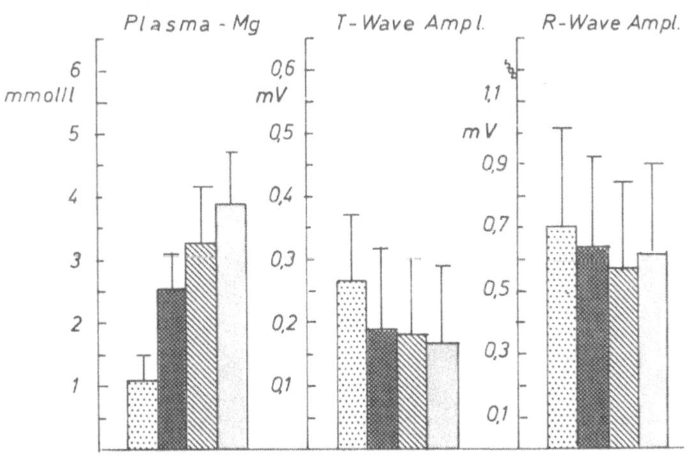

Fig. 5. Magnesium concentration in plasma, *T*- and *R*-wave amplitudes in rabbits before (░), 60 minutes (■), 90 minutes (▧), and 120 minutes (□) after hemodialysis against high dialysate magnesium concentration. (┬ = S.D.)

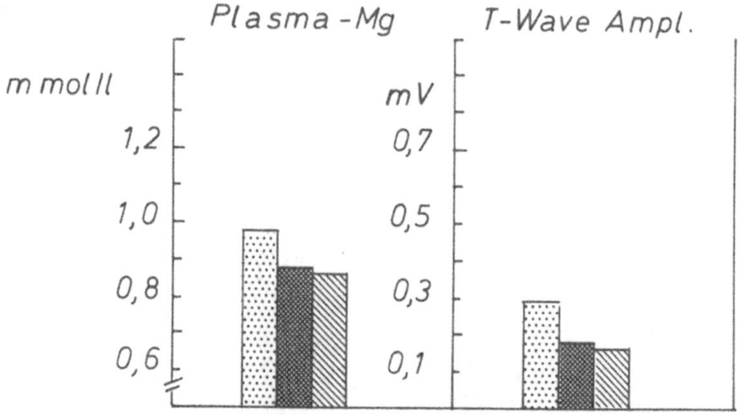

Fig. 6. Magnesium concentration in plasma and *T*-wave amplitude before ( ), during ( ), and after ( ) hemodialysis. (n = 33)

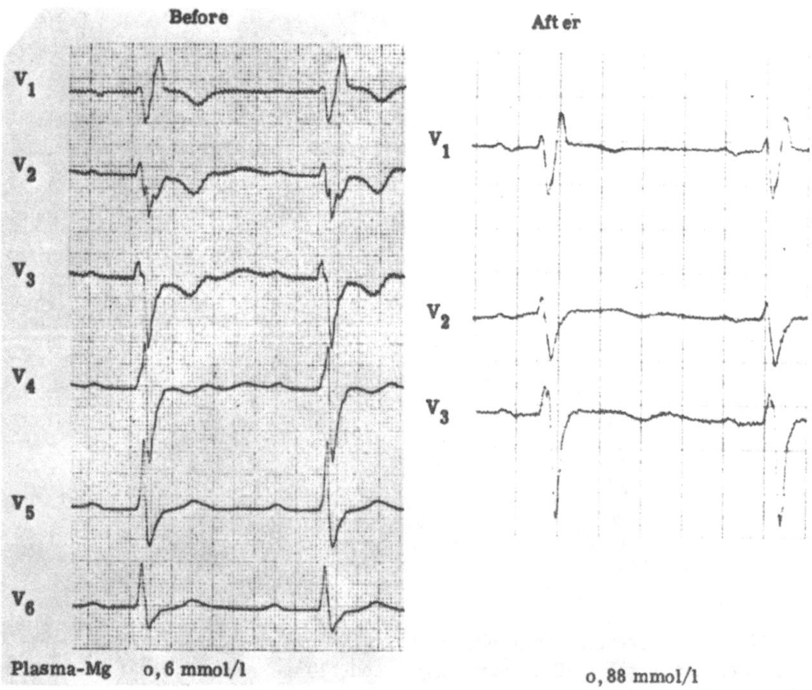

Fig. 7. ECG before and after treatment with magnesium in a patient with digitalis intoxication and hypomagnesemia.

A patient with digitalis intoxication and hypomagnesemia showed considerable improvement of the ECG after normalization of plasma Mg concentrations (Fig. 7).

DISCUSSION

These clinical and animal experimental studies have shown that deviations of plasma Mg concentrations can lead to ECG abnormalities. Increased *T*-wave amplitude and decreased *R*-wave amplitude were produced by increasing plasma Mg concentrations by oral magnesium loads. Under the same conditions other ECG parameters remained normal. Only the ECG of rabbits, pretreated with rauwolfia alkaloids, showed an increasing *T*-wave amplitude and simultaneously a decreasing *R*-wave amplitude after induced hypermagnesemia. The ECGs of animals which were not pretreated with rauwolfia alkaloid showed decreasing *T*- and *R*-wave amplitudes.

Prolonged PQ, QT, and QRS intervals in animal experiments were dependent on decreasing pulse rate. *T*- and *R*-wave amplitude deviations were not dependent on changes in the concentrations of other electrolytes. Simultaneously measured sodium, potassium, and calcium concentrations in plasma and red blood cells (RBC) were normal. Mg RBC concentrations increased after oral Mg load in patients.

The ECG deviations of patients on chronic intermittent hemodialysis may be an indication that the observed *T*- and *R*-wave amplitude deviations depend on the plasma Mg concentrations. At the same time we found decreased *T*-wave amplitude when there was a decrease of Mg concentration under dialysis (Zumkley and Wadynski, 1973).

In animal experiments we could not observe any ECG alterations due to acute hypomagnesemia (Lison et al., 1976). There were no significant abnormalities in the ECG of rabbits under hemodialysis with a magnesium-free dialysate. In the ECG of a digitalized patient suffering from hypomagnesemia we found digitalis intoxication-like alterations, which improved in a few days with Mg therapy.

At first sight it seems difficult to explain why significant alterations of *T*- and *R*-wave amplitude in cases of acute hypermagnesemia could be observed only in animal experiments after pretreatment with rauwolfia alkaloids. But it has to be considered that adrenalin depletion of the heart muscle under rauwolfia alkaloids therapy may cause an increased sensitivity to Mg ions. Antoni et al. (1963) have reported similar findings for potassium ions. These authors found a significantly increased potassium sensitivity of isolated arterial and patellar muscle in guinea pigs, by adrenalin and noradrenalin depletion, after rauwolfia alkaloid therapy for several days.

CONCLUSIONS

After oral Mg load in six patients there was a significant increase of the plasma Mg concentration, usually accompanied by an increase of the *T*-wave amplitude and simultaneous decrease of the *R*-wave amplitude as shown in the ECG. Acute hypermagnesemia of rabbits was induced by hemodialysis-induced increased *T*-wave amplitude, combined with the occurrence of decreased *R*-wave amplitude only in rabbits pretreated with rauwolfia alkaloids. Possibly adrenalin depletion in the myocardium might cause an increased myocardial sensitivity to Mg ions.

After hemodialysis with a Mg-free dialysate there were no typical ECG deviations in animal experiments which could be regarded as being caused by hypomagnesemia. In one case we were able to show that there exists an intensified sensitivity for digitalis in cases of hypomagnesemia.

REFERENCES

Antoni, H., Herkel, K., and Fleckenstein, A. Die Restitution der automatischen Erregungsbildung in kaliumgelähmten Schrittmacher-Geweben durch Adrenalin. *Pfluegers Arch.* 277, 633–649 (1963).

Lison, A.E., Knoll, O., Ahlbrand, P.E., and Zumkley, H. Tierexperimentelle Störungen des Magnesium-Haushaltes. *Verh. dtsch. Ges. inn. Med.* 82, 912–915 (1976).

Seller, R.H., Cangino, J., Kim, K.E., Mendelssohn, S., Brest, A.N., and Schwarz, C. Digitalis toxicity and hypomomagnesemia. *Am. Heart J.* 3, 57–79 (1970).

Wacker, W.E.C., and Vallee, B.L. Study of magnesium metabolism in acute renal failure employing multichamel flame spectrometer. *N. Eng. J. Med.* 257, 1254–1256 (1957).

Zumkley, H., and Wadynski, A. Beziehungen zwischen EKG und intra-extrazellulärer Elektrolytkonzentration während Hämodialyse. *Verh. Dtsch. Ges. inn. Med.* 79, 738–741 (1973).

Zumkley, H., Wessels, F., Winter, R., and Palm, D. Magnesiumintoxikation bei Niereninsuffizienz. *Med. Klin.* 69, 587–590 (1974).

19

Myocardial Protein Synthesis in Magnesium Deficiency: Effects of Morphine

WALTER B. ESSMAN
ERIC J. ESSMAN

INTRODUCTION

The interdependency of magnesium (Mg) and myocardial function has been established on several grounds. One major issue is that potassium (K) loss represents a major factor in the susceptibility and pathogenesis of cardiomyopathy, and the likelihood of K loss is increased with Mg deficiency. Cellular loss of K in Mg deficiency may be brought about by a decreased maintenance of a concentration gradient through decreased microsomal Mg, Na,K-ATPase activity. This appears to be the case with hypercalcemia and its resultant cardiotoxicity, and inhibition or cardiotonic agents by Mg-dependent ATPase. Digitalis toxicity is associated with myocardial Mg loss (Hochrein et al., 1967), and such toxicity is reversed by Mg (Szekely and Wynne, 1951). Mg-deficient animals are also more susceptible to the effects of cardiac glycosides (Kleiger et al., 1966). Another possible basis for the maintenance of myocardial K by Mg resides in a K efflux through the mitochondrion mediated by histone; K efflux and mitochondrial swelling may be prevented by Mg. (Schwartz, 1966; Johnson et al., 1967). Mg deficiency results in a disruption of myocardial mitochondria and the efflux of K.

Myocardial Mg loss has also been associated, as a dependent variable, with cardiomyopathies. Significant loss of myocardial Mg has been reported with an electrolyte-steroid-induced cardiac necrosis (Du Ruisseau and Mori, 1959). Myocardial Mg loss in cardiac necrosis is caused by phosphate loading of parathyroidectomized animals or with isoproterenol (Lehr et al., 1966; Lehr, 1969). Mg loss was earlier and greater than myocardial K loss. In clinical studies the infarcted segment of tissue in an acute myocardial infarction had approximately 26 percent less Mg content than a noninfarcted segment; the latter, however, still had approximately 36 percent less Mg than myocardium from patients without heart disease (Iseri et al., 1952). An extensive review of the interrelationship of Mg to ischemic heart disease has appeared (Seelig and Heggtveit, 1974), and some of the clinical factors basic to hypomagnesemia and their effect upon cardiolytic drugs has also been considered (Essman, 1978).

The rather consistent evidence that myocardial metabolism is altered in Mg deficiency has warranted consideration of the effects of morphine upon this metabolopathy (Essman, 1978). Although a Ca dependency for the myocardial effects of morphine has been indicated, little data have been available for Mg, which undoubtedly is altered with changes in Ca availability. Myocardial protein and RNA synthesis might be expected to decrease with hypomagnesemia, particularly in view of the mitochondrial and microsomal effects of such a deficiency state.

MATERIALS AND METHODS

In our studies, male CF-Is strain mice, at 35 days of age, were maintained on a low-Mg test diet (Nutritional Biochemicals) or a balanced diet of Purina lab chow for 16 days. Food and water (double-glass-distilled) were provided ad. lib. One group of Mg-deficient mice, was placed on an ad. lib. Purina lab chow diet with ad. lib. tap water for two weeks. Prior to the diet change, blood samples were obtained, via the caudal vein, for Mg assay. The myocardial tissue was removed, as were blood samples obtained from the abdominal aorta. The latter were collected in heparinized tubes containing NaF, and the plasma was assayed for Mg concentration, using atomic absorption spectroscopy. A similar assay was carried out for extracts of fresh myocardium, and the remaining tissue was utilized for in vitro studies of protein synthesis. Subcellular fractions were prepared from freshly excised myocardium, utilizing differential and sucrose density gradient centrifugation; this yielded a nuclear, mitochondrial, and microsomal fraction. Myocardial tissue or derived subcellular fractions obtained from hypomagnesemic or from control mice was incubated under physiologic conditions in a tris-KCl-sucrose buffer for 60 minutes with C^{14}-leucine (1.66 μCi/ml). Either 0.9 percent NaCl or morphine sulfate (10^{-7}, 10^{-6}, or 10^{-5} *M*) were added to the incubation mixture. The reaction was stopped by cooling and proteins were precipitated and/or extracted and the tissue or fraction protein concentration was determined. The solubilized fractions were counted in a liquid scintillation counter and the specific activity of the incorporated isotope was determined.

Table 1. Mean ($\pm \sigma$) Rate of C^{14}-Leucine Incorporation (mM mg $protein^{-1}$ hr^{-1}) into Mouse Myocardium: Effects of Morphine on Hypomagnesemic, Normomagnesemic, and Mg-supplemented Mice

Condition	*Hypomagnesemia*	*Normomagnesemia*	*Hypomagnesemia + Diet*
NaCl (0.9%)	0.261 (0.04)	0.516 (0.07)	0.253 (0.08)
Morphine (10^{-7} M)	0.226 (0.04)	0.359 (0.02)[a]	0.323 (0.04)[b]
Morphine (10^{-6} M)	0.278 (0.03)	0.344 (0.09)[a]	0.283 (0.04)
Morphine (10^{-5} M)	0.260 (0.04)	0.373 (0.06)[a]	0.279 (0.01)

[a] $p < .01$.
[b] $p < .02$.

RESULTS

Blood Mg levels among hypomagnesemic mice were appreciably lower (2.37 ± 0.41 mg percent) than for control animals (3.20 ± 0.16 mg percent), and after 14 days of a normal diet, previously hypomagnesemic mice did show increased blood levels (2.92 ± 0.19 mg percent). Myocardial Mg concentration was lower in the experimental mice (14.21 ± 0.68 mEq/kg), and hypomagnesemic mice, after two weeks on a normal diet, did show increased myocardial Mg content (17.63 ± 0.56 mEq/kg).

The effects of myocardial Mg deficiency and the influence of morphine upon myocardial protein synthesis are summarized in Table 1. Protein synthesis by the hypomagnesemic mouse myocardium was reduced by 49 percent, and partial restoration of myocardial Mg with a normal diet, failed to provide for any increase in the depressed rate of synthesis. In the normomagnesemic myocardium, morphine at all concentrations caused a significant decrease ($p < .01$) in myocardial protein synthesis, whereas in the hypomagnesemic myocardium, morphine had no further effect upon the already reduced rate of myocardial protein synthesis. In the minimally hypomagnesemic myocardium (Mg-deficient + normal diet) morphine increased protein synthesis significantly ($p < .02$) only at the lowest concentration (10^{-7} M)–27 percent, whereas the increments at high concentrations (10 and 12 percent, respectively) did not approximate statistical significance. Changes in protein synthesis by subcellular fractions from Mg-deficient myocardium, and effects of morphine are summarized in Table 2. Significant increases in protein synthesis were most notable in the mitochondrial fraction, as a result of morphine. Although the protein synthesis rates for mitochondria were somewhat higher for hypomagnesemic and diet-supplemented mouse myocardium, the augmentation of mitochondrial protein synthesis by morphine was related to the Mg status of the myocardium. Augmentation of mitochondrial protein synthesis by morphine increased as a function of a decrease in myocardial Mg. Therefore,

Table 2. Mean (± σ) Rate of C^{14}-Leucine Incorporation (m*M* mg $protein^{-1}$ hr^{-1}) into Subcellular Fractions from Myocardium: Effects of Morphine in the Mouse Under Differing Mg Disposition

	Subcellular Fraction								
	Nuclei			Mitochrondria			Microsomes		
Condition	*H*[a]	*N*[b]	*D*[c]	*H*	*N*	*D*	*H*	*N*	*D*
NaCl (0.9%)	0.312 (0.02)	0.411 (0.08)	0.399 (0.08)	0.414 (0.02)	0.304 (0.14)	0.416 (0.17)	0.266 (0.10)	0.297 (0.22)	0.369 (0.03)
Morphine (10^{-7} *M*)	0.312 (0.02)	0.490 (0.04)	0.319 (0.04)	0.550[d] (0.17)	0.339[f] (0.05)	0.519[e] (0.09)	0.266 (0.05)	0.358[f] (0.12)	0.341 (0.07)
Morphine (10^{-6} *M*)	0.398 (0.14)	0.540 (0.01)	0.301 (0.11)	0.607[d] (0.05)	0.367[f] (0.19)	0.661[e] (0.22)	0.269 (0.11)	0.218 (0.03)	0.401 (0.17)
Morphine (10^{-5} *M*)	0.305 (0.02)	0.397 (0.03)	0.364 (0.01)	0.640[d] (0.01)	0.425[e] (0.13)	0.525[e] (0.02)	0.287 (0.17)	0.252 (0.09)	0.387 (0.17)

[a]H = hypomagnesemic mice.
[b]N = hormomagnesemic mice.
[c]D = Mice fed Mg-supplemented diet.
[d]$p < .001$.
[e]$p < .01$.
[f]$p < .05$.

in whole myocardium (where morphine does not gain ready access to the mitochondrion) hypomagnesemia (and reduced protein synthesis) is not affected by morphine. The mitochondrion from hypomagnesemic myocardium is, however, sensitive to the effects of morphine, which stimulate protein synthesis in this organelle. The decrease in protein synthesis observed in the whole myocardium appears to be accounted for by reduced synthesis in the nucleus and microsomes.

Mg deficiency resulted in a decreased rate of incorporation of labeled amino acid into nuclear and microsomal proteins, but mitochondrial protein synthesis was significantly increased (37 percent) by the Mg deficiency. Morphine did not alter the already reduced protein synthesis measured for the nuclear and microsomal fractions. At concentrations of morphine above 10^{-5} *M*, mitochondrial protein synthesis in hypomagnesemic myocardium was increased (increments of 28 percent and 14 percent above control levels by morphine at 10^{-6} and 10^{-5} *M*, respectively).

CONCLUSION

It is apparent that the effects of morphine upon the myocardium depend upon the nutritional and metabolic integrity of such tissue. Changes that alter its synthetic machinery, either through limitations upon endogenous metabolic pathways, or by causing structural and/or permeability changes in the membranes of subcellular organelles, appear consistently to alter the metabolic effects of morphine upon the myocardium.

REFERENCES

Du Ruisseau, J.P., and Mori, K. Biochemical studies on experimental cardiomyopathy: Electrolytes in rat tissues. *Br. J. Exp. Path.* 40, 250–254 (1959).

Essman, W.B. Morphine action in myocardial metabolopathies, in *Factors Affecting the Action of Narcotics.* M.W. Adler, L. Manara, and R. Samanin, eds. Raven Press, New York (1978), pp. 681–702.

Hochrein, H., Kuschke, H.J., Zaqqa, Q., and Fahl, E. Das Verhalten der intracellularen magnesium–konzentration in Myocard bei Insuffezienz, Hypoxie und Kammerflimmern. *Lin. Wochschr.* 45, 1093–1096 (1967).

Iseri, L.T., Alexander, L.C., McCarghey, R.S., Boyle, A.J., and Myers, G.B. Water and electrolyte content of cardiac and skeletal muscle in heart failure and myocardial infarction. *Am. Heart J.* 43, 215–227 (1952).

Johnson, C.J., Mauritsen, C.M., Starbuck, W.C., and Schwartz, A. Histones and mitochondrial ion transport. *Biochemistry* 6, 1121–1127 (1967).

Keliger, R.E., Seta, K., Vitale, J.J., and Lown, B. Effects of chronic depletion of potassium and magnesium upon the action of acetylstrophanthidin on the heart. *Am. J. Card.* 17, 520–527 (1966).

Lehr, D. Tissue electrolyte alteration in disseminated myocardial necrosis. *Ann. N.Y. Acad. Sci.* 156, 344–378 (1969).
Lehr, D., Krukowski, M., and Colon, R. Correlation of myocardial and renal necrosis with tissue electrolyte changes. *JAMA* 197, 105–112 (1966).
Schwartz, A. The effect of histones and other polycations on cellular energetics. 1. Mitochondrial oxidative phosphorylation. *J. Biol. Chem.* 241, 1122–1127 (1966).
Seelig, M., and Heggtveit, H.A. Magnesium interrelationships in ischemic heart disease: a review. *Am. J. Clin. Nut.* 27, 59–79 (1974).
Szekely, P., and Wynne, N.A. The effects of magnesium on cardiac arrhythmias caused by digitalis. *Clin. Sci.* 10, 241–247 (1951).

20

Chelated and Complexed Magnesium: Its Effects on Lipoproteins and Blood Coagulation

ALEXANDER J. STEINER

INTRODUCTION

One of the early events associated with the development of atherosclerosis is the deposition of low-density lipoproteins (LDL) in the intima and superficial media of arteries. It has long been stressed that intimal injury, with formation of mural thrombi is the causative or initiating event (Virchow, 1856). A detailed review of arterial damage related to deficiency of magnesium (Mg) has been reported by Seelig and Haddy (1980). It is possible that marginal Mg deficiency might also contribute to atherogenesis via abnormalities in lipid metabolism and coagulopathy due to Mg deficiency, and that excess fat intake might be one of the pathways which lead to these decreased Mg levels. This pilot study describes the effects of daily oral intake of small doses of various forms of chelated and complexed Mg on plasma lipids and Factor V. Our ultracentrifugation studies show that Mg administration is associated with lowering of plasma lipoprotein levels, more specifically the level of very-low-density lipids (VLDL), by about 45 percent (see Fig. 1). Factor V formation was suppressed to about the same degree. This observation may help to decrease the gap among the various theories on the roles of lipids, mural thromosis, and Mg deficiency in the pathogenesis of atherosclerosis.

METHODS

Eleven patients were kept on a reduced-fat diet (35 percent of the total calories as fat) for one month and then were started on a regime of Mg

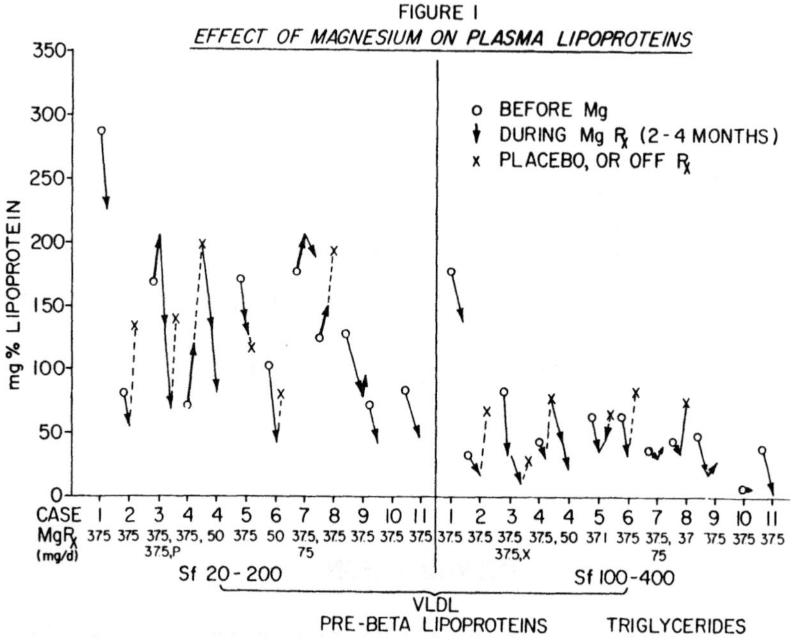

Fig. 1. Effect of magnesium on plasma lipoproteins.

supplementation in the form of tablets (12.5 mg total per tablet), containing a mixture of Mg glycinate (100 mg), Mg-ascorbic acid complex (100 mg), and Mg paraminobenzoate (10 mg)[a].

Complete data are available on these 11 patients, whose blood lipoproteins were analyzed by analytical ultracentrifugation, and whose Factor V levels were determined.[b] The serum lipoproteins were grouped according to the following Svedberg flotation (S_f) units for lipoprotein quantitation: S_f 0 to 12, 12 to 20, 20 to 100, and 100 to 400 fractions.[c] Factor V levels were assayed, utilizing artifically produced Factor-V-deficient plasma as the substrate.

[a]Three tablets contained 37.5 mg of magnesium, which was composed of 100 mg magnesium-ascorbic acid complex, 100 mg magnesium glycinate, and 10 mg magnesium paraminobenzoate. Tablets were manufactured by J.J. Miller Pharmaceutical Co., St. Louis, Mo. The commercial preparation, which was not used in these experiments, contained, in addition, the following vitamins: A–5000 units; D–400 units; E–10 mg; B_1–20 mg; B_2–3 mg; B_6–5 mg; and B_{12}–9 mcg.

[b]Factor V analyses were done by Dr. John D. Bouhasin, hematologist, Cardinal Glennon Memorial Hospital for Children, St. Louis, Mo.

[c]Determined by the Institute of Medical Physics (Belmont, Calif.).

Table 1. Effect of Chelated Magnesium as a Plasma Lipid Lowering Agent*

Case Study #1

Male J.M.–Age 26–Ht. 69½ in–Wt. 246 lbs
10/29/64

S_f^o	*Normal (mg%)*	*Before Mg*	*37½ mg Mg*	*Decrease (%)*
0–12	305	402	445	↑
12–20	50	72	59	±
20–100	87	286	224	22
100–400	29	179	139	22

Case Study #2

Male A.J.S.–Age 60–Ht. 65½ in–Wt. 148 lbs
9/24/64

S_f^o	*Normal (mg%)*	*Before Mg*	*37½ mg Mg*	*Placebo*	*Decrease (%)*
0–12	360	299	301	272	±
12–20	67	27	29	38	±
20–100	104	80	54	136	33
100–400	67	32	16	67	50

Case Study #3

Male H.B.–Age 46–Ht. 72¾ in–Wt. 186 lbs

S_f^o	*Normal (mg%)*	*8/1/64 Before Mg*	*10/7/64 After 37½ mgMg*	*11/14/64 37½ mg Mg*	*12/19/64 37½ mg Mg*	*2/27/65 27 Days Placebo*	*Decrease (%)*
0–12	364	166	209	185	242	228	–
12–20	68	27	45	37	32	43	–
20–100	109	168	206	131	67	139	60
100–400	83	83	32	32	5	29	94

Case Study #4

Female E.LaR.–Age 55–Ht. 62 in–Wt. 130 lbs

S_f^o	*Normal (mg%)*	*10/5/64 Before Mg*	*4/19/65 50 mg Mg*	*5/26/65 Placebo*	*6/26/65 50 mg Mg*	*7/24/65 50 mg Mg*	*Decrease (%)*
0–12	363	635	543	630	549	674	↓±
12–20	90	88	64	88	72	91	↓±
20–100	99	71	120	198	136	80	+13
100–400	52	43	30	77	43	24	50

Case Study #5

Female F.H.–Age 51–Ht. 64½ in–Wt. 176 lbs

S_f^o	*Normal (mg%)*	*9/12/64 Before Mg*	*5/1/65 37½ mg Mg*	*6/1/65 37½ mg Mg*	*6/30/65 Placebo*	*Decrease (%)*
0–12	357	358	367	312	291	↓±
12–20	84	64	56	56	53	↓±
20–100	121	171	136	126	118	26
100–400	62	62	35	43	64	31

Table 1 (Continued)

Case Study #6

Male G.C.–Age 65–Ht. 72 in–Wt. 193 lbs

$\overset{\circ}{Sf}$	*Normal (mg%)*	*8/27/64 Before Mg*	*1/19/65 After 50 mg Mg*	*5/8/65 Off Mg 2/1/65*	*Decrease (%)*
0–12	360	540	535	606	± ↑ off Mg
12–20	67	51	48	43	↓
20–100	105	102	43	80	58
100–400	67	64	32	83	50

Case Study #7

Female H.E.–Age 48–Ht. 65½ in–Wt. 104½ lbs

$\overset{\circ}{Sf}$	*Normal (mg%)*	*3/13/65 Before Mg*	*7/3/65 37½ mg Mg*	*1/29/66 75 mg Mg*	*Decrease (%)*
0–12	364	513	486	437	–
12–20	92	45	35	40	–
20–100	106	177	206	187	+6
100–400	55	35	32	40	+14

Case Study #8

Female B.H.–Age 56–Ht. 62¾ in–Wt. 161 lbs

$\overset{\circ}{Sf}$	*9/5/64 Pretest*	*11/7/64 37½ mg Mg*	*3/6/65 Placebo*	*Normal (mg%)*	*Decrease (%)*
0–12	524	478	445	362	↓
12–20	110	112	91	90	↓
20–100	125	152	192	97	+21
100–400	43	35	72	52	19

Case Study #9

Male A.N.–Age 50–Ht. 72 in–Wt. 196 lbs

$\overset{\circ}{Sf}$	*Normal (mg%)*	*1/25/65 Pre Mg*	*3/27/65 37½ mg Mg*	*4/24/65 37½ Mg*	*Decrease (%)*
0–12	365	323	304	342	–
12–20	68	43	37	51	–
20–100	110	128	78	91	29
100–400	78	48	16	26	46

Case Study #10

Female L.W.–Age 56–Ht. 65 in–Wt. 184 lbs

$\overset{\circ}{Sf}$	*Normal (mg%)*	*1/4/65 Before Mg*	*2/6/65 37½ Mg*	*Decrease (%)*
0–12	364	255	190	–
12–20	92	32	32	–
20–100	106	72	43	40
100–400	55	6	5	16

Table 1 (Continued)

Case Study #11

Female D.O.–Age 39–Ht. 66 in–Wt. 127 lbs

S_f^o	*Normal (mg%)*	*9/5/64 Before Mg*	*1/10/65 37½ Mg*	*Decrease (%)*
0–12	325	348	445	–
12–20	61	29	53	–
20–100	70	83	48	42
100–400	33	38	3	92

*Blood taken for lipoprotein analysis by analytical ultracentrifugation was sent to The Institute of Medical Physics, 1020 Sixth Avenue, Belmont, California, and reported in mg percent of S_f^o 0–12, 12–20, 20–100, 100–400 fractions. After one to three months of therapy it was found that the S_f^o 20–100 and S_f^o 100–400 fractions were lowered; these contain most of the triglycerides.

The series of 11 patients studied were part of a double-blind study, and a part of the blood was analyzed by a one stage Factor V assay utilizing artificially produced Factor-V-deficient plasma as the substrate. Most of the patients in this study were given one tablet three times daily (37.5 mg Mg/day) for two to four months, while some were given 50 mg Mg/day, or 75 mg Mg/day. In some case studies a "placebo" period was followed which in essence meant no Mg supplementation, as in the first phase of the study (control period). Blood samples were taken for analyses at no less than monthly intervals.

RESULTS

Effects on Plasma Lipids

The effect of the Mg supplementation was notable only in the VLDL or pre-β-lipoprotein fractions (S_f^o of 20 to 100 and 100 to 400 fractions; see Fig. 1, Table 1). Eight of the 11 patients showed reductions of 15 to 75 mg/100 ml in the S_f^o 100 to 400 fraction, in which most of the endogenously produced triglyceride is found. Nine subjects showed decreases of 30 to 120 mg/100 ml in the S_f^o 20 to 100 fraction; a few showed slight increases in that portion of the VLDL fraction. The average percent decrease in S_f^o 20 to 100 fraction was 24 percent. The average percent decrease in S_f^o 100 to 400 fraction was 42 percent. Note: the larger molecular weight triglyceride fraction (S_f^o 100 to S_f^o 400) is lowered most. By increasing the intake of magnesium to 50 or 80 mg per day, changes occur with greater

Table 2. Effect of Chelated Magnesium On Factor V Concentration Levels

Case Study No.	*Name*	*Age*	*Date*	*Factor V (%)*	*Comment*
1	J.M.	26	10/29/64	100	Control
			2/6/65	40	37½ mg Mg
2	A.J.S.	61	1/19/65	53	37½ mg Mg
3	H.B.	46	8/1/64	100	Control
			10/7/64	52	37½ mg Mg
			2/27/65	75	Placebo
			3/27/65	33	75 mg Mg
4	E.LaR.	55	10/5/64	62	Control
			4/19/65	54	50 mg Mg
			5/26/65	125	Placebo
			7/24/65	50	62½ mg Mg
5	F.H.	51	9/12/64	82	Control
			5/1/65	63	37½ mg Mg
			6/1/65	70	37½ mg Mg
6	G.C.	65	8/27/64	73	Control
			1/19/65	26	50 mg Mg
			5/8/65	97	Placebo
7	H.E.	48	9/2/64	120	Control
			7/3/65	100	37½ mg Mg
			1/29/66	56	75 mg Mg
8	B.H.	56	9/5/64	100	Control
			11/7/64	84	37½ mg Mg
			3/6/65	164	Placebo
9	A.N.	50	1/25/65	61	Control
			3/27/65	47	37½ mg Mg
			4/24/65	50	37½ mg Mg
10	L.W.	56	1/4/65	76	Control
			2/6/65	68	37½ mg Mg
			3/6/65	53	37½ mg Mg
			4/3/65	78	Placebo
11	D.O.	39	9/5/64	125	Control
			1/10/65	51	37½ mg Mg

rapidity. Several patients who were given 50 to 75 mg Mg/day showed decreases in the VLDL fractions (S_f^o 20 to 100 and 100 to 400) more rapidly than did those given the 37.5 mg Mg/day dosage. The above data show that magnesium at physiologic concentrations normalized hypertriglyceridemia in about 40 percent of 11 patients.

Table 3. Summary of the Effect of Chelated Magnesium on Factor V Levels

Case No.	*Patient's Name*	*Factor V Control (%)*	*Lowest Factor V After Concentration Mg Administration (%)*
1	J.M.	100	40
2	A.J.S.	100	53
3	H.B.	100	33
4	E.LaR.	62	50
5	F.H.	82	63
6	G.C.	73	26
7	H.E.	120	56
8	B.H.	100	84
9	A.N.	61	48
10	L.W.	76	53
11	D.O.	125	51
Average[a]		91	50

[a]It was found that untreated patients showed a base line for Factor V which varied from 61 to 125 percent and averaged 91 percent. After taking Chelated Magnesium for one to five months, a prolongation of clotting was found due to Factor V deficiency. The average of 11 determinations was 41 percent below normal. (91–50 = 41).

Effects on Blood Coagulation, as Measured by Factor V Levels

The same 11 patients reported above were studied for changes in Factor V levels (Tables 2 and 3) after having taken the Mg tablets for 2 to 4 months. The data suggest that the subjects had prolongation of clotting time caused by Factor V deficiency. Comparable patients who had not been given Mg supplements, had baseline Factor V levels of 61 to 125 percent, with an average of 99, in contrast to the average of 50, among the lowest Factor V values after Mg administration (Table 2 and 3).

DISCUSSION

The use of Mg to alter components of the blood that have been implicated in atherogenesis has received intermittent attention. These components are: (1) blood lipids; and (2) factors that increase intravascular coagulation. Malkiel-Shapiro et al. (1956) reported that patients with ischemic heart disease (IHD) exhibited decreased β-lipoproteins while they were being treated with intramuscular (i.m.) $MgSO_4$ injections. Parsons (1958) confirmed this observation, and further reported that in such patients the pre-β-lipoprotein bands were eliminated, their low lecithin/cholesterol ratios were reversed, and their plasmin (fibrinolysin) inhibition values were reduced. Huntsman et al.

(1960) found that orally administered Mg citrate with peptone or glutamic acid produced short-term increased thrombingeneration time. Lieber (1961) reported that an orally administered Mg–aluminum silicate preparation lowered the β-lipoprotein/α-lipoprotein ratio, and Steiner (1962) found that oral administration of chelated and complexed Mg (as in this presentation) decreased the β_2-lipoprotein fraction.

Emphasis has long been placed on the importance of elevated levels of blood cholesterol in the formation of atherosclerotic plaques; recently atheromatous changes in primates have been reversed by feeding low-fat, low-cholesterol diets (Wissler and Vesselinovitch, 1977). It is of interest that Mg administration has also decreased the arterial damage caused by atherogenic diets in dogs (Bunce et al., 1962) and rats (Vitale et al., 1957; Hellerstein et al., 1960), and that long-term Mg-supplementation of rabbits fed an atherogenic diet significantly reversed the arterial lipid deposition (Nakamura et al., 1965). Further insight was provided by Rademeyer and Booyens (1965) who showed that addition of 25 percent butterfat to the diet of rats lowered their serum Mg levels substantially. This observation is not surprising, since it was first shown in 1918 (Sawyer et al., 1918) that high-fat intakes interfered with the absorption of Mg (and of calcium).

More than 125 years ago at the time of writing, Virchow (1856) implicated mural thrombus formation on damaged intima as an initiating lesion in atherosclerosis, a theory reiterated more recently (Duguid, 1946; Pickering, 1963). It is provocative that experimental atherogenic diets are also coagulopathic, and that Mg administration corrects the decreased coagulation time and increased prothrombin consumption caused by fat loads (Szelenyi et al., 1967), and protects against damage produced by a hyperlipemic thrombogenic diet (Savoie, 1972).

The clinical laboratory findings presented here suggest that low Mg doses, given in a form that may be better absorbed and utilized than are inorganic salts, appear to exert a beneficial effect both on blood lipids and on the tendency toward increased thrombus formation in hyperlipidemic subjects. The major effect of the Mg was on the VLDL (S_f^0 20 to 400) fraction, the lipoproteins associated with increased risk for atherogenesis. Investigation of the effect of Mg on blood coagulation was undertaken when a patient who had been taking 37.5 mg Mg/day for a year suffered from oozing of blood from an operative wound for 48 hours. When he was found to have a deficiency of Factor V [a factor that is necessary for thrombin formation (Owren, 1947); Factor V is also a substrate for plasmin (Biggs and MacFarlane, 1962), and might be platelet Factor I (Biggs, 1976); Factor V deficiency being an uncommon abnormality], the status of Factor V in the other patients receiving Mg was investigated. Significantly subnormal values were found in Mg-treated patients, as compared with values in comparable patients not receiving Mg therapy. The Factor V deficiency may have been contributory to bleeding only in three patients during a 10-year study period. In addition to the patient noted above, we observed a man who developed hematuria from a previously undiagnosed bladder cancer, and a woman who had vaginal bleeding from a cervical polyp.

CONCLUSIONS

This study suggests that only moderate Mg supplementation may correct two abnormalities of blood constituents that are linked to the development of atherosclerosis. It lowers the VLDL, and decreases the level of a coagulation Factor V. These effects might mediate the antiatherosclerotic effect of Mg administration in the experimental model, and possibly in human beings.

ACKNOWLEDGMENTS

The author gratefully acknowledges the help of Mildred S. Seelig, M.D., F.A.C.N., New York University, and Muriel I. Jobe, coagulation technologist at Missouri Baptist Hospital, St. Louis, Mo., who proofread the section of this chapter dealing with human blood coagulation.

REFERENCES

Biggs, R. *Human Blood Coagulation,* 1st ed. Blackwell Scientific Publications, Oxford (1972) (1976).

Biggs, R., and MacFarlane, R.G. *Human Blood Coagulation and Its Disorders,* 1st ed. Blackwell Scientific Publications, Oxford (1962).

Bunce, G.E., Chiemchaisra, Y., and Phillips, P.H. The mineral requirements of the dog. IV. Effect of certain dietary and physiologic factors upon the magnesium deficiency syndrome. *J. Nut.* 76, 23–29 (1962).

Duguid, J.B. Thrombosis as a factor in the pathogenesis of coronary atherosclerosis. *J. Path. Bact.* 58, 207–212 (1946).

Hellerstein, E.E., Nakamura, M., Hegsted, D.M., and Vitale, J.J. Studies on the interrelationships between dietary magnesium, quality and quantity of fat, hypercholesterolemia and lipidosis. *J. Nut.* 71, 339–346 (1960).

Huntsman, R.G., Hurn, B.A.L., and Lehman, H. Observations on the effect of magnesium on blood coagulation. *J. Clin. Path.* 13, 99–101 (1960).

Lieber, I.I. Colosterol y aterosclerosis. Traitmiento de la hipercolosterolemia en la aterosclerosis con catalizadores metalicos. *Prensa Med. Argent.* 48, 44–52 (1961).

Malkiel-Shapiro, B., Bersohn, I., and Terner, P.E. Parenteral magnesium sulphate therapy in coronary heart disease. A preliminary report on its clinical and laboratory aspects. *Med. Proc.* 2, 455–462 (1956).

Nakamura, M., Torii, S., Hiramatsu, M., Hirano, J., Sumiyoshi, A., and Tanaka, K. Dietary effect of magnesium on cholesterol-induced atherosclerosis of rabbits. *J. Atheroscler. Res.* 5, 145–158 (1965).

Owren, P.A. Parahemophilia. Hemorrhagic diathesis due to absence of a previously unknown clotting factor. *Lancet* 1, 446–448 (1947).

Parsons, R.S. The biochemical changes associated with coronary artery disease treated with magnesium sulphate. *Med. J. Austral.* 1, 883–884 (1958).

Pickering, G. Arteriosclerosis and atherosclerosis. The need for clear thinking. *Am. J. Med.* 34, 7–18 (1963).

Rademeyer, L.J., and Booyens, J. The effects of variations in the fat and carbohydrate content of the diet on the levels of magnesium and cholesterol in the serum of white rats. *Br. J. Nut.* 19, 153–162 (1965).

Savoie, L.L. Production de necroses cardiaques non-occlusives chez le rat par un régime thrombogène. *Path. Biol.* 20, 117–125 (1972).

Sawyer, M., Baumann, L., and Stevens, F. Studies of acid production. II. The mineral loss during acidosis. *J. Biol. Chem.* 33, 103–109 (1918).

Seelig, M.S., and Haddy, F.J. Magnesium and the arteries. I. Effects of magnesium deficiency on arteries and on the retention of sodium, potassium, and calcium, in *Magnesium in Health and Disease.* Proceedings of the 2nd International Symposium on Magnesium. Montreal, Canada, 1976. M. Cantin and M.S. Seelig, eds. SP Medical and Scientific Books, Jamaica, N.Y. (1980), pp. 605–638.

Steiner, A.J. Atherosclerosis and the enigma of blood cholesterol. *J. Appl. Nut.* 15, 240–246 (1962).

Szelenyi, I., Rigo, J., and Ahmed, B.O. The role of Mg in blood coagulation. *Throm. et Dia. Haemorr.* 18, 626–633 (1967).

Virchow, R. *Phlogose und Thrombose im Gefassystem. Gesammelte Abhandlungen zur Wissenschaftlichen Medizine.* Meidinger Sohn, Frankfurt, Germany 458–000 (1856).

Vitale, J.J., White, P.L., Nakamura, M., Zamchek, N., and Hellerstein, E.E. Interrelationships, between experimental hypercholesterolemia, magnesium requirement, and experimental atherosclerosis. *J. Exp. Med.* 106, 757–766 (1957).

Wissler, R.W., and Vesselinovitch, D. Regression of atherosclerosis in experimental animals and man. *Mod. Con. Card. Dis.* 46 (6), 27–32 (1977).

21

Magnesium and Thrombosis: Interrelations with Latent Tetany, Cirrhosis, and Cancer

PHILIPPE COLLERY
PIERRE COUDOUX
HENRI GEOFFROY

INTRODUCTION

Thromboses can be macroscopic or microscopic, disseminated or localized, and occult or overt. Stasis or hypercoagulability contribute to venous thromboses and microthromboses; endothelial lesions play a more important role in arterial thromboses (Collery, 1976). Hypercoagulability itself is influenced by many factors, among which is magnesium (Mg) deficiency (Tonks, 1966; Szeleny et al., 1967; Herrman et al., 1970; Giafferi, 1972; Collery et al., 1977). Patients with latent tetany (spasmophilia) caused by primary Mg deficiency, have exhibited thromboses (Durlach, 1967a, b; Dupont et al., 1969; Maurat, 1976). Mg deficiency secondary to disease (such as cancer or cirrhosis) and treatment seems to play a major role in disseminated or localized consumption coagulopathy. There is evidence that consumption-coagulopathy can play a role in the evolution of cancer or cirrhosis (Tytgat et al., 1971; Liehr et al., 1972; Boneu et al., 1974; Rocha and Lopez Borrasca, 1975; Blasco, 1975; Boureille et al., 1975; Ficquet, 1975; Heene, 1975; Testart et al., 1975; Collery et al., 1976). In this study we examined the association of Mg and thrombosis among spasmophilia, cirrhosis, and cancer patients.

METHODS

Our study included 65 spasmophilic patients, 61 chronic alcoholics, among whom 32 had decompensated cirrhosis, and 27 cancer patients. Con-

Table 1. Signs of Latent Tetany (Spasmophilia) in 65 Patients[a]

Depression (16)
Lipothymia (10)
Pain (Abdominal, Pelvic) (13); (Low-Back) (3)
Cardiorespiratory symptoms (7)
Paresthesias (6)
Vertigo (2)
Cephalea (2)
Gynecologic disorders (2)
Raynaud's disease (1)

[a]Numbers in parenthesis refer to number of patients.

sumption coagulopathy was detected biologically with snake venom (reptilase test) and by measuring circulating fibrinogen-degradation products (FDP). Reptilase values (controls = 20 to 24 seconds) were considered moderately increased at 27 to 35 seconds, severely increased at 35 to 40 seconds, and extremely high when over 40 seconds. A rise of FDP between 10 and 20 μg/ml was considered moderate, between 20 and 40 μg/ml severe, and above 40 μg/ml extremely high. When consumption coagulopathy is disseminated, blood platelets and fibrinogen decrease, as does Quick's test; Howell's test and cephalin kaolin test increase.

Mg was measured by atomic absorption spectrophotometry. Our normal values are: plasma Mg: 18 to 22 mg/liter and RBC (Red Blood Cell) Mg: 50 to 62 mg/liter.

In several patients, the effect of Mg repletion was tested.

RESULTS

Latent Tetany (Spasmophilia)

The manifestations of the neuromuscular irritability of primary Mg deficiency have been described by Durlach (1972) and Durlach and Cordier (1973), and were identified in 65 patients (Table 1): 55 women and 10 men, in most of whom the diagnosis was verified by electromyogram (EMG) or electrotroencephalogram; Chvosteck's and Trousseau's signs are unreliable indices of this disorder. Excluded were patients with organic disease, although their histories often included at least one surgical operation. We also excluded patients with chronic alcoholism, which causes Mg loss (Durlach and Cachin, 1967), and those taking neuroleptic, cardiotonic, or diuretic drugs. We did not consider the patients' use of contraceptive or anxiolytic drugs. The diagnosis was made only when there were low plasma or RBC Mg levels, despite the fact that the Mg deficiency of some spasmophilic patients can be revealed only by dynamic test (Durlach and Pechery, 1973).

Table 2. Plasma and RBC Magnesium in Spasmophilic Patients

In 65 spasmophilic patients:
- 46 had low RBC Mg levels.
- 14 had both low RBC and plasma Mg levels.
- 5 had low plasma Mg levels without disorders of hemostasis.

Low RBC Mg levels alone were seen in 46 patients, low plasma and RBC levels in 14, and low plasma levels in only 5 (15 to 18 mg/liter) (Table 2). The decrease of RBC Mg was often moderate (46 to 49 mg/liter in 26 patients). It was severe in 12 cases (42 to 45 mg/liter), and marked in 6 (patients whose RBC Mg was below 42 mg/liter, 2 patients having RBC Mg below 38 mg/liter).

Among these 65 spasmophilic patients with Mg deficiency, only one had thrombosis. This 58-year-old man who had had three pulmonary embolisms within two years had a low RBC Mg level (48 mg/liter).

We observed no disorders of hemostasis, even among patients with a severe Mg deficiency, but we did not explore platelet adhesiveness or aggregability.

Chronic Alcoholism and Compensated Cirrhosis

Mg levels were measured in chronic alcoholism, with and without hepatic involvement (Table 3); hepatitis and cirrhosis, which are considered together because hepatic biopsies were not available for all. Of 29 patients, 10 showed moderate biological signs of hepatocellular insufficiency, and only 3 had a Quick's test below 50 percent. Magnesium deficiency was present in 25 of the 29 alcoholics. On the other hand, the remaining four patients had elevated RBC Mg levels; all four were suspected of having cancer. The plasma Mg level was low in 24 cases: 15 were equal to or below 16 mg/liter and 1 was severely hypomagnesemic (12.5 mg/liter). Low RBC Mg levels were associated with low plasma levels in ten cases.

A significantly increased reptilase test was obtained in four patients who suffered from pronounced hepatocellular insufficiency.

Table 3. Plasma and RBC Magnesium in Chronic Alcoholism and Compensated Cirrhosis

In chronic alcoholism and compensated cirrhosis, 29 patients were studied:
- 25 had Mg deficiency:
  - 24 with low plasma Mg levels.
  - 10 with both low RBC and plasma Mg levels.
- 4 had elevated RBC Mg levels (and a suspicion of cancer).

Table 4. Studies of Decompensated Cirrhosis[a]

Plasma Mg and RBC Levels	*Signs of Consumption Coagulopathy*
12 patients had low plasma Mg levels:	
at 16 or 17 mg/liter (in 5 cases)	Moderate
at 14 or 15 mg/liter (in 6 cases)	Severe
at 13 mg/liter (in one case)	Extremely high
3 patients had low RBC Mg levels	Moderate
8 patients had low plasma and RBC Mg levels	Severe or extremely high
9 patients had normal or high plasma and RBC Mg levels	Severe or extremely high

[a]32 patients were studied.

Decompensated Cirrhosis

Plasma and RBC Mg levels were studied in 32 patients with icteric decompensation, edema, and ascitis (Table 4). Mg deficiency was found in 23 patients.

Twelve patients with hepatocellular insufficiency with a Quick's test between 30 and 70 percent, had hypomagnesemia. Low plasma Mg levels were correlated with signs of consumption coagulopathy: moderate in five patients with plasma Mg levels at 16 to 17 mg/liter, severe in six patients with 14 to 15 mg/liter, and extremely marked in one patient with a plasma Mg level at 13 mg/liter (this 29-year-old patient had clinically severe cirrhosis with epistaxis and purpura).

Low RBC Mg levels were seen only in three patients who had no or only moderate signs of consumption coagulopathy, and in whom hepatic disorders were not severe.

Both low plasma (13 to 17 mg/liter) and RBC Mg levels (very low in three patients, as low as 36 mg/liter in one patient) were found in eight patients who had signs of severe hepatocellular insufficiency, and in many patients clear signs of consumption coagulopathy.

In nine patients, no Mg deficiency was found. Among these nine patients, two died rapidly in a state of disseminated intravascular coagulation (DIC). Among the remaining seven patients, we strongly suspected degenerative cirrhosis in five cases.

Effects of Magnesium Therapy in Decompensated Cirrhosis

There was a clear difference in outcomes in patients, depending on whether or not they were given Mg. The influence of Mg on coagulation and on hepatic function was notable. It was seen in a patient with Mg deficiency who had severe signs of decompensated cirrhosis, very high reptilase

Table 5. Plasma and RBC Magnesium Levels in Cancer Patients

Plasma Mg levels are normal or low.
RBC Mg levels are often high.
Signs of consumption coagulopathy are very frequent.

levels, and Quick test results of 35 percent. His clinical and laboratory evidence of hepatic failure improved with very small doses of calcium heparinate (0.1 to 0.2 ml t.i.d.), but his hemostatic tests remained abnormal: Quick test results of 40 percent, moderate increase of reptilase values, and of circulating FDP. Plasma Mg remained low. Parenteral Mg therapy for 25 days, followed by oral Mg supplements, resulted in a rise in Quick test results to 90 percent, and a drop in reptilase to normal with disappearance of circulating FDP. In another patient who had hematemesis, 75,000 platelets/mm^3, and high FDP, parenteral Mg therapy was followed by cessation of bleeding episodes and normal platelet count. She discontinued Mg therapy when she left the hospital, and was readmitted five months later, (having resumed drinking) with cirrhotic decompensation, metrorrhagic flooding, epistaxis, purpura, and thrombophlebitis in a leg. A third patient with hypomagnesemia (13 mg/liter plasma Mg and 41 mg/liter RBC Mg), 65 percent Quick test, and thrombocytopenia (65,000 platelets mm^3) responded to parenteral Mg with correction of abnormal tests, including an increased placelet count to 140,000 platelets/mm^3 within two weeks. This patient continued taking Mg orally and was in good condition six months later. Another patient's Quick test rose from 30 to 50 percent after a month of oral Mg therapy; the reptilase test became normal.

Cancer

We have found increased RBC Mg levels in 26 of 43 patients with cancer (Table 5); these levels increased cyclically (Collery et al., 1979 in press). The periodicity and amplitude or RBC Mg changes varies with the rapidity of the growth of the cancer. Among those patients not exhibiting elevated RBC Mg levels, there has often been found long-term magnesiuresis (usually in response to diuretics), parenteral nutrition, alcoholism, cirrhosis, and severe undernourishment or cachexia, all of which decrease availability to the body of exogenous Mg. We have also studied patients with early tumor, predominantly hepatic localization, or marked hypercalcemia. Effective antineoplastic therapy may also result in decreased RBC Mg, or in lengthened cycles. When the tumor is not growing, the curve may be flat. Similarly, patients with a slowly advancing tumor, albeit one that is large and old, may all show no rise in RBC Mg levels.

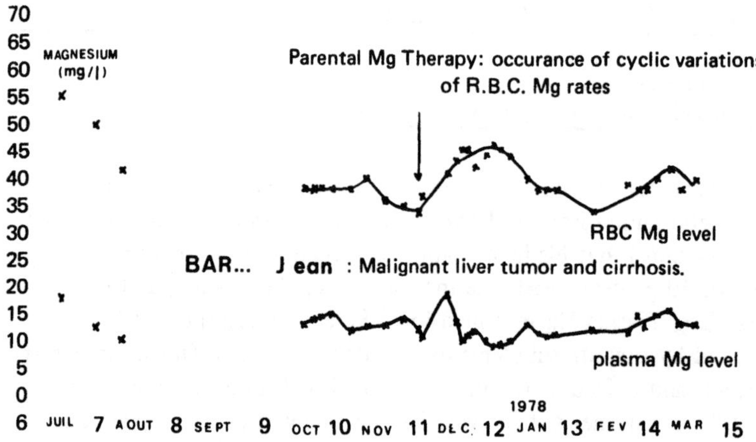

Fig. 1.

Unlike RBC Mg, plasma Mg is not high where there is no renal failure. It is often normal during some periods of the evolution, and low at other periods, with sometimes very low rates (10 to 15 mg/liter). Plasma Mg levels do not follow a cyclic pattern.

In the course of cancer, there are often signs of consumption coagulopathy (Boneu et al., 1974; Blasco, 1975; Collery, 1976).

Effects of Magnesium Therapy in Cancer

Parenteral Mg was given to one patient suffering from tongue cancer, whose plasma and RBC Mg levels were very low because of an associated hypercalcemia. This treatment was soon followed by a worsening of primitive cancer and the occurrence of bone metastasis.

In B.J., another patient suffering from malignant liver tumor and cirrhosis, Mg deficiency was voluntarily maintained for a long time, whereas under the effect of heparin and chemotherapy the tumor remained at rest (Fig. 1). In spite of heparin given at small doses, an infectious syndrome provoked the occurrence of DIC with multiple hemorrhages and marked biological signs of consumption coagulopathy. Magnesium levels were then very low (plasma Mg level 10 mg/liter; RBC Mg level 36 mg/liter). The parenteral administration of Mg allowed us to counteract consumption coagulopathy, but this was followed by the resuming of tumor growth and the occurrence of cyclic variations of RBC Mg rates.

COMMENTS

Variations in Mg levels—that is, variations in plasma Mg, which represents extracellular Mg, or in RBC Mg, which represents intracellular Mg—may be in the same direction or in opposite directions. We have observed that in spasmophilia the deficiency has been principally of RBC Mg. In chronic alcoholism, with or without hepatic involvement, the Mg deficiency was noted in plasma; in patients with decompensated cirrhosis, there can be both plasma and RBC Mg deficiencies. Patients with cancer have increased RBC Mg levels with a cyclic pattern, and plasma Mg levels are low or normal. Paradoxically, in patients with both cirrhosis and cancer, RBC Mg levels are liable to be normal.

Thus, the lack of RBC Mg deficiency in cirrhotic patients might be an indication of cancer. Mg levels in all these conditions may be modified, particularly by hypercalcemia, renal failure, or under the influence of treatment.

Consumption coagulopathy is very frequent, or even constant, in patients with cirrhosis (Fisher, 1976; Delmont, 1976) or cancer. It may be localized in the liver, in the case of cirrhosis (Ficquet, 1975), or in the tumor in the case of cancer (Collery, 1976; Collery et al., 1976). The plasma Mg deficiency seen in these diseases may be contributory to the genesis of consumption coagulopathy, but other processes may also participate. In cancer, the Stuart-factor-activating procoagulant factors might be synthesized by the malignant cell (Collery, 1976). During cirrhosis, there may be an insufficiency of purification of coagulation-activated factors, as a result of stasis in the liver, release of procoagulant factors from lysed hepatic cells and from hemolysed RBC (Ficquet, 1975).

Consumption coagulopathy worsens as the erythrocytes fragment in the clots (Collery et al., 1980). In course of thrombotic microangiopathy, thromboplastin is released. Blood stasis is more important in the cirrhotic liver, or in the malignant tumor, because of the slowed circulation caused by clots; coagulation-activated factors then remain stagnant, instead of being inactivated.

The consequences of this consumption coagulopathy may be severe. They may jeopardize the life of the patient in the course of an acute crisis of DIC, as coagulation factors are consumed and fibrinolysis predominates. Hypercoagulability, which is the first stage of consumption coagulopathy, may be responsible for multilocalized, main-vessel thrombosis. Finally consumption coagulopathy makes the preexistent cancer (Collery, 1976) or cirrhosis (Ficquet, 1975) worse.

Unlike spasmophilic patients, cirrhotic or cancerous patients have markedly low plasma Mg levels, so we may wonder whether thrombosis might not essentially be linked with extracellular Mg deficiency. While plasma Mg appears to play an important part in thrombogenesis (Durlach and Cachin, 1967a), RBC Mg might reflect cellular pathology. Possibly Mg deficiency in the hepatic cell might intensify the cellular damage in the case of cirrhosis, whereas increased Mg levels in the malignant cells might encourage their growth. It is possible that induced Mg depletion in tumor cells might retard their development (Collery et al., in press). On the other hand, a too-severe drop of plasma Mg increases the risk of DIC, and a too-severe drop of RBC Mg levels may worsen hemolysis, which causes anemia and procoagulant factor release, and may also increase the organism's immunologic deficiency. Insofar as we may judge from our cancer patients, plasma Mg levels should not go below 15 mg/liter and RBC Mg levels should not go below 40 mg/liter.

CONCLUSIONS

In the course of treatment of spasmophilia, Mg therapy is useful, since it counteracts neuromuscular hyperexcitability and an hypercoagulability factor.

In the course of cirrhosis, Mg may improve coagulation, thereby favorably influencing hepatic function activity. Thus, it seems desirable to add Mg therapy to the heparinotherapy proposed by others (Coleman et al., 1975; Ficquet, 1975; Klein et al., 1975; Braunstein et al., 1976; Fischer et al., 1976). While raising hepatic cellular Mg levels, we might improve their functions, since Mg influences various enzymatic reactions, energy transfer reactions and protein and nucleic acid synthesis.

On the other hand, Mg therapy appears to be undesirable in the treatment of cancer, since it might increase the growth of primary tumor and of metastases. However, Mg depletion might increase consumption coagulopathy. Thus, heparinotherapy is even more desirable in the course of cancer if Mg depletion is maintained or instituted as a therapeutic modality.

REFERENCES

Blasco, A. Contribution à l'étude du devenir du fibrinogène marqué chez les cancéreux. Essai d'interprétation. *Thèse Méd.* Toulouse (1975), No. 249.

Boneu, A., Armand, J.P., Blasco, A., Bugat, R., Boneu, B., Lucot, H., Pris, F., and Combes, P.F. Demi-vie du fibrinogène marqué à l'iode 131 chez les cancéreux. Effets de l'héparine. *Nouv. Presse Méd.* 5, 415–418 (1974).

Boureille, J., Hayet, M., Joram, F., and Bentot, G. Coagulation intravasculaire chez le cirrhotique. 6 observations. *Nouv. Presse Méd.* 4 (17), 1267–1276 (1975).

Braunstein, K.M. Minimal heparin cofactor activity in disseminated intravascular coagulation and cirrhosis. *Am. J. Clin. Path.* 66 (3), 488–494 (1976).

Coleman, M., Finlayson, N., Bettigole, R.E., Sadula, D., Cohn, M., and Pasmentier, M. Fibrinogen survival in cirrhosis: improvement by "Low-dose" heparin. *Ann. Int. Med.* 83 (1), 79–81 (1975).

Collery, P. Etude clinique et pathologique des thromboses veineuses et embolies pulmonaires au cours des cancers bronchiques et pulmonaires. Déductions thérapeutiques. *Thèse Med.* Reims (1976), No. 29, p. 181.

Collery, P., Coudoux, P., and Geoffroy, H. Maladie thromboembolique et cancer bronchopulmonaire. *J. Méd. Nord Est* 1 (11), 10–19 (1976).

Collery, P., Coudoux, P., and Geoffroy, H. Role of Mg in venous thrombogenesis in cancer. Changes in Mg levels in neoplastic diseases, in *Nutrition and Cancer.* Proceedings of the 18th Annual Meeting of the American College of Nutrition, Houston, Texas, 1977. J. Van Eys, B.L. Nichols, and M.S. Seelig, eds. SP Medical and Scientific Books, Jamaica, N.Y. (1979), pp. 213-231.

Collery, P., Coudoux, P., Bonnet, D., and Geoffroy, H. Intérêt de l'étude des variations dynamiques du magnésium plasmatique et érythrocytaire au cours des états cancéreux. Proceedings of the 5th Annual French Colloquium on Mg, Paris, France, 1977. *Rev. Fr. End. Cl. Met. Nut.* 19 (2), 133–149 (1978).

Collery, P., Coudoux, P., Boy, J., Kochman, S. Cancer et tests inflammatoires. Interprétation des résultats en fonchon de la crase sanguine. *Conc. Med.* 102 (33), 4697–4699 (1980).

Delmont, J., Bisset, J., Rampal, P., Camous, J.P., and Faure, X. Métabolisme du fibrinogène chez le cirrhotique. Etude dynamique par méthode isotopique. *Nouv. Presse Med.* 5 (25), 1567-1569 (1976).

Dupont, B., Pony, J.C., Le Bihan, G., and Leborgne, P. Maladie phlébothrombosante et magnésium. *Sem. Hôp* 48, 3048-3054 (1969).

Durlach, J. Magnésium et thrombose. *Conc. Méd.* 89 (38), 5967–5977 (1967b).

Durlach, J. Le rôle antithrombosique physiologique du magnésium à propos d'une maladie phlébothrombosante par déficit magnésien. *Coeur Méd. Int.* 6, 213–232 (1967c).

Durlach, J. Intérêt du magnésium en médecine. *Gaz. Méd. de France* 79 (8), 1179–1191 (1972).

Durlach, J., and Cordier, M.L. Magnésium, système neuro-musculaire et psychisme. *Vie Méd.* 35 (2), 4317–4324 (1973).

Durlach, J., and Cachin, M. Magnésium et alcoolisme chronique. *Revue Alcool.* 13 (1), 3–40 (1967a).

Durlach, J., and Pechery, C. Mode d'exploration pratique du magnésium chez l'homme. *Vie Méd.,* 35 (2), 4307-4312 (1973).

Ficquet, R. Intérêt de la surveillance de la coagulation plasmatique chez le cirrhotique: incidences thérapeutiques. *Thèse Méd.* Reims (1975).

Fischer, M., Falkensammer, C., Klein, H.J., Irsigler, K., Bruneder, H., and Schack, H. Therapeutische Möglichkeiten bei verbrauchskoagulopathien aktiver leberzirrhosen: Niederdosierte Heparintherapie. *Wien. Klin. Wochenschr.* 88, 488 494 (1976).

Giafferi, D. Le rôle du magnésium vis à vis de la coagulation sanguine. *Gaz. Méd. France* 79 (24), 4168–4172 (1972).

Heene, D.L. Verbrauchskoagulopathie bei leberrerkrankungen. *Diagnostische Kriterien. Méd. Welt.* 26, 47, 2133-2136 (1975).

Herrman, R.G., Lacefield, W.B., and Crowe, V.G. Effect of ionic calcium and magnesium on human platelet agregation. *Proc. Soc. Exp. Biol. Méd.,* 135 (1), 100–103 (1970).

Klein, H.J., Falkensammer, C., Gauss, P., and Fischer, M. Heparintherapie bei leberzirrhose. *Acta. Med. Austriaca* 2 (3), 99–100 (1975).

Liehr, H., Gruen, M., and Thiel, H. Different stimuli to disseminated intravascular coagulation in liver diseases. *Thromb. Diath. Haemorrh.* 28 (2), 325-332 (1972).

Maurat, J.L. Magnésium et pathologie cardiovasculaire. *Méd. Hyg.* 1193, 693–695 (1976).

Rocha, E., and Lopez Borrasca, A. Niveles circulantes de productos de degradacion on del fibrinogeno y monomeros de fibrina de cirrhosis hepatica. *Rev. Méd. Univ. Navarra* 18 (3–4), 143–147 (1974).

Szeleny, I., Rigo, J., Ahmed, B.O., and Sos, J. The role of magnesium in blood coagulation. *Thromb. Diath. Haemorrh.* 18 (3-4), 626-633 (1967).

Testart, J., Hemet, J., and Metayer, P. Gastrite hémorragique par coagulation intramusculaire localisée au cours de l'évolution d'une cirrhose inflammatoire cryptogénétique. *Sem. Hôp.* 51 (18), 1235-1241 (1975).

Tonks, R.S. Magnésium, adénosine diphosphate et plaquettes sanguines. *Nature* 210, 106-107 (1966).

Tytgat, G.N., Collen, D., and Verstraete, M. Metabolism of fibrinogen in cirrhosis of the liver. *South. Méd. J.* 64 (10), 1690-1701 (1971).

22

Recommendations of the Magnesium Intervention Trial

H. L. JOHANSEN
L. C. NERI

INTRODUCTION

The possible role of magnesium (Mg) deficiency in cardiovascular disease (CVD) has been stressed and reviewed in the literature (Szelenzi, 1973; Seelig and Heggtveit, 1974; Birch and Giles, 1977; Neri and Johansen, 1978). These and other articles have stimulated a new interest in the relationship between Mg and CVD, and it was in this context that the World Health Organization (WHO) Collaborating Center for Reference on Studies of Cardiovascular Disease in Relation to Water Quality of the Department of Epidemiology, at the University of Ottawa, Ottawa, Canada and the Bureau of Epidemiology, National Health, and Welfare of Canada, cosponsored a workshop March 9th and 10th; 1978 to study the feasibility, practicality, and modality of magnesium intervention trials. The participants were Profs. T. Anderson and D. Hewitt from Toronto, Dr. H.L. Johansen, Mr. J.R. Marier, and Prof. L.C. Neri from Ottawa, Prof. G. Fodor from Newfoundland, Dr. M. Seelig from New Jersey, and Dr. R. Sharrett from Bethesda, Maryland. In the initial review of the available evidence, the following points were stressed.

Perhaps the strongest epidemiologic evidence for a magnesium effect on CVD is its concentration differences found in heart muscle of residents of hard- and soft-water towns, and between cardiac and accident victims from the same town (Chipperfield and Chipperfield, 1973; Anderson et al., 1975; Chipperfield et al., 1976). The apparent lack of support in the second of the Chipperfields' reports (Chipperfield and Chipperfield, 1976) militates against full acceptance of this data; however, waters from both towns they studied had extremely low concentrations of Mg. As the water supplies were classified as "hard" and "soft" mainly on the basis of their calcium content, the results are very unlikely to provide a sensitive test of any association between Mg and CVD. In their 1977 review, the Chipperfields again advocated Mg as the element most likely responsible for the "water effect" (Chipperfield and Chipperfield, 1977).

In Ontario, the study of Mg concentration in the myocardia of accident victims in hard and soft water areas was repeated (Anderson, 1978) to determine if the initial deficiencies found in the previous study could be confirmed, and indeed, magnesium concentrations were found lower in the hearts of people living in soft-water areas, where a higher incidence of heart disease was known to exist. This finding supports the hypothesis that myocardial magnesium deficiency precedes the insult. The geographic comparison of accident cases also gives support to Seelig's claim that our modern diet is in many instances inadequate in Mg (Seelig, 1964), and that Mg content in very hard water may compensate for this inadequacy.

In face of this evidence, the need to confirm the cause-and-effect relationship was evident. Two main investigative thrusts were therefore proposed: intervention trials and prospective observational studies.

The major problem with prospective studies is the difficulty in identify ing individuals with deficient Mg levels. Serum magnesium concentrations do not reflect a person's magnesium status and have shown no geographical differences (Anderson, 1972). Hair Mg determinations are extremely unreliable, and Mg in the nails is washed out very readily in the preparation of specimens. In urine, a single 24-hour collection would vary, either because the individual is a Mg waster or is Mg-deficient, so this method also fails to provide a reliable estimate of Mg status. A more reliable alternative is to accurately estimate how much an individual retains of a Mg load given to him or her. Normally a person should retain no more than 10 to 15 percent of the injected Mg; if an individual retains 40 to 50 percent, it is evidence that he or she is Mg deficient. In addition, a deficient electrolyte concentration in the heart muscle can be suspected if certain electrocardiogram (ECG) changes are found (Seelig, 1969). It was obvious to the group that more work is needed on techniques to determine a person's magnesium status.

An easier approach would be to identify geographic areas where the inhabitants could be Mg-deficient. Two ways are available: one is to measure the Mg concentration of the autopsy tissues, another is a dietary estimation of magnesium intake. One advantage of this approach is that by choosing an area of natural Mg deficiency, there is very little risk of toxic effects with the supplementation. This would obviate, for example, risk of toxicity for people with severe renal damage.

Consideration was then given to the form of magnesium and the type of vehicle by which it can be delivered. Magnesium aspartate-HCl has been shown to be well absorbed and therapeutically effective. The way in which supplementation can be done also has its own problems. It was considered impractical to provide more magnesium by adding it to public water supplies. Possible options would be Mg supplementation in bread, salt, or tablets (or in an after-dinner mint!).

The next major question the workshop addressed itself to was whether or not to advocate trials at the secondary or primary prevention levels. If you seek secondary prevention, you are looking at essentially clinical trials. Two clinical trials, one in Czechoslovakia (Fodor, private communication), and one in Russia (Stepan et al., 1967) were described as examples. Militating against the use of trials at the primary prevention level is the fact that it usually calls for large sample sizes. For example, considering death rates of 6 percent in middle-aged men with a five-year follow-up, an estimated 24,000 people would be needed. Another proposal was to restore Mg to bread in Newfoundland: enrichment of the diet is common in Newfoundland because of its low mineral levels. However, if this is done, a control group must be very carefully chosen so that the result can be related to the intervention.

Using a high-risk group, it would be possible to have a smaller sample size. Among groups that can conceivably provide definitive data are youngsters with congenital cardiac anomalies or children of families with hyperlipidemia. Another group are patients going to have corrective cardiac surgery. Myocardial infarction (MI) survivors might be brought into a trial which could be relatively inexpensive, or one could use individuals with a history of heart disease who are being administered digitalis (which pulls Mg out of the heart) or on diuretics (which causes its excretion in the urine). In this regard, hypertensives are of particular interest, because many of them are on diuretics and because of their increased risk of heart disease. Two other groups to be considered are diabetics and individuals with frequent ectopic beats.

Considering alternative end-points for primary prevention trials where periodic follow-up can be prohibitively expensive, hard end points obtainable from hospital records, such as sudden death, documented MI, or all deaths, may have to be used. However, where there usually is continuing contact with the individual patient, one could consider a number of additional parameters, such as the disappearance of angina, the number of nitroglycerin tablets required, exercise stress tests, or electrocardiographic evaluation, as end-points.

In conclusion, two different approaches to the ultimate objective can be considered: a small trial with a high-risk group or a larger primary prevention trial. Both trials must be double-blind. Most investigators are enthusiastic about studying high-risk groups because of the low sample size requirement and low costs. In the case of magnesium, however, these types of studies may conceivably be inappropriate for testing the hypothesis. A trial on the primary prevention level in the general population might be better because of the greater likelihood of the anticipated benefits.

The following studies were considered by the workshop:

I. *Non-Intervention*

A. Confirm ECG (electrocardiogram) as indicator of magnesium deficiency. Match males aged 35 to 47 in two areas, one high-magnesium, one low-magnesium. Study the duration of QRS complex, ST voltage, serum Ca and Mg, dietary records, and results of a physical examination.

B. Obtain the incidence of MI in people taking Mg containing drugs for other causes, for example, ulcers and kidney stones. Compare to a suitable control group.

II. *Clinical*

A. Cardiac surgery–add Mg to intravenous fluid for a selected group, check Mg concentration of heart muscles and/or angina after surgery.

B. Changes in ECGs with Mg supplementation.

C. Metabolic studies–for example: Do a 24-hour urine Mg analysis before and after a Mg load in children from hyperlipidemia families, or children with cardiac anomalies.

D. Consider patients who have a known or likely Mg deficiency and see if heart symptoms are changed with Mg supplementation.

  a. Multiparous teenagers with preeclampsia or toxemias and their children (cord blood at birth).

  b. Diuretics and/or digitalis users.

  c. Diabetics.

E. Ectopic-beats population: examine clinically; do an exercise stress test.

F. Genitourinary (GI) resections.

III. *Intervention*

The following groups of people were suggested as being suitable for an intervention trial (see Table). [Sample-size is based on a five-year follow-up (Halperin et al., 1968)].

Group	*End Point*	*Sample Size*
A. Hypertensives	First coronary event	1,000
B. Healthy 40- to 59-year-old white males	MI and coronary death	14,000
C. Entire population through food	Deaths from all causes	Newfoundland and Nova Scotia
D. Post-IHD (surviving greater than 6 months)	Effect on angina, MI, and death	1,000
E. Poorly controlled diabetics	First coronary event	
F. Ectopic-beats population	New coronary event	2,000

Group B, healthy males, is the most desirable group, but it would be difficult due to the large population required. Group F, the ectopic-beats population, would call for a difficult screening process to identify the population. Post-ischemic-heart-disease (IHD) individuals (Group D) look like the most promising group, and Groups A and E are also possible, although they may need to be stratified by the type of medication used. Supplementing the entire population through its food supply (Group C above) should not be done until studies using Groups, A, D, and/or E are mounted, so that popular opinion is not polarized.

Given the above information, the following composite study was recommended.

INTERVENTION TRIAL RECOMMENDED

In order to increase the chances of obtaining an effect, and in order to reduce costs, a composite trial of white males aged 40 to 59 from the following two high-risk groups was recommended. (As well as being at high risk of CHD, hypertensives are Mg wasters.)

Group	*Sample Size (Case and Control)*
Hypertensives	1,000
Post-IHD (greater than 6 months)	1,000

One advantage of using these groups is that compliance is likely to be good, as these groups are used to taking medication and are more aware of their health. Alcoholics and people with renal damage or Addison's disease are to be excluded. The trial would be double-blind, with possibly one person monitoring so that the trial may be terminated if problems develop or significant results are obtained. Minimum patient follow-up should be every six months by a doctor and every three months by a nurse. All medications used should be recorded.

Magnesium aspartate hydrochloride is the drug of choice. Dosage should be on a weight basis (5 mg/kg), which would mean approximately 150 mg of elemental Mg twice a day.

End points measured should include death from myocardial infarction, sudden death not otherwise explained, and frequency of anginal attacks.

Centers should be located in soft-water areas, as it is more likely that a magnesium-deficient population will be found in these areas.

REFERENCES

Anderson, T.W. Serum electrolytes and skeletal mineralization in hard and soft water areas. *Canad. Med. Assoc. J.* 107, 34–37 (1972).

Anderson, T.W., Neri, L.C., Schreiber, G.B., Talbot, F.D.F., and Zdrojewski, A. Ischemic heart disease, water hardness and myocardial magnesium. *Canad. Med. Assoc. J.* 113, 199–203 (1975).

Anderson, T.W. Private communication (1978).

Birch, G.E., and Giles, T.P. The importance of magnesium deficiency in cardiovascular disease. *Am. Heart J.* 94-5, 649–657 (1977).

Chipperfield, B., and Chipperfield, J.R. Heart muscle magnesium, potassium and zinc concentration after sudden death from heart disease. *Lancet* 2, 293 (1973).

Chipperfield, B., and Chipperfield, J.R. Magnesium and the heart. *Am. Heart J.* 93–96, 679–682 (1977).

Chipperfield, B., Chipperfield, J.R., Behr, G., and Burton, P. Magnesium and potassium content of normal heart muscle in areas of hard and soft waters. *Lancet* 1, 121–122 (1976).

Fodor, J.G. Private communication (1900).

Halperin, M., et al. Sample sizes for medical trials with special reference to long-term therapy. *J. Chron. Dis.* 21, 13–24 (1968).

Neri, L.C., and Johansen, H.L. Water hardness and cardiovascular mortality. *Ann. N.Y. Acad. Sci.* 304, 203–219 (1978).

Seelig, M.S. The requirements of magnesium by the normal adult: Summary and analysis of published data. *Am. J. Clin. Nut.* 14, 342–390 (1964).

Seelig, M.S. Electrographic patterns of magnesium depletions appearing in alcoholic heart disease. *Ann. N.Y. Acad. Sci.* 162, 609–617 (1969).

Seelig, M.S., and Heggtveit, H.A. Magnesium interrelationships in ischemic heart disease– A review. *Am. J. Clin. Nut.* 27, 59–79 (1974).

Stepan, T., Schitz, G., and Frohlich, E. Vorlaufige mitteilung uber verwendung sogenannter elektrolytschlepper bei myokardinfarct. *Wein Med. Wochschr.* 117, 884–889 (1967).

Szelenzi, I. Magnesium and its significance in cardiovascular and gastro-intestinal disorders. *World Rev. Nut. Diet.* 17, 189–224 (1973).

23

Sodium-Potassium Pump Activity in Volume-expanded Hypertension

F.J. HADDY
M.B. PAMNANI
D.L. CLOUGH

It has long been known that increased dietary sodium chloride exacerbates human hypertension. Furthermore, it is now clear that the normal human being also responds to increased dietary sodium chloride with increased arterial pressure. For example, Luft et al. (1978) showed that 800 mEq/day sodium chloride for three days significantly increases mean arterial blood pressure in normal male black subjects, and that 1200 mEq/day for three days does the same in normal male white subjects.

The mechanism of this effect is not known (Haddy and Overbeck, 1976). It clearly does not result from an immediate direct effect of the sodium chloride, or of the volume expansion, because intravenous infusion of an amount of saline equivalent to that retained does not immediately raise blood pressure. It will raise blood pressure with time, however, suggesting some unknown slowly acting indirect effect. One possibility is that the volume expansion somehow leads to inhibition of Na^+,K^+-ATPase and hence sodium-potassium pump activity in vascular and cardiac muscle. Such inhibition, with ouabain for example, is known to increase the contractility of cardiac and vascular smooth muscle. This possibility was suggested by the observation that the vasodilator action of potassium is subnormal in dogs with one-kidney, one-wrapped hypertension (Overbeck and Haddy, 1967; Overbeck, 1972), a type of experimental hypertension which is thought to be volume expanded. Potassium dilates by stimulating membrane Na^+,K^+-ATPase, and hence the electrogenic sodium-potassium pump in vascular smooth muscle (Chen et al., 1971, 1972). Therefore, we decided to examine sodium-

Table 1. Na^+, K^+-ATPase and Na^+-K^+ Pump Activities in Cardiovascular Tissues of Animals with Experimental Volume-expanded Hypertension

Type of Hypertension	*Species*	*Cardiac Na^+, K^+-ATPase Activity*	*Vessel Rubudium Uptake*[a]	*Reference*
One-kidney, one-wrapped	Dog	–	Decreased	Overbeck et al. (1976)
One-kidney, one-clip	Rat	Decreased	Decreased	Pamnani et al., unpublished Clough et al. (1977a) Clough et al. (1977b)
One-kidney, DOCA-salt	Rat	Decreased	Decreased	Pamnani et al. (1978a) Clough et al. (1978)
Acute renoprival	Rat	Decreased	–	Nivatpumin et al. (1973)
Acute volume expansion	Rat	–	Decreased	Pamnani et al. (1978b)

[a]Ouabain-sensitive uptake, which reflects Na^+-K^+ pump activity.

potassium pump activity in the blood vessels of dogs with one-kidney, one-wrapped hypertension. We adapted the rubidium uptake technique for measuring sodium-potassium pump activity in myocardial tissue to blood vessels, and measured ouabain-sensitive rubidium uptake. Rubidium is known to substitute for potassium in the operation of the sodium-potassium pump. The ouabain-sensitive rubidium uptake is that uptake related to active transport, because ouabain inhibits the sodium-potassium pump, which is responsible for active transport.

Mesenteric arteries and veins were removed from paired normotensive and hypertensive animals and immediately placed in cold, potassium-free Krebs-Henseleit solution to suppress the pump (Overbeck et al., 1976). The pump was then stimulated by transferring the vessels to a warm solution containing nonradioactive rubidium. Two minutes later, radioactive rubidium was added and its uptake measured after exactly 16 minutes. Uptake by ouabain-treated vessels was subtracted from this value to give ouabain-sensitive uptake, which reflects sodium-potassium pump activity.

Ouabain-sensitive rubidium uptake was significantly decreased in the hypertensive artery (Table 1). Ouabain-insensitive uptake, which probably reflects distribution in extracellular water and passive penetration into cell water, was normal. Ouabain-sensitive uptake was also reduced in the mesenteric veins, where the pressure is not elevated. Again, ouabain-insensitive uptake was normal.

Pamnani also examined ouabain sensitive rubidium uptake in the tail artery of the rat with one-kidney, one-clip hypertension, another form of experimental volume-expanded hypertension. Here too it was reduced (Pamnani et al., unpublished observation).

These studies suggested that the sodium-potassium pump is in fact suppressed in animals with experimental one-kidney renal hypertension, and that this suppression is not secondary to the increased pressure. Since operation of the sodium-potassium pump is intimately associated with membrane Na^+,K^+-ATPase activity, we decided to examine this parameter next. Like sodium-potassium pump activity in intact cells, Na^+,K^+-ATPase activity of isolated cell membranes is inhibited by ouabain and removal of potassium. Residual activity is due to a Mg^{2+}-ATPase. Na^+,K^+-ATPase activity is then the difference between total ATPase and Mg^{2+}-ATPase activities. There are practical difficulties in the measurement of Na^+,K^+-ATPase activity in blood vessels, but this is not the case for myocardium. Therefore, Clough, working in our laboratory, first measured Na^+,K^+-ATPase activity in cell membranes from the left ventricle of rats with one-kidney, one-clip hypertension (Clough et al., 1977a). He found it significantly suppressed relative to that in appropriate control animals. Mg^{2+}-ATPase activity, on the other hand, was slightly increased. The activity of 5'-nucleotidase was normal (5'-nucleotidase is a cell membrane marker).

We next wondered whether the change in Na^+,K^+-ATPase activity was secondary to increased pressure. We therefore prepared a new series of rats with one-kidney, one-clip hypertension, and Clough measured Na^+,K^+-ATPase activity in both the right and left ventricles (Clough et al., 1977b). As in the previous series, Na^+,K^+-ATPase activity was decreased, and Mg^{2+}-ATPase activity was increased in left ventricular membranes. The same was the case for right ventricular membranes. Sialic acid, another membrane marker, was not different in the membranes of the hypertensive and normotensive animals, either in the right or left ventricle.

Still more recently, we extended our studies to one-kidney, DOCA, salt hypertension in the rat, another form of volume-expanded hypertension. The findings were similar to those in the dog with one-kidney, one-wrapped hypertension, and to findings in the rat with one-kidney, one-clip hypertension, both with respect to blood vessel rubidium uptake and cardiac Na^+,K^+-ATPase activity. Ouabain-sensitive rubidium uptake in the tail artery was decreased, whereas ouabain-insensitive uptake was increased (Pamnani et al., 1978a). Na^+,K^+-ATPase activity of left ventricular cell membranes was decreased, whereas Mg^{2+}-ATPase activity was increased (Clough et al., 1978). Thus, here too there appears to be decreased sodium-potassium pump activity.

Decreased Na^+,K^+-ATPase activity has also been observed in the heart of the rat with acute renoprival hypertension (Nivatpumin et al., 1973).

Pamnani et al. (1978a, 1979) have also examined two forms of hypertension in the rat not considered to be volume expanded [spontaneously hypertensive rats (SHR) and dexamethasone], and here did not find decreased rubidium uptake by the tail artery.

If the decreased pump activity in volume-expanded hypertension is in fact related to volume expansion, acute volume expansion of the normal animal with saline should reproduce the findings. Thus in his latest series of experiments, Pamnani (1978b) infused enough saline intravenously in the normal rat to raise extracellular fluid volume by 30 percent and measured rubidium uptake by the tail artery. This suppressed rubidium uptake to the same extent as seen in the hypertensive animal, that is, about 30 percent. Furthermore, supernates of boiled plasma from the volume-expanded animal suppressed rubidium uptake by the tail artery harvested from another rat. Thus suppression seems to result from a heat-stable humoral agent.

Bioassay studies indicate that the blood of animals with volume-expanded hypertension contains a heat-stable slowly acting pressor and sensitizing agent (Haddy and Overbeck, 1976; Haddy et al., 1979). Other studies indicate that volume expansion produces a heat-stable natriuretic factor in plasma which inhibits sodium transport by the renal tubule (Haddy and Overbeck, 1976). Studies should now be performed to determine whether these observations are related to those reported in this paper.

CONCLUSIONS

In summary, dietary sodium chloride can induce or exacerbate hypertension. The mechanism of these effects are unknown. One possibility is that the associated increase in volume inhibits Na^+,K^+-ATPase, and hence the sodium-potassium pump in vascular and cardiac muscle. Such inhibition (with ouabain, for example) is known to increase the contractility of these tissues. We have therefore examined Na^+,K^+-ATPase and sodium-potassium pump activities in blood vessels and heart in several types of experimental volume-expanded hypertension. Na^+,K^+-ATPase activity was assayed in microsomal fractions of rat left ventricular myocardium. Sodium-potassium pump activity was determined by the radioactive rubidium uptake technique in mesenteric arteries of the dog and the tail artery of the rat. One-kidney perinephritic hypertension in the dog, one-kidney Goldblatt hypertension in the rat, and one-kidney, DOCA, salt hypertension in the rat were studied. In all cases, Na^+,K^+-ATPase and sodium-potassium pump activities were suppressed relative to those in appropriate control animals. The changes do not appear to be secondary to the hypertension, since sodium-potassium pump and Na^+,K^+-ATPase activities were also suppressed in mesenteric veins (perinephritic hypertension) and right ventricle (Goldblatt hypertension), respectively, where the pressure is not elevated. Suppressed arterial pump activity was reproduced in the normal rat during acute saline volume expansion, and plasma supernates from these animals suppressed pump activity when applied to arteries from normal rats. These studies show that sodium-potassium pump activity of cardiovascular muscle is suppressed in experimental volume-expanded hypertension, that suppression also occurs following acute volume expansion, and that this is associated with a ouabainlike substance in the plasma. Thus volume expansion, presence of humoral agent, suppressed pump activity, and elevated pressure may be related in experimental volume-expanded hypertension.

REFERENCES

Chen, W.T., Anderson, D.K., Scott, J.B., and Haddy, F.J. The mechanism of the vasodilator effect of potassium. *J. Lab. Clin. Med.* 78, 797 (1971).

Chen, W.T., Brace, R.A., Scott, J.B., Anderson, D.K., and Haddy, F.J. The mechanism of the vasodilator action of potassium. *Proc. Soc. Exp. Biol. Med.* 140, 820–824 (1972).

Clough, D.L., Pamnani, M.B., and Haddy, F.J. Decreased Na, K-ATPase activity in left ventricular myocardium of rats with one-kidney DOCA-saline hypertension. *Clin. Res.* 26, 361 (1978).

Clough, D.L., Pamnani, M.B., Overbeck, H.W., and Haddy, F.J. Decreased myocardial Na, K-ATPase in rats with one-kidney Goldblatt hypertension. *Fed. Proc.* 36, 491 (1977a).

Clough, D.L., Pamnani, M.B., Overbeck, H.W., and Haddy, F.J. Decreased Na, K-ATPase in right ventricular myocardium of rats with one-kidney Goldblatt hypertension. *Physiologist* 20, 18 (1977b).

Haddy, F.J., and Overbeck, H.W. The role of humoral agents in volume expanded hypertension. *Life Sci.* 19, 935–948 (1976).

Haddy, F.J., Pamnani, M.B., and Clough, D.L. Humoral factors and the sodium-potassium pump in volume expanded hypertension. *Life Sci.* 24, 2105–2118 (1979).

Luft, F., Block, R., Weyman, A., Murray, R., and Weinberger, M. Cardiovascular responses to extremes of salt intake in man. *Clin. Res.* 26, 365 (1978).

Nivatpumin, T., Scheuer, J., Bhan, A.K., and Penpargkul, S. Effects of acute uremia on myocardial function in rats. *Clin. Res.* 21, 952 (1973).

Overbeck, H.W. Vascular responses to cations, osmolality, and angiotensin in renal hypertensive dogs. *Am. J. Physiol.* 223, 1358–1364 (1972).

Overbeck, H.W., and Haddy, F.J. Forelimb vascular responses in renal hypertensive dogs. *Physiologist* 10, 270 (1967).

Overbeck, H.W., Pamnani, M.B., Akera, T., Brody, T.M., and Haddy, F.J. Depressed function of a ouabain-sensitive sodium-potassium pump in blood vessels from renal hypertensive dogs. *Circ. Res.* 38, (suppl. II), 48–52 (1976).

Pamnani, M.B., Clough, D.L., and Haddy, F.J. Altered activity of the Na^+-K^+ pump in arteries of rats with steroid hypertension. *Clin. Sci. Mol. Med.* 55, 41s–43s (1978a).

Pamnani, M.B., Clough, D.L., Steffen, R.P., and Haddy, F.J. Depressed Na^+-K^+ pump activity in tail arteries from acutely volume expanded rats. *Physiologist* 21, 88 (1978b).

Pamnani, M.B., Clough, D.L., and Haddy, F.J. Na^+-K^+ pump activity in tail arteries of spontaneously hypertensive rats. *Jap. Heart J.* 20, (suppl. I), 228–230 (1979).

Index

GPSR Compliance

The European Union's (EU) General Product Safety Regulation (GPSR) is a set of rules that requires consumer products to be safe and our obligations to ensure this.

If you have any concerns about our products, you can contact us on ProductSafety@springernature.com

In case Publisher is established outside the EU, the EU authorized representative is:

Springer Nature Customer Service Center GmbH
Europaplatz 3
69115 Heidelberg, Germany

Batch number: 10607212

Printed by Printforce, the Netherlands